Blepharisma

The facing page illustrates several of the variations in morphology and pigmentation found in *Blepharisma japonicum* v. intermedium. All pictures show living, unstained cells. The organisms were held in place by a Rotocell compressor during photography, and for this reason they appear somewhat flatter and broader than they actually are when swimming freely. All were photographed with an Exacta camera using a Wild microscope with a 20 × objective and a 10 × ocular, except the lower left, which was taken with a 100 × objective and a 10 × ocular. All photographs except the last by Robert Grainger. In general, because of the color process used, the pictures have a sharper blue tint than would be evident in the actual cells; the reds are fairly true to life.

Upper left: A normal vegetative cell; the pink color is characteristic. The peristome and membranellar band are visible at the upper right, and the contractile vacuole shows clearly at the posterior end. *Upper middle:* A cannibal giant of *B. japonicum* v. intermedium feeding on *B. americanum*. When fed on its own species, the giant increases at least twofold in linear dimensions. A still-living *Blepharisma* is curled up in the large central food vacuole; two other vacuoles contain the concentrated pigment and other undigested residue from blepharismas ingested some time previously. *Upper right:* A laboratory-grown albino mutant, showing the macronucleus, two large food vacuoles filled with bacteria, and the contractile vacuole. The membranellar band (upper right) was in motion when this picture was taken, and four metachronal beats may be seen passing in waves down the membranelles. The tonguelike undulating membrane is clearly visible at the posterior end of the peristome. This cell is somewhat more compressed and flattened than the normal pigmented cell in the upper left picture. *Middle left:* A small blue cell compared with a larger reddish cell. The blue pigmentation was produced by exposing the cell's blepharismin to low-intensity visible light. The larger cell has extruded a good deal of its pigment and developed numerous vacuoles because of rough handling during photography. *Middle right:* A very much flattened red *Blepharisma* photographed by phase optics. Note the six metachronal beats of the membranelles, the five prominent food vacuoles, and the lateral stripes (kineties) that converge toward the anal pore. *Lower left:* The array of pigment granules in a "blue" organism photographed by oil immersion. About six rows of granules are visible between each two ciliary stripes. Some granules have been extruded even under the dim lighting used for the picture. *Lower right:* A cell from which most of the pigment has been extruded by immersion in medium at 0° C for 2 minutes. The photograph here is grayer in tone than a living cell, which usually retains more of its pinkish tinge.

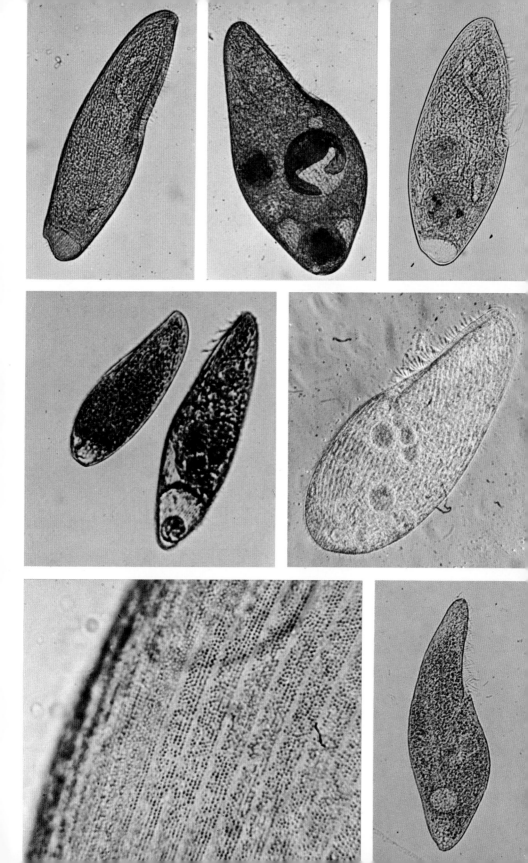

Blepharisma

The Biology of a Light-Sensitive Protozoan

By ARTHUR C. GIESE

With the Collaboration of Shōichirō Suzuki, Robert A. Jenkins,
Henry I. Hirshfield, Irwin R. Isquith, and Ann M. DiLorenzo

STANFORD UNIVERSITY PRESS
Stanford, California, 1973

Stanford University Press
Stanford, California
© 1973 by the Board of Trustees of the
Leland Stanford Junior University
Printed in the United States of America
ISBN 0-8047-0817-7   LC 73-190525

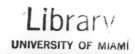

To S. C. Brooks and C. V. Taylor
who first aroused my interest
in cells and unicellular organisms

Preface

The genus *Blepharisma*, created by the Swiss protozoologist Perty in 1852, includes infusorians with a number of distinctive characteristics in common, most notably the presence of a pink pigment. Another prominent character, which gives the genus its name, is a set of membranelles that flutter like lashes on an eyelid (Gk. *blepharon*, an eyelid; *blepharidos*, an eyelash). *Blepharisma* is widely distributed in both fresh and salt waters but is not easily found in nature, even though it is possible to see pigmented members of the larger species with the naked eye. It was in 1929, in a collection from a pond on the Stanford campus, that I found my first blepharismas, which proved to have many desirable properties for classroom use. *Blepharisma* is large, self-stained, and much slower in movement than *Paramecium*, the most common organism used to illustrate the ciliate protozoans. Also, the pigment blepharismin, which induces light-sensitivity, has proved highly suitable for photobiological research.

Since the genus was first described it has been studied by investigators in many parts of the world. The literature is large and widely scattered, and it has never been collected or reviewed. The present book is therefore an attempt to summarize the available information on *Blepharisma* and to describe the biology of the genus in a form readily available to investigators, teachers, and students, many of whom have in the past asked me to refer them to a source of this nature.

A few other protozoan genera have received comprehensive treatment—e.g., *Paramecium* (Wichterman, 1953), *Stentor* (Tartar, 1961), and *Euglena* (Wolken, 1961, 1967; Buetow, 1968). There are several volumes on *Amoeba*, and a treatise on *Tetrahymena* is in preparation. Considering the widespread use of protozoans in research and teaching, it is surprising that studies of this kind are so infrequent. Especially in view of the present explosion of specialized literature, a general summary is perhaps the best way to obtain basic information quickly, along with a guide to the relevant literature.

My treatment of this genus is admittedly incomplete in several crucial areas, but only because the appropriate information in these areas is lacking. Numerous opportunities for further investigation are clearly apparent, and some of these are suggested in Chapter 13.

I am particularly grateful for the willingness of several colleagues to contribute their expertise on special topics to this volume. Drs. Henry I. Hirshfield, Irwin R. Isquith, and Ann M. DiLorenzo review the taxonomy of the genus; Dr. Robert A. Jenkins considers the fine structure of representative species; and Dr. Shōichirō Suzuki surveys morphology, nuclear behavior, and morphogenesis. To all, I am indebted.

I am also indebted to a host of students, both undergraduate and graduate, who have shown interest in *Blepharisma* and whose reports and theses form the substance of much of the published and unpublished work cited in this book.

Work on *Blepharisma* in our laboratory has been supported by grants from the National Institutes of Health, the American Cancer Society, the Atomic Energy Commission, and the Rockefeller Foundation, to all of whom I am grateful.

I am indebted to Dr. Sharon Smith, Mrs. Barbara McCaw, Dr. J. Nilsson, and Dr. K. C. Smith for critical reading of some of the chapters, and to various investigators for permission to use their figures and data. I am also indebted to Miss Pauline Schimberg and Miss Gertrude Zilske for expert typing, and to Mrs. Juliana Spranza for much of the original art work. Most of all, I am indebted to my wife Raina, whose patience is exceeded only by her careful, critical reading of the entire manuscript.

A.C.G.

Contents

Blepharisma

CHAPTER ONE

Introduction and General Morphology

Blepharisma is a ciliate protozoan genus belonging to the class Ciliata, subclass Spirotricha, order Heterotricha. A spirotrich ciliate has complex buccal ciliature with an extensively developed membranellar band on the left side of the oral area and an undulating membrane on the right side (Fig. 1.1). The membranelles and the undulating membrane, both concerned with food intake, are made up of rows of interdigitated, or "fused," cilia. In heterotrichs the whole cell is also covered with simple, unmodified cilia, and only the feeding organelles contain complex fused cilia.

The classification of species in the genus *Blepharisma* is still under intensive study, and the number of definite species is not fully ascertained (see Chapter 12). The individual species can be differentiated largely by their macronuclear characters, although cytoplasmic characters are often distinctive enough to be of some use. The macronucleus of a *Blepharisma* takes one of four shapes: compact and often spherical, as in *B. seculum*; binodal (dumbbell-shaped, clubbed, or halteriform), as in *B. undulans*; multinodal (moniliform or beaded), as in *B. americanum*; and filiform (filamentous), as in *B. japonicum*. Although a number of species have been found for each of these macronuclear types (megakaryotypes), the species just listed have perhaps been those most extensively used in experimental studies. *B. japonicum*, in particular, is large, deeply pigmented, and vigorous, and has therefore been used extensively even in the United States (however, no species with a filiform macronucleus has yet been reported as native to this country).

Blepharisma is not often encountered in ponds during routine collections (see Chapter 4), but it is widespread in distribution, having been reported from North and South America, Europe, Asia, Africa, and Australia. And if sought, some species could most likely be found on many

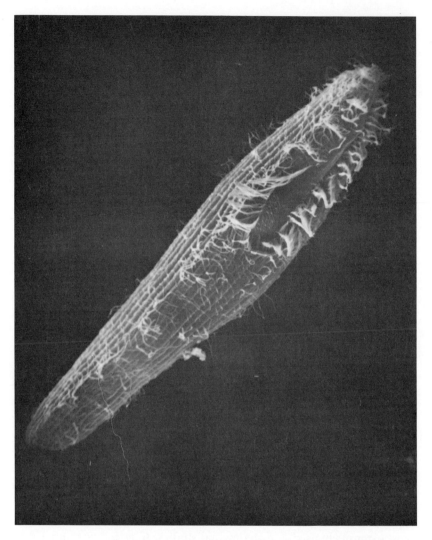

Fig. 1.1. Micrographs of *Blepharisma* taken by various methods. Above: a scanning electron micrograph taken at low power, showing the ciliary rows on the cell surface and the peristome. *Opposite.* Top: a scanning micrograph at higher magnification, showing details of the ciliary rows and peristomal structure. Scanning micrographs courtesy of Dr. Eugene Small and The American Microscopical Society (Trans. **90**: Figs. 37, 38). Center: *B. japonicum* v. intermedium, photographed by phase optics; the contractile vacuole shows clearly, and contributing vacuoles are clustered at the posterior end. The macronucleus appears as a dark filament. Bottom: a light micrograph in which the macronucleus appears as a lighter body; the food vacuoles are out of focus, but the membranelles and ciliary rows are evident.

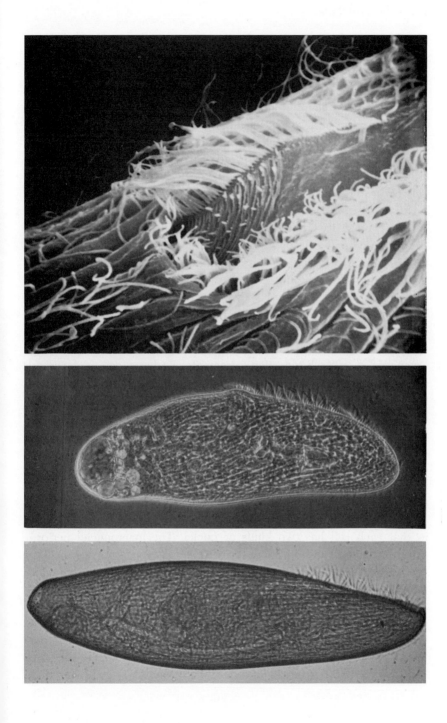

islands from which the genus has not yet been reported. The widespread occurrence of a species presupposes some effective method of distribution. It is difficult to see how the vegetative stages of *Blepharisma* could be distributed, since the cells are relatively fragile and sensitive to small changes in a variety of conditions; possibly, they are carried by some host, as *Paramecium* is by snails (McGuire and Belk, 1967). However, many species have been found to form cysts, at least under some conditions (see Chapter 10), and could easily travel in that form.

Because of the very complexity of most ciliates (and some flagellates), it is sometimes argued that protozoans are not single cells but animals in which cellularity failed to develop. Although cilia or flagella are present on some tissue cells of almost all multicellular animals, they do not form membranelles, undulating membranes, cirri, and the like as they do in ciliates. The grouping of these organelles into a complex peristome for feeding, the presence of a cytopyge for voiding indigestible residues, and the presence of a contractile vacuole for voiding excess fluid certainly imply that a ciliate may be a complex, though small, animal rather than a cell. In fact, Ehrenberg's "The Infusorians as complete organisms" (1838) listed ciliate organelles as homologues of various organs in higher animals. When microscopy improved to the point that these organelles could be seen in detail, Ehrenberg's view in its extreme form was set aside, although objections to regarding protozoans as single cells have nonetheless continued to appear for many years. Electron microscopy, however, has dispelled all real doubt. No matter how complicated, the organelles of ciliates prove to be no more than elaborations of the organelles found in all cells, both plant and animal (see Chapter 3).

Ciliates possess a nuclear system distinct from that of other organisms in that each cell has two kinds of nuclei. The macronuclei perform trophic functions, and the micronuclei transfer genetic information. This vastly complicates ciliate genetics: not only are two types of nuclei present, but both may be multiple. The macronucleus normally arises anew from the zygotic nucleus during sexual reproduction; but in some cases the old macronucleus continues to function, further confusing the issue (see Chapter 2). To this extent, a ciliate is an aberrant cell, and hardly one that a geneticist would choose for his research. On the other hand, although Sonneborn's investigations demonstrate that inheritance in protozoans is essentially like that in metazoans, some interesting information not obtainable with other organisms has come from genetic studies of a few ciliates (Preer, 1969). But *Blepharisma* has figured little in these studies, and the data are too scant for review at the present time.

The very presence of complex, readily visible organelles has led to the extensive use of *Blepharisma* and other ciliates in experiments on regeneration. It is presumed that all cells can regenerate to some extent, but the organelles of most cells are too small to see under low-power light microscopy. (In many nerve cells the extensive fibers are a readily visible organelle, but these regenerate very slowly.) Therefore, almost all experiments on animal regeneration at the cellular level have been performed with ciliates, and there are many parallels between what is found in such experiments with a single-celled ciliate like *Blepharisma* and those with a multicellular organism (see Chapters 8 and 9).

Perhaps the most interesting feature of *Blepharisma* is its possession of blepharismin, a photosensitizing pigment somewhat like hypericin. If this pigment were found only in a mutant *Blepharisma* it would not be as unusual, since the mutants of many other organisms accumulate pigments—e.g., the porphyrins are found in the erythrocytes of a person suffering from erythropoietic porphyria. Only a few types of bacteria are known to accumulate a photosensitizing pigment (porphyrin) in the wild type. In *Blepharisma* the photosensitizing system itself is unique even among cells that possess a photosensitizing pigment, in that blepharismin, under strong light, reacts lethally on the cell carrying it (see Chapter 11). This raises questions about *Blepharisma*'s evolution and genetic survival, especially since colorless mutants have appeared but have not populated natural pools.

General Morphology

Although the species of *Blepharisma* differ from one another in many respects, they are generally pyriform (spindle-shaped) and pink in color with a well-defined peristome and a cytopyge.* The body of *Blepharisma* is not highly contractile, although contraction is evident during defecation and when a cell is cut. However, blepharismas are

---

* The remainder of this chapter was contributed by Shōichirō Suzuki, Yamagata University, Japan.

remarkably flexible, as can be seen when one forces its way through a small aperture.

The size of blepharismas bacteria-fed in the laboratory varies in different species from approximately 50 μm,* the minimum size in *B. undulans*, to 450 μm, the maximum size in *B. japonicum*. Some marine forms are said to be even larger but were not available for measurement. The size of a *Blepharisma* is greatly affected by nutrition, and if unstable nutritional dwarfs or cannibal giants are included in the measurements, the variation in size is even greater—approximately 35 to 750 μm (Stolte, 1924; Giese, 1938; Suzuki, 1954; Hirshfield et al., 1962).

The shape of *Blepharisma* is also variable, depending on nutrition. Generally, the anterior half of the body is flattened laterally, and the posterior half is expanded and almost circular in cross section. Well-nourished cells usually assume a pyriform shape, expanded posteriorly, and underfed organisms have an elongate spindle shape. The ventral (oral) surface is readily distinguishable from the dorsal (aboral) surface of the body by the presence of the peristome, an oral groove extending from the anterior body for almost one-half the body length. The peristome is broadened and deepened posteriorly, and twisted to some degree as well (Fig. 1.2).

The color of blepharismas also presents great variations, from almost colorless to deep pink. Some species are reported to be colorless (e.g., *B. lateritium* v. hyalinum), and still others are greenish blue in color (*B. coeruleum*. Suzuki, 1954; Hirshfield et al., 1965; Isquith et al., 1965). The coloration is caused by subpellicular pigment granules, which are arranged in longitudinal rows between each pair of ciliary rows (Fig. 1.3). Because the color is affected by light, it should be determined from cultures grown in darkness (see Chapter 11).

Feeding Organelles

The peristome is provided on the right margin with an undulating membrane, and on the left with a band of membranelles (Figs. 1.2 and 1.5). (These structures will be used to define right and left throughout this book.) The undulating membrane is composed of the cilia arising from the posterior half of the peristomal margin interconnected with

---

* The nm, or nanometer, is a unit of length equal to 10^{-9} meter. The micrometer, abbreviated μm, is 10^{-6} meter and is equivalent to the older term μ, the micron. Nanometers and micrometers are used throughout this book, since they have been adopted as the preferred terms by microscopists.

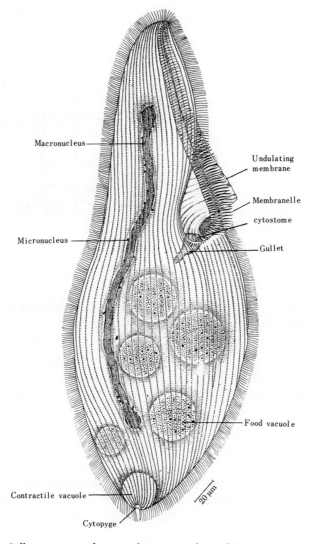

Fig. 1.2. Cell structures in the normal vegetative form of *B. japonicum*.

one another by interdigitating projections. The membrane can easily be observed while the cell is alive, but it breaks up into its component cilia during fixation and staining. In the anterior half and posterior terminal region of the peristome the cilia do not fuse but remain separated as a simple ciliary row fringing the peristomal margin.

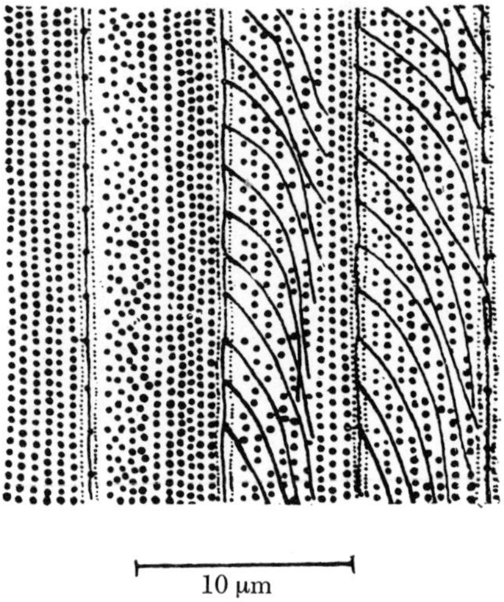

Fig. 1.3. Arrangement of cilia and pigment granules in *B. japonicum*.

|———————————————|
10 μm

The membranellar band (also called the adoral zone of membranelles, AZM) is a longitudinal row of membranelles that spirals from the anterior tip of the cell to the cytostome, where it ends in a "terminal spiral." The number of membranelles composing the band varies between species and individuals; for example, it is 28–30 in *B. seculum* (Hirshfield et al., 1965) and 95 in *B. japonicum* (Suzuki, 1951, 1954). Although a membranelle appears to be a large cilium on first inspection, it is actually a flat, triangular structure composed of three transverse rows of fused cilia—except anteriorly, where it may be composed of two rows of cilia, or terminally, where it may have only one row.

The floor of the peristomal groove itself is covered with cilia arranged in transverse rows. The posterior region of the groove forms a broad, concave vestibulum opening posteriorly into the cytostome, which leads into a funnel-shaped depression, the cytopharynx (gullet).

The Cilia and Fibrils

In *Blepharisma* the body cilia are arranged in longitudinal rows on the cell's surface, arising from shallow depressions in the pellicle; they run parallel to the peristomal margin on the right side, forming an acute angle with the left margin of the peristome. The rows vary in number within a species, depending on the size of the organism: 10–14 on one side in *B. seculum*, 10–16 in *B. undulans*, 12–22 in *B. musculus* v. giesei,

18–25 in *B. americanum,* and 25–38 in *B. japonicum* (Suzuki, 1954; Inaba et al., 1958; Bhandary, 1959, 1962; Hirshfield et al., 1965; Isquith et al., 1965). Cannibal giants of any species develop extra rows as they increase in girth (see Chapter 5).

If blepharismas are impregnated with silver or stained with haematoxylin, various fibrillar systems can be observed in association with the ciliary rows and the other ciliary organelles; these were first revealed by light microscopy in *B. japonicum* (Suzuki, 1954, 1957). Cilia arise from the kinetosomes, which are embedded in the ectoplasm in longitudinal rows corresponding to the ciliary rows. Along the right side of each kinetosomal row there is a longitudinal fiber, the kinetodesma; in addition, a short, fine fibril arises from each kinetosome and runs posteriorly and to the right to join with the kinetodesma (Fig. 1.3). The body kineties in general run parallel from their starting points toward the cytopyge, making loose counterclockwise spirals. But in the V-zone (the V-shaped area posterior to the peristome) the kineties branch proximally from the posterior end of the body (Fig. 1.4).

All the body kineties, including those of the V-zone, join at the cell's posterior terminal with the circumanal fibril that surrounds the cytopyge. This fibril seems to be contractile, since the cytopyge is able to form a large opening during defecation. The kinetosomes of each membranelle give off numerous delicate fibrils toward the interior of the cell to form a triangular, flattened bundle, which tapers into a thick, thread-

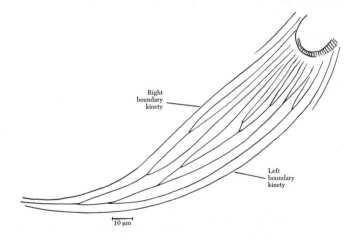

Fig. 1.4. The pattern of kineties in the V-area of *B. japonicum.*

like bundle extending transversely to connect with a kinetosome of the undulating membrane. Thus the floor of the peristome is lined with numerous transverse fibrils running parallel to one another (Fig. 1.5). In the posterior region of the peristome these peristomal fibrils run obliquely toward the rear from the right margin, forming curves that surround the circular depression of the vestibulum, and also forming a dense fibrillar band that runs parallel to the posterior portion of the membranellar band (Fig. 1.6).

Because the floor of the vestibulum lacks subpellicular fibrils like those associated with the peristome, it is not a very strong structure and is often everted or burst when *Blepharisma* is fixed for study. However, the formation of the peroral cone and cytoplasmic bridge that appear during conjugation is dependent on this same structural weakness. The floor of the vestibulum is covered with a ciliary membrane (Suzuki, 1957) whose component cilia arise from the right margin of the peristome and curve toward the cytostome. Thus the posterior portion of the right peristomal margin is provided with two membranes, the undulating membrane and the less conspicuous membrane overlapping the floor of the vestibulum.

The membranelles extend into the cytostomal region but do not enter deeply into the cytopharynx. However, a bundle of fibrils does enter the cytopharynx, forming tight clockwise spirals at first and then spreading loosely into numerous slender fibrils that pass into the cytoplasm. Although the origin of the pharyngeal fibrils is obscure, they are most likely an extension from the kineties found in the posterior terminal spiral of the membranellar band.

The Nuclei

The macronucleus of *Blepharisma* varies in shape as previously mentioned, depending on the species; four types are recognizable in vegetative cells (trophonts). The nodes of the moniliform (beaded) type vary in number from two in *B. undulans* to twelve in *B. musculus* v. multinodatum, though in a few marine forms 25 or more nodes have been reported.

The ground substance of the macronucleus presents an alveolar appearance, with scattered spherules of various sizes surrounded by dense chromatin (Fig. 1.7). In nuclei stained with Heidenhain's hematoxylin these spherules appear as achromatic vacuoles with or without an in-

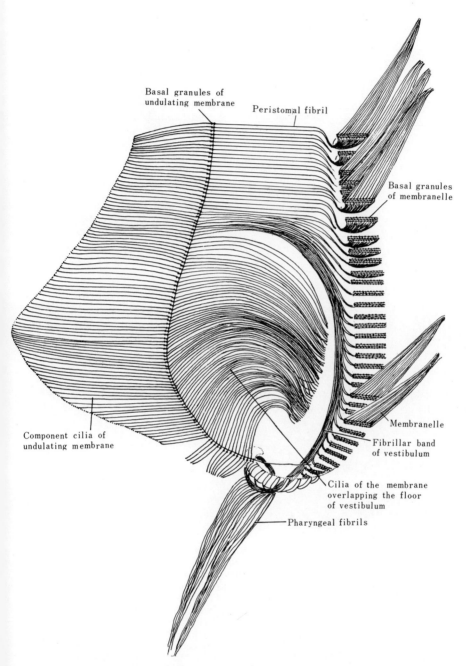

Fig. 1.5. The major fibrillar systems related to the peristome of *B. japonicum*.

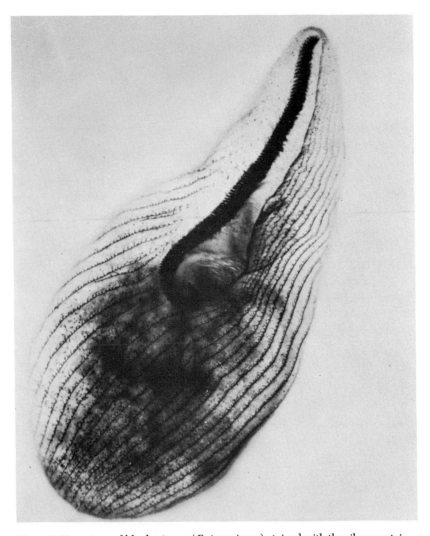

Fig. 1.6. Two views of blepharismas (*B. japonicum*) stained with the silver-protein method (Protargol) of Dregesco, as modified by J. Frankel and M. Dziadosz. The cells are fixed in equal parts of Bouin and saturated mercuric chloride; thereafter they are treated successively with methyl alcohol, formalin, potassium permanganate, oxalic acid, and Protargol. A final treatment with hydroquinone/sodium sulfite solution and oxalic acid is necessary before the cells are dehydrated, cleared, and mounted (Permount). This method is especially suitable for bringing out the kinetosomes and fiber systems of ciliates (compare the peristomal fibers in the photo above with the schematic drawing of the same structures in Figure 1.5). Sometimes, as in the photo opposite, Protargol will also stain the macronucleus. Staining and microphoto by Heywood R. Sawyer, Jr., University of Wyoming.

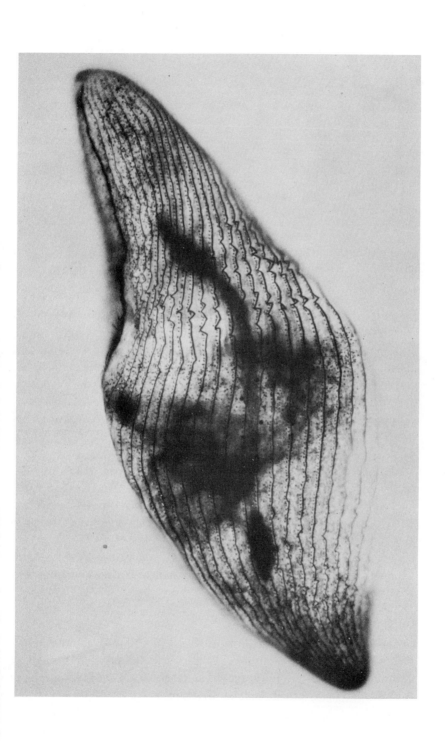

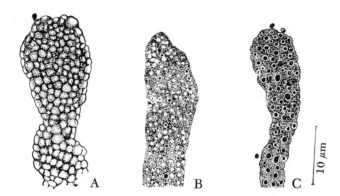

Fig. 1.7. Terminals of the vegetative nucleus of *B. japonicum*, stained with Feulgen preparation (*A*), Heidenhain's hematoxylin (*B*), and Borrel mixture (*C*). From Suzuki, 1957.

tensely stained outer wall. They are variously referred to as nucleoli (Stolte, 1924), spherules (Young, 1939; Suzuki, 1951), or "large bodies," and apparently correspond to the nucleoli of other ciliates (Seshachar, 1964). Young (1939), who reported that the spherules are cyclic in occurrence and disappear during division, considered them to be storage products used up during division. Kennedy (1965), on the basis of cytochemical tests, regarded them as carbohydrate-protein complexes. It is possible that they are nucleoli discharging ribosomal RNA, like those in other cells.

The micronuclei of *Blepharisma* are small ovoid bodies located near or in contact with the macronuclear membrane. They are densely packed with chromatin and may be stained homogeneously by various nuclear stains. The micronuclei vary in number, depending on the species and the individual cell: e.g., 2–12 in *B. undulans*, 2–30 in *B. americanum*, 2–25 in *B. japonicum*, and 6–30 in *B. japonicum* v. intermedium (Suzuki, 1954; Bhandary, 1959, 1962; Hirshfield et al., 1965; Isquith et al., 1965).

Cytoplasm

The inner cytoplasm, or endoplasm, of *Blepharisma* is granular in texture, with a variety of inclusions: Golgi bodies, mitochondria, pigment granules, glycogen granules, fat droplets, food vacuoles, a contractile vacuole, and many other vacuoles of various sizes.

The Golgi bodies of *Blepharisma* were first described by Moor (1931) as ring-shaped structures scattered through the cytoplasm (for fine structure, see Chapter 3).

The mitochondria occur throughout the endoplasm as small spherical, ovoid, or rod-shaped bodies of various sizes. They are also densely distributed in the outer cytoplasm, or ectoplasm, in close proximity to the pigment granules.

The pigment granules are small spherical bodies stainable by hematoxylin or pyronin but negative to the Feulgen reaction and to Janus green B (Suzuki, 1951). Weisz (1950), on the basis of staining reactions, reported that the pigment granules of *Blepharisma* were mitochondria. This was questioned by Utsumi and Yoshizawa (1955), and by Inaba et al. (1958). Kennedy (1965) eventually demonstrated by electron microscopy that they are separate entities of quite a different structure (see Chapter 3).

The glycogen granules and fat droplets, which can be detected by cytochemical methods, are reserve substances (Utsumi, 1956a, 1956b; Kennedy, 1965). The glycogen (paraglycogen) granules are particularly numerous around the macronucleus and the food vacuoles. The fat droplets appear in various sizes, varying in number with the nutritive condition of the cell.

The food vacuoles, large and numerous in well-fed blepharismas, usually circulate only in the posterior half of the body. Indigestible matter is ejected from the cytopyge (anus) alternately with the discharge of the posteriorly located contractile vacuole. The cytopyge is oblong, extending from the posterior-dorsal end of the body to the left side; when very full, it expands to form a large bowl-shaped opening. In healthy blepharismas only a single contractile vacuole is present. Under unfavorable conditions, however, several small vacuoles appear in the posterior region, where each unites successively with the one next posterior to form a large vacuole.

LITERATURE CITED

Bhandary, A. V. 1959. Cytology of an Indian race of *Blepharisma undulans* Stein. J. Protozool. **6**: 333–39.
———— 1962. Taxonomy of genus *Blepharisma* with special reference to *Blepharisma undulans*. J. Protozool. **9**: 435–42.

Ehrenberg, C. G. 1838. Die Infusionsthierchen als volkommene Organismen. Leipzig, 547 pp.

Giese, A. C. 1938. Cannibalism and gigantism in *Blepharisma*. Trans. Am. Micros. Soc. **57**: 245–55.

Hirshfield, H. I., L. Chunosoff, and A. V. Bhandary. 1962. Macronuclear variability of *Blepharisma* associated with growth. Intern. Soc. Cell Biol. **2**: 27–56.

Hirshfield, H. I., I. R. Isquith, and A. V. Bhandary. 1965. A proposed organization of the genus *Blepharisma* Perty and description of four new species. J. Protozool. **12**: 136–44.

Inaba, F., R. Nakamura, and S. Yamaguchi. 1958. An electron-microscopic study on the pigment granules of *Blepharisma*. Cytologia **23**: 72–79.

Isquith, I. R., A. J. Repak, and H. I. Hirshfield. 1965. *Blepharisma seculum*, sp. nov., a member of the subgenus (*Compactum*). J. Protozool. **12**: 615–18.

Kennedy, J. R. 1965. The morphology of *Blepharisma undulans* Stein. J. Protozool. **12**: 542–61.

McGuire, B., Jr., and D. Belk. 1967. *Paramecium* transport by land snails. J. Protozool. **14**: 445–47.

Moor, I. 1931. Reaction of *Blepharisma* to Golgi impregnation methods. Proc. Soc. Exp. Biol. Med. **28**: 805–6.

———— 1934. Morphology of the contractile vacuole and cloacal region in *Blepharisma undulans*. J. Exp. Zool. **69**: 59–104.

Preer, J. R., Jr. 1969. Genetics of the Protozoa. *In* Research in protozoology (T. T. Chen, ed.), III, 128–278. New York.

Seshachar, B. R. 1964. Observations on the fine structure of the nuclear apparatus of *Blepharisma intermedium* Bhandary (Ciliata: Spirotricha). J. Protozool. **11**: 402–9.

Seshachar, B. R., and A. V. Bhandary. 1962. Observation on the life cycle of a new race of *Blepharisma undulans* from India. J. Protozool. **9**: 265–70.

Stolte, H. A. 1924. Morphologische und physiologische Untersuchungen an *Blepharisma undulans* Stein. Arch. Protist. **48**: 245–301.

Suzuki, S. 1951. Morphological study of *Blepharisma undulans* from Japan. Bull. Yamagata Univ. Nat. Sci. **3**: 275–80.

———— 1954. Taxonomic studies on *Blepharisma undulans* with special reference to macronuclear variation. J. Sci. Hiroshima Univ. (Ser. B., Div. 1) **15**: 205–20.

———— 1957. Morphogenesis in the regeneration of *Blepharisma undulans japonicus* Suzuki. Bull. Yamagata Univ. Nat. Sci. **4**: 85–192.

Utsumi, K. 1956a. Cytochemical study on ciliated protozoa, 3. Med. and Biol. **41**: 143–46.

———— 1956b. Cytochemical study on ciliated protozoa, 4. Med. and Biol. **41**: 226–30.

Utsumi, K., and K. Yoshizawa. 1955. Fibrous organelles of *Blepharisma*. (Japanese) Saibokagaku-Symposium **5**: 139–50.

——— 1957. Intracellular structure of *Blepharisma* as revealed by electron microscope. Zool. Mag. **66**: 234–39.

Weisz, P. B. 1950. On the mitochondrial nature of pigment granules in *Stentor* and *Blepharisma*. J. Morph. **86**: 177–84.

——— 1951. An experimental analysis of morphogenesis in *Stentor coeruleus*. J. Exp. Zool. **116**: 231–57.

Young, D. 1939. Macronuclear reorganization in *Blepharisma undulans*. J. Morph. **64**: 297–347.

CHAPTER TWO

Nuclear Behavior

Nuclear functions in *Blepharisma*, as in most ciliates, are divided between the micronucleus (of which several may be present) and the macronucleus, the former being active in sexual processes and the latter in trophic. The behavior of micronuclei and macronuclei is well correlated in both sexual and asexual processes; but in *Blepharisma* it appears especially complex because of the number of micronuclei and the changes in form of the macronucleus. The macronucleus varies in shape in different species, four interphase types being present: compact, halteriform (clubbed or binodal), moniliform (multinodal or beaded), and filiform (filamentous).

Nuclear Behavior During Binary Fission

The sequence of macronuclear events during binary fission is not always the same, and depends on the macronuclear configuration of the species. In blepharismas with halteriform, moniliform, or filiform interphase macronuclei, the macronucleus condenses to form a spherical central mass midway during division but reelongates before the cell splits into two daughter cells (Weisz, 1949; Suzuki, 1951, 1954; McLoughlin, 1957; Bhandary, 1959, 1962; Helson et al., 1959; Seshachar and Bhandary, 1962). When a primary compact macronucleus is already present (as in *B. seculum*; Isquith et al., 1962), it elongates until it is divided between the two daughter cells and then contracts to assume the interphase shape.

During cell division a filiform macronucleus (as in *B. japonicum*) contracts to form a straight, thick, dumbbell-shaped body. As the connecting strand shortens, the terminal masses increase in size and approach each

By Shōichirō Suzuki, Yamagata University, Japan.

other until they fuse into a single compact mass (Fig. 2.1). In rare cases, however, the connecting strand adjacent to either terminal mass diminishes and almost disappears. The central condensed macronuclear mass later reelongates first into a thick rod shape and then into the characteristic elongate filiform shape. This splits and separates equally into the two daughter cells.

A moniliform macronucleus behaves differently in different species. In *B. undulans*, which has a two-noded moniliform macronucleus, the sequence of events during division is essentially like that of the filiform macronucleus. The terminal masses of the macronucleus gradually increase in size and approach each other to fuse into a single compact mass. In *B. americanum*, which has a multinodal macronucleus, the macronuclear condensation shows considerable individual variability. For example, preceding the formation of a central condensed mass, the macronuclear nodes fuse to form two to four nodal masses, with or without internodal strands. Usually, the middle nodes fuse with the terminal nodes, forming enlarged anterior and posterior terminal nodes (Fig. 2.2, C–D); but they may also fuse into one or two masses lying between the terminal masses. When two terminal masses are connected with a nuclear strand, or when three or four nuclear masses with or without internodal strands are formed, the "bimacronucleated" stage observed by Young (1939) and Weisz (1949) is not seen (Fig. 2.2, A–B, E–F). In still other species with moniliform macronuclei (as in *B. musculus* v. giesei) the macronuclear nodes either condense into two terminal masses or condense directly into a central nuclear mass. In these cases, the internodal strands connecting the nuclear masses are usually maintained (Suzuki, unpublished).

A few observers have noted the complete dissolution of the nuclear nodes or nodal masses during condensation in *B. americanum* and other species (McLoughlin, 1957; Suzuki, 1954). But such examples are not common, unlike the contrary observations of Young (1939) and Weisz (1949). And in all cases the nodal masses, whatever their number, eventually unite to form a single condensed, spherical mass.

Renodulation, followed by the reelongation of the condensed macronuclear mass, precedes the cytoplasmic division in several species of *Blepharisma* (Bhandary, 1959; Weisz, 1949; McLoughlin, 1957; Helson et al., 1959; Hirshfield et al., 1962, 1965), including *B. musculus* v. giesei (Suzuki, unpublished). It occurs after the separation of daughter cells

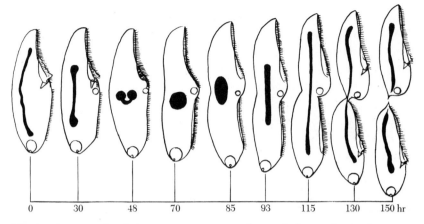

Fig. 2.1. Macronuclear behavior at various times during the binary fission of *B. japonicum*. From Suzuki, 1957a.

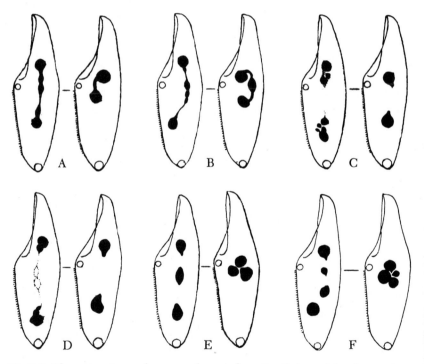

Fig. 2.2. The various types of macronuclear condensation that may take place before the formation of a single condensed mass in a dividing cell of *B. japonicum*. *A–B*, condensation without dissolution of the nuclear nodes or connecting strand. *C–F*, condensation into isolated nuclear masses. From Suzuki, 1954.

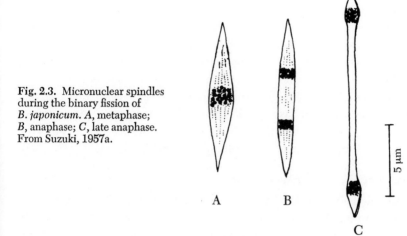

Fig. 2.3. Micronuclear spindles during the binary fission of *B. japonicum. A,* metaphase; *B,* anaphase; *C,* late anaphase. From Suzuki, 1957a.

in *B. americanum* (Suzuki, 1954). The interphase macronucleus often presents a bifurcated or duplicated form. These abnormalities are usually produced as the result of incomplete or unsuccessful coalescence of the macronuclear anlagen during the reorganization after conjugation; otherwise, they are derived from macronuclear masses isolated during division (Helson et al., 1959).

Micronuclear division is correlated with macronuclear division. When macronuclear contraction begins, the micronuclei swell, forming vesicular bodies containing chromatin granules. The minute size and close packing of these granules make them difficult to count accurately (approximately eight were counted in Feulgen preparations). Suzuki (1957a–b) regards these granules as chromosomes, though they could be "chromosome aggregates" (see Chapter 3). Micronuclear mitosis begins after the macronucleus contracts into its short dumbbell shape and is completed just before the fully condensed macronuclear mass begins to reelongate. Metaphase micronuclear spindles are scattered in the cytoplasm around the macronucleus; and in Feulgen preparations red granular chromosomes, already duplicated to sixteen, are visible at this time in the middle of each spindle (Fig. 2.3). During micronuclear anaphase the chromosomes separate into two groups of eight, which migrate toward opposite poles.

In micronuclear telophase, the spindle elongates into a filiform body with expanded terminals containing the dense chromatin. In Stage IV of division the micronuclei, which have already completed mitosis and are distributed around the ends of the macronucleus, are divided unequally between the two prospective daughter cells. The micronuclei then migrate toward the macronucleus, and have come to rest near it at the position characteristic of interphase by the time its reelongation is completed. Occasionally, micronuclear division is so delayed that metaphase and telophase spindles are still evident when the macronucleus is already halfway through the reelongation process, as observed in *B. tropicum* (Seshachar and Bhandary, 1962).

Reorganization and Regeneration

Detailed observations have been made of nuclear behavior in *B. japonicum* during oral replacement (formerly called physiological reorganization) and regeneration (Suzuki, 1957). The macronucleus contracts into a spherical mass midway in the process and then reelongates to resume its vegetative configuration. The micronuclei undergo mitosis, just as in cell division, shortly before or during macronuclear condensation (Fig. 2.4). However, during physiological reorganization and regeneration the macronucleus does not divide, nor is a fission line formed (Weisz, 1949). The timing of macronuclear events during regeneration in *B. japonicum* v. intermedium (Parker and Giese, 1966) and its change under experimental conditions are considered in Chapter 10.

Conjugation

Bütschli (1876), Calkins (1912), Stolte (1924), Moore (1924), Giese (1938), Young (1939), and Weisz (1950a–b) have all made observations on restricted aspects of conjugation in *Blepharisma*. More complete morphological and cytological studies of conjugation are those by Suzuki (1957a–b), Bhandary (1959, 1960), and Seshachar and Bhandary (1962), working with *B. japonicum, B. musculus* v. seshachari, *B. americanum*, and *B. tropicum*. Some of these investigators, however, paid no attention to the stages of pregamic and postgamic divisions, which are illustrated in detail only for *B. japonicum* (Suzuki, 1957a–b). Accordingly, this chapter discusses nuclear behavior during conjugation only in *B. japonicum*.

Prior to conjugation two blepharismas pair up, adhere to one another near their anterior ends by the peristomal region, and then attach by

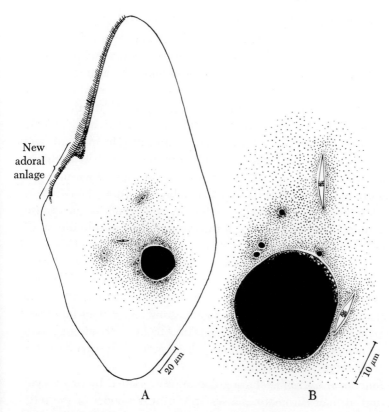

New
adoral
anlage

A   B

Fig. 2.4. Oral replacement in an anterior fragment of *B. japonicum*. *A* shows the complete fragment, and *B* the immediate area of the nuclei. The condensed macronucleus, the metaphase spindles of the micronuclei, and the developing adoral zone are all visible. From Suzuki, 1957a.

their peroral cones as well (i.e., by the cytoplasmic projections that arise from the posterior peristomal region). Thus each conjugant forms two temporary connections with its partner, but fusion subsequently occurs along the full length of the peristome. Fusion is followed by three pregamic divisions, syngamy, and three postgamic divisions.

The macronucleus. Soon after conjugation has begun, the macronucleus starts to degenerate. During the first and second pregamic micronuclear divisions it contracts to an irregular tangle, and sometimes breaks into two pieces (see Fig. 2.10, *A–D*). It then condenses into one of various fairly regular shapes (e.g., S-shaped) by the end of the third postgamic division. Eventually, by the time the new macronuclear anlagen begin to differentiate (Fig. 2.10, *E–N*), the old macronucleus becomes a ring-shaped or horseshoe-shaped mass enclosed in a well-defined membrane. At this time it contains some achromatic spherules and has an unstable area along its inner margin. After the conjugants separate, the old encapsulated macronucleus condenses to a compact spherical mass, still reacting strongly to the Feulgen test (see Fig. 2.11).* When the macronuclear anlagen in the exconjugant become slightly positive to the Feulgen stain, resorption of the old macronucleus begins. The macronucleus loses its alveolar structure, and the chromatin granules at its center no longer absorb Feulgen stain: the decrease in stainability then proceeds peripherally until it reaches the outer membrane of the macronucleus.

Pregamic divisions. A few hours after the conjugants begin to fuse, the micronuclei leave the vicinity of the macronuclear membrane, swell, and gather in the midbody of the *Blepharisma*. About half of the 3–29 micronuclei (16 is the most common number) of a conjugant are functional and destined to undergo the first pregamic division; these swell to form vesicular bodies, each showing reticular chromatin within. The other micronuclei, destined to degenerate, grow larger than functional ones, become negative to the Feulgen stain (though retaining a strong affinity to hematoxylin), and gradually disintegrate and disappear during the later stages of conjugation.

The functional micronuclei are gradually surrounded by dense cytoplasm, and distinct chromatin masses appear at the nodes of the reticular chromatin. As the reticular structure disappears, the chromatin masses organize into eight granular chromosomes. The spindles of the first pregamic division elongate in the anaphase and become somewhat dumbbell-shaped, with unequal-sized terminal expansions, each enclosing one set of eight chromosomes. The larger half of the anaphase spindle develops into a functional nucleus, whereas the smaller is cast away at the end of telophase as a small body enclosing a compact chromatin mass (Fig. 2.5; Fig. 2.10, *A–B*). Thus only one product of the first pregamic division is viable.

The micronuclei left after the first pregamic division then undergo the second pregamic division, forming typical spindles. The number of the micronuclei taking part in the second division is usually 5–10, though it ranges from one to 16. Each metaphase spindle contains four double

---

* Stolte (1924) and Young (1939) mistook these encapsulated old macronuclear masses for developing macronuclear anlagen and consequently identified the young macronuclear anlagen as the degenerating old macronucleus.

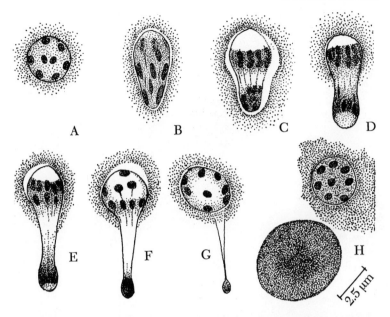

Fig. 2.5. Division stages of a micronucleus in the first pregamic division during conjugation in *B. japonicum*. *A–B*, prophase; *C–E*, anaphase; *F–G*, telophase. From Suzuki, 1957b.

chromosomes. In anaphase, the double chromosomes separate into two groups of four and move toward opposite poles, finally disjoining to form haploid micronuclei. In late anaphase the spindle becomes a rod-shaped body, and the chromosomes disintegrate into chromatin masses that occupy both ends of the spindle (Fig. 2.6, Fig. 2.10, *C*). One of the haploid nuclei in each conjugant now becomes the functional one and migrates toward the peroral region. This functional micronucleus is distinguishable from the others by its special location, larger size, and dense enclosing cytoplasmic sphere.

As the functional micronucleus undergoes the third pregamic division, all the nonfunctional micronuclei begin to disintegrate. The spindles of the third pregamic division are similar in external features to those of the second pregamic division but are much smaller. The chromosomes gather on the equatorial plane of the metaphase spindle and split to form two groups of four chromosomes, each group migrating toward an opposite pole of the anaphase spindle (Fig. 2.7; Fig. 2.10, *C*). Thus two haploid gametic pronuclei are produced in each conjugant.

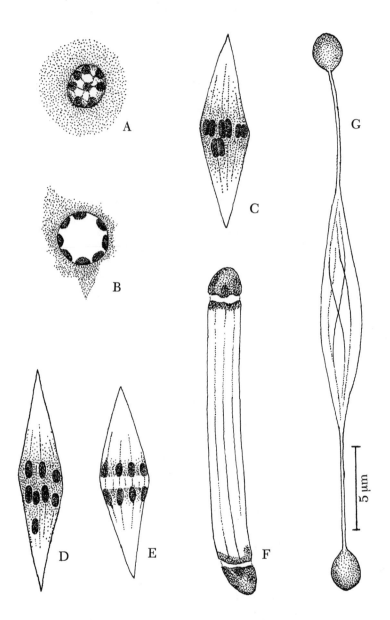

Fig. 2.6. Stages in the second pregamic division of *B. japonicum. A–B*, prophase;
the eight chromosomes of a functional micronucleus assume a peripheral position.
C, metaphase; four double chromosomes are arranged on the equatorial plane.
D–F, anaphase; two groups of four chromosomes migrate toward opposite poles of
the spindle. *G*, telophase; the sister nuclei are separated, with a long connecting
strand. From Suzuki, 1957b.

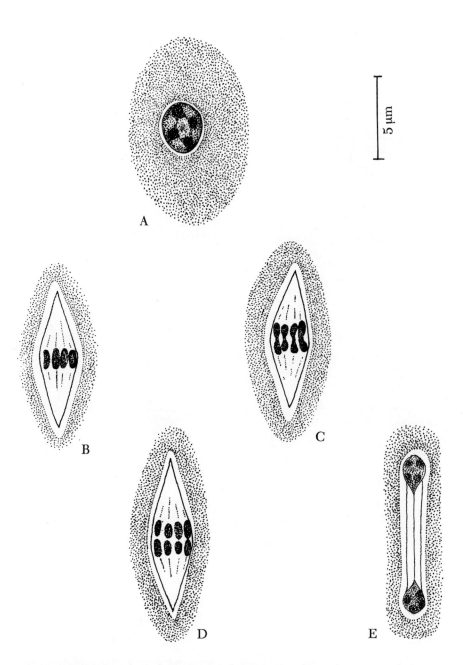

Fig. 2.7. The third pregamic division in *B. japonicum*. *A*, early prophase. *B–C*, metaphase. *D–E*, anaphase. From Suzuki, 1957b.

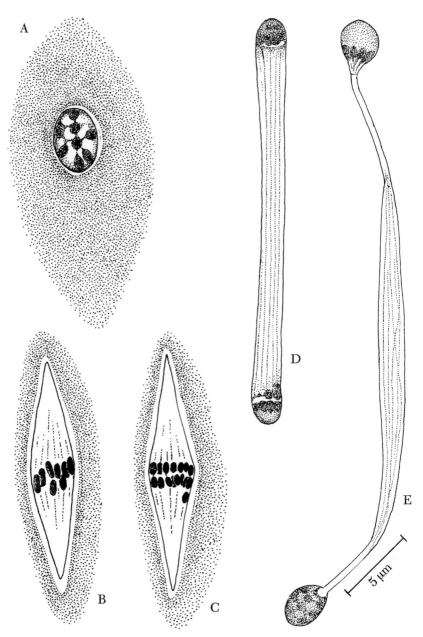

Fig. 2.8. The first postgamic division in *B. japonicum*. *A*, resting stage of synkaryon after fertilization. *B*, metaphase spindle. *C–D*, early and late anaphase. *E*, telophase. From Suzuki, 1957b.

Fusion of pronuclei, postgamic division, and formation of anlagen. The pronuclei in each conjugant are differentiated functionally—not morphologically—into stationary and migratory nuclei. Reciprocal migration and fusion of the pronuclei between the two conjugants now begin while the pronuclei are still in the vesicular state, but they assume a spindle shape just before fusion is completed (Fig. 2.10, *F–G*).

The synkaryon formed in this manner in each conjugant next undergoes three successive postgamic divisions to produce eight nuclei (Fig. 2.10, *H–M*). These divisions are characterized by two sets of eight chromosomes observable in the metaphase and anaphase spindles, and by a long connecting strand between the daughter nuclei in the telophase (Fig. 2.8). Typically, six of the eventual eight micronuclei increase in size and become macronuclear anlagen; the other two continue to divide, producing additional micronuclei. Usually, two of the macronuclear anlagen grow larger than the others, but sometimes only one grows larger; in still other cases, from three to five, and occasionally all six develop into large macronuclear anlagen (Fig. 2.10). The number of macronuclear anlagen (including the additional ones from later micronuclear divisions) thus varies in different conjugants, ranging from one to thirteen (six is most common). The micronuclei usually multiply until eight are produced, but they may also vary in number (2–15).

The conjugants separate after the macronuclear anlagen are differentiated but while they are still Feulgen-negative. The macronuclear anlagen, at first, are achromatic spherical bodies, including one or two deeply staining granules; but as they increase in size, the granules swell into vesicular spherules and become negative to the Feulgen stain, like those observed in the interphase macronucleus (Fig. 2.9). The macronuclear anlagen become intensely positive to the Feulgen reaction only after the disintegration of the old macronucleus (Fig. 2.11).

Post-conjugation cell division. Prior to the division of the exconjugants the macronuclear anlagen assume a longitudinal position, the large anlagen usually distal and the small anlagen lying between them. The two opposite groups of large and small anlagen then fuse to form two large masses; rarely, the anlagen fuse into three masses. When the anlagen are equal-sized they first form longitudinal connections, producing a moniliform nuclear chain that closely resembles the interphase macronucleus of *B. musculus* v. giesei and other species. This chain divides at midlevel and condenses into two terminal masses.

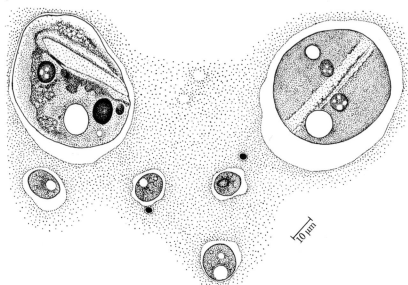

Fig. 2.9. Developing macronuclear anlagen in *B. japonicum*, drawn from a hematoxylin preparation. Two large and four small anlagen appear, as well as two micronuclei. Some spherules in the anlagen are stained intensely, but others have lost their staining capacity or are vacuolating. From Suzuki, 1957b.

In any case, the exconjugant *B. japonicum* eventually presents a "bi-macronucleate" appearance analogous to that observed in the division of *B. americanum*. Each of the nuclear masses forms an elongate projection from its proximal end and fuses with the other to form a single macronucleus. The macronucleus then elongates and the exconjugant divides soon afterward.

The durations of the major events during conjugation and reorganization in *B. japonicum* are presented in Table 2.1.

Conjugation in Other Species

Details of the nuclear events during conjugation are not identical in different species of the genus. On the basis of macronuclear behavior and formation, conjugation in *Blepharisma* may be divided into two general types, each of which includes two subtypes.

Type 1. Macronuclear anlagen begin to differentiate before the separation of conjugating pairs and subsequently unite to form a single macronucleus in each exconjugant. Examples are *B. japonicum* and *B. americanum*. However, the formation of the vegetative macronu-

TABLE 2.1

Duration of Stages in the Conjugation of *B. japonicum*

Stages	Time after union
First pregamic division	4–7 hr
Second pregamic division	8–14
Third pregamic division	15–18
Postgamic division	18–23
Macronuclear anlagen appear	24–48
Separation of conjugants	38–68
Terminal anlagen masses form	125+
Terminal anlagen masses fuse	165+
First division of exconjugant	174+

cleus differs in these species. In *B. japonicum* the macronuclear anlagen fuse to form two masses, which elongate and unite into a single macronucleus. In *B. americanum* they become connected by slender strands to form a moniliform macronucleus. Another example of the second subtype is *B. americanum* v. trinodatum.

Type 2. The macronuclear anlagen, before beginning to differentiate, are segregated into separate cells by exconjugant division. Examples are *B. tropicum* and *B. musculus* v. seshachari. Again, the two differ in their formation of the vegetative macronucleus. In *B. tropicum* the old macronucleus condenses into a single mass, and the macronuclear anlagen are formed while the conjugants are still attached. In *B. musculus* v. seshachari the old macronucleus breaks into nodes, and the macronuclear anlagen are formed only after the separation of the conjugants. *B. musculus* v. giesei is another example of the second type.

The four characteristic subtypes are summarized in Table 2.2.

Nuclear Reorganization Other than Conjugation

Nuclear behavior during encystment and excystment is dealt with in Chapter 10.

Autogamy. Giese (1938) reported multiconjugation in *B. americanum*, as did Weisz (1950a) for two undetermined species having moniliform macronuclei, one from Woods Hole and the other from North Carolina. Since nuclear change occurs synchronously in all participants regardless of the attachment pattern, and since these changes are identical in nature and duration to those in normal conjugation, Weisz considered multiconjugation to be evidence for autogamy in these

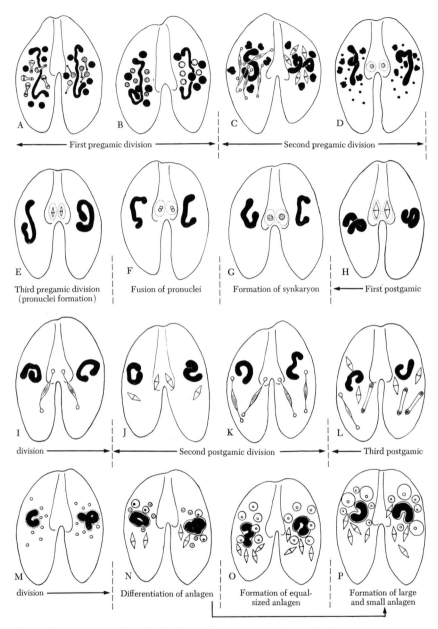

Fig. 2.10. Sequence of nuclear behavior during conjugation in *B. japonicum.* Light figures represent functional nuclei. Dark circles or masses are degenerating nuclei and are shown only in the stage during which they arise, except for the unused degenerative nuclei of the first pregamic division. From Suzuki, 1957b.

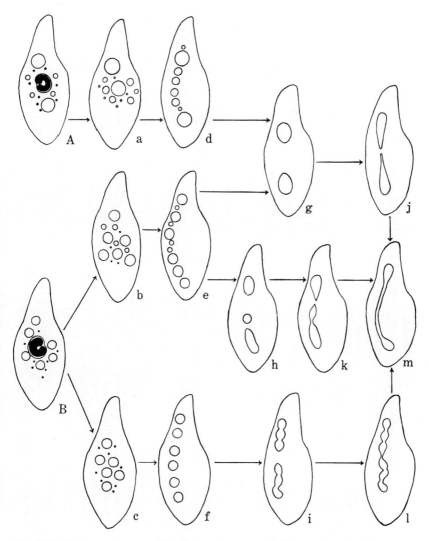

Fig. 2.11. Various sequences of forming new macronuclei in exconjugants of *B. japonicum*. *A*, an exconjugant containing two large and four small macronuclear anlagen, eight micronuclei, and an old macronucleus; the small anlagen fuse with the large ones to form two terminal masses. *B*, an exconjugant containing six equal macronuclear anlagen, eight micronuclei, and an old macronucleus. In sequences *a* and *b* additional anlagen are produced. In *c* the micronuclei do not develop into additional anlagen. In *d*, *e*, and *f* the anlagen form a rough line (micronuclei are not shown in these and subsequent drawings). In the third stage the anlagen fuse to form two spherical masses (*g*), three smaller masses (*h*), or two moniliform masses (*i*). These masses then fuse (*j–l*) and finally form a new macronucleus (*m*). From Suzuki, 1957b.

TABLE 2.2

Conjugation Types Exemplified in Four Species of *Blepharisma*

Phenomenon	B. musculus v. seshachari (Bhandary, 1959)	B. tropicum (Seshachar & Bhandary, 1962)	B. americanum (Bhandary, 1962)	B. japonicum (Suzuki, 1957a)
Ma behavior	forms nodes	condenses to single mass	condenses to single mass	condenses to single mass
Pregamic divisions: Mi undergoing 1st division	7–8	6–10	4–16	half or more of 3–29 Mi
Products undergoing 2d division	5–8	6–10	6–8	usu. 4–11
Products undergoing 3d division	1	2[a]	1	1
Postgamic divisions	2	2–3	3	3
Products of postgamic divisions	4 (3 Ma anl. and 1 Mi anl. that divides thrice, producing 8 Mi); Mi divide again, making 18 bodies	4 (2 Ma, 1 Mi, and 1 degenerative nucleus); or 8 (3–4 Ma, rest Mi)	8 (3–7 Ma anl., rest Mi anl.); divide to increase Mi	usu. 8 (6 Ma anl., 2 Mi anl.); Mi anl. divide to increase Mi or produce extra Ma
Formation of Ma anl.	uniform anl. form after conjugation	uniform anl. form before separation of conjugants	uniform anl. form before separation	unequal anl. form before separation
Formation of vegetative nuclei	exconjugant division segregates nuclei; 1 Ma anl. and 4–8 Mi in each daughter	exconjugant div. segregates nuclei; 1 Ma anl. and variable Mi in each daughter	Ma anl. form before separation	Ma anl. form before separation
Time before separation	24–30 hr	24 hr	24 hr	38–68 hr
Time of entire process	5–6 days	—	5–6 days	7 days

[a] Two of the 2d-division products move toward the peroral cone: one enters the peroral region and again divides; the other divides outside and its products degenerate.

species. Inaba (1965) also studied multiconjugation between two strains of *Blepharisma* that are somewhat different from each other in external morphology but resemble each other closely in macronuclear configuration. In this case cytological observations revealed the simultaneous development of macronuclear anlagen in all three participants, suggesting autogamy in one member of the multiconjugate. However, in both cases the researcher's failure to observe the syngamy of gametic nuclei and the related mitotic divisions renders the evidence for autogamy inconclusive.

Parthenogenetic conjugation. Moore (1924), observing the formation of macronuclear anlagen in split conjugants, suggested that parthenogenetic reorganization (endomixis) is perhaps a normal periodic phenomenon in *Blepharisma*. Suzuki (1957b) has reported that under certain circumstances conjugation in *B. japonicum* is parthenogenetic. Observations both on intact pairs and on conjugants experimentally split indicated that the micronuclei in parthenogenetic conjugation develop as follows. The second micronuclear division corresponding to the second pregamic division in conjugation is not reductional and produces diploid nuclei. One of the products of this division, a diploid nucleus equivalent to the synkaryon in conjugation, then undergoes three divisions in succession, producing eight nuclei. From three to six (typically four) of these develop into macronuclear anlagen, which may increase in number through subsequent divisions. Half the macronuclear anlagen pass into daughter cells of the first division of the parthenogenetic exconjugants. The fusion of the macronuclear anlagen, as seen in true conjugation, may or may not occur before cell division. Inasmuch as the third pregamic division and syngamy are omitted, parthenogenetic conjugation is abbreviated, and the time required for its completion is considerably less than that for conjugation.*

Regardless of when the cells of a parthenogenetic conjugating pair are separated, the nuclei complete their divisions, forming macronuclear anlagen and micronuclei without forming a synkaryon. Normal vegetative cells, each with a macronucleus and multiple micronuclei, are thus produced. Occasionally, 33 or 34 equal-sized premature macronuclear anlagen are formed, not only in parthenogenetic conjugants split at an

---

* Parthenogenetic development of gametic nuclei during conjugation has also been observed in *Paramecium bursaria* (Chen, 1940a–b, 1946) and *P. trichium* (Diller, 1948).

early stage of conjugation but also in paired conjugants. This suggests that the parthenogenetic nuclei resulting from the second division are equivalent to a synkaryon in nature; and they do occasionally begin synchronous divisions to form numerous macronuclear anlagen.

Parthenogenetic conjugation differs from autogamy (or "cytogamy" as it is sometimes called). In autogamy there are three pregamic divisions, producing haploid gametic nuclei as in true conjugation, but no nuclear exchange occurs between the members of the "conjugating" pair; instead the gametic nuclei produced in a given individual fuse to form the synkaryon (self-fertilization).

Although the term parthenogenetic conjugation has been commonly applied to anlagen formation without syngamy, in the broadest sense parthenogenesis means that a "female" gamete develops without fertilization by a "male" gamete. Accordingly, aberrant types of conjugation in *Blepharisma* and *Paramecium* are not true examples of parthenogenesis. The development of micronuclei into nuclear anlagen in these cases should therefore be regarded as apomixis without gametogenesis and fertilization, or as apomictic conjugation, in contrast to amphimictic (normal cross-fertilizing) or autogamous (self-fertilizing) conjugation.

LITERATURE CITED

Bhandary, A. V. 1959. Cytology of an Indian race of *Blepharisma undulans* Stein. J. Protozool. **6**: 333–39.

———— 1960. Conjugation in *Blepharisma undulans americanus*. J. Protozool. **7**: 250–55.

———— 1962. Taxonomy of genus *Blepharisma* with special reference to *Blepharisma undulans*. J. Protozool. **9**: 435–42.

Bütschli, O. 1876. Studien über die ersten Entwicklungsvorgänge der Einzelle, die Zellteilung und Konjugation der Infusorien. Abhandl. Senckenb. Naturforsch. Ges. **10**: 1–250.

Calkins, G. 1912. The paedogamous conjugation of *Blepharisma undulans*. J. Morph. **23**: 667–86.

Chen, T. T. 1940a. Polyploidy and its origin in *Paramecium*. J. Hered. **31**: 175–84.

———— 1940b. Conjugation in *Paramecium bursaria* between animals with diverse nuclear constitutions. J. Hered. **31**: 185–96.

———— 1946. Varieties and mating types in *Paramecium bursaria*, 1: New variety and types from England, Ireland, and Czechoslovakia. Proc. Nat. Acad. Sci. **32**: 173–81.

Christie, S. L., and H. I. Hirshfield. 1967. Macronuclear variation during the life cycle of *Blepharisma dawsoni* n. sp. and *B. wardsi*. J. Protozool. **14**: 759–62.

Dembitzer, H. M., and H. I. Hirshfield. 1966. Some new cytological observations in the heterotrichous ciliate *Blepharisma*. J. Cell Biol. **30**: 201–7.

Diller, W. F. 1948. Nuclear behavior of *Paramecium trichium* during conjugation. J. Morph. **82**: 1–52.

Giese, A. C. 1938. Size and conjugation in *Blepharisma*. Arch. Protistenk. **91**: 125–234.

Helson, L., P. Pecora, and H. I. Hirshfield. 1959. Macronuclear change in a strain of *Blepharisma undulans* during the divisional cycle. J. Protozool. **6**: 131–35.

Hirshfield, H. I., and A. V. Bhandary. 1963. Macronuclear variability of *Blepharisma* associated with growth. *In* "Cell Growth and Cell Division," Symp. Intern. Soc. Cell Biol. **2**: 27–56.

Hirshfield, H. I., I. R. Isquith, and A. V. Bhandary. 1965. A proposed organization of the genus *Blepharisma* Perty and description of four new species. J. Protozool. **12**: 136–44.

Inaba, F. 1965. Conjugation between two strains of *Blepharisma*. J. Protozool. **12**: 145–51.

Isquith, I. R., and H. I. Hirshfield. 1968. Non-Mendelian inheritance in *Blepharisma intermedium*. J. Protozool. **15**: 513–16.

Isquith, I. R., A. J. Repak, and H. I. Hirshfield. 1965. *Blepharisma seculum*, sp. nov., a member of the subgenus (*Compactum*). J. Protozool. **12**: 615–18.

McLoughlin, D. K. 1957. Macronuclear morphogenesis during division of *Blepharisma undulans*. J. Protozool. **4**: 150–53.

Minutoli, F., and H. I. Hirshfield. 1968. DNA synthesis cycle in *Blepharisma*. J. Protozool. **15**: 532–35.

Moore, E. L. 1924. Regeneration at various phases in the life history of the infusorians *Spathidium spatula* and *Blepharisma undulans*. J. Exp. Zool. **39**: 249–315.

Padmavathi, P. B. 1959. Studies on the cytology of an Indian species of *Blepharisma* (Protozoa: Ciliata). Vest. Ceskoslov. Spol. Zool. **23**: 193–99.

Parker, J. W., and A. C. Giese. 1966. Nuclear activity during regeneration in *Blepharisma*. J. Protozool. **13**: 617–22.

Repak, A. J., and H. I. Hirshfield. 1967. A triple staining technique for buccal cilia, pigment, and nucleus of *Blepharisma*. Trans. Amer. Micros. Soc. **86**: 341–42.

Saxena, D. M. 1966. Isolation of macronuclei from the ciliates *Blepharisma intermedium* and *Spirostomum ambiguum*: The role of digitonin. Indian J. Exp. Biol. **4**: 182–84.

———— 1968. Cytochemistry of *Blepharisma intermedium* and *Spirostomum ambiguum* (Ciliata: Spirotricha). Ann. Histochem. **13**: 291–300.

Seshachar, B. R. 1960. Effect of centrifugation on the macronucleus of *Spirostomum* and *Blepharisma*. Nature **186**: 333–34.

———— 1964. Observations on the fine structure of the nuclear apparatus of *Blepharisma intermedium* Bhandary (Ciliata: Spirotricha). J. Protozool. **11**: 402–9.

———— 1966. Further observations on the chromosomal filaments of the ciliate macronucleus. Cytologia **31**: 77–79.

Seshachar, B. R., and A. V. Bhandary, 1962. Observation on the life cycle of a new race of *Blepharisma undulans* from India. J. Protozool. **9**: 265–70.

Stolte, H. A. 1924. Morphologische und physiologische Untersuchungen an *Blepharisma undulans* Stein. Arch. Protist. **48**: 245–301.

Suzuki, S. 1951. Morphological study on *Blepharisma undulans* from Japan. Bull. Yamagata Univ. Nat. Sci. **3**: 275–80.

———— 1954. Taxonomic studies on *Blepharisma undulans* with special reference to macronuclear variation. J. Sci. Hiroshima Univ. (Ser. B., Div. 1) **15**: 205–20.

———— 1957a. Conjugation in *Blepharisma undulans japonicus* Suzuki with special reference to the nuclear phenomena. Bull. Yamagata Univ. Nat. Sci. **4**: 43–68.

———— 1957b. Parthenogenetic conjugation in *Blepharisma undulans japonicus* Suzuki. *Ibid.* **4**: 69–84.

Utsumi, K. 1956a. Cytochemical study on ciliated protozoa, 3. Med. and Biol. **41**: 143–46.

———— 1956b. Cytochemical study on ciliated protozoa, 4. Med. and Biol. **41**: 226–30.

Weisz, P. B. 1949. The role of the macronucleus in the differentiation of *Blepharisma undulans*. J. Morph. **85**: 503–18.

———— 1950a. Multiconjugation in *Blepharisma*. Biol. Bull. **98**: 242–46.

———— 1950b. On the morphogenetic role of the macronucleus during conjugation in *Blepharisma undulans*. J. Exp. Zool. **114**: 293–304.

Woodruff, L. L. 1927. Studies on the life history of *Blepharisma undulans*. Proc. Soc. Exp. Biol. Med. **24**: 769–70 and **25**: 683–86.

Woodruff, L. L., and H. Spencer. 1922. Racial variation in *Blepharisma undulans*. Proc. Soc. Exp. Biol. Med. **19**: 339–40.

Young, D. 1939. Macronuclear reorganization in *Blepharisma undulans*. J. Morph. **64**: 297–347.

CHAPTER THREE

Fine Structure

Ciliates of the genus *Blepharisma* have been the subjects of numerous studies in fine structure, and their general ultrastructure is perhaps better known than that of their closer relatives among the heterotrichs (e.g., *Stentor, Spirostomum,* or *Condylostoma*). Studies of other genera have been mainly concerned with identifying the structures responsible for the pronounced contractility of those organisms.

The most comprehensive electron-microscope study of *Blepharisma* is that of Kennedy (1964), which describes essentially all the features of vegetative cells. Dembitzer and Hirshfield (1966) have added information on the cortical fibrous system and the intracytoplasmic membranes. Dembitzer (1968) utilized electron-microscope cytochemistry to elucidate the fate of the food vacuoles and the relationship of the previously observed intracytoplasmic membrane system and Golgi bodies to digestion. The nuclear apparatus has been examined by Seshachar (1964), micronuclear division by Jenkins (1967), and nuclear division during binary fission, in particular the changes in macronuclear chromatin, by Inaba and Sotakawa (1968). Other recent work has been concerned with the effects of light-bleaching and strychnine on pigment granules and their extrusion (Kennedy, 1966) and with the ultrastructure of the resting cysts of *B. stoltei* (Repak and Pfister, 1967). Work over the last three or four years has served to clarify earlier studies of cytoplasmic inclusions (Utsumi and Yoshizawa, 1957), the cortex (Utsumi and Yoshizawa, 1957; Borysko and Dembitzer, 1958), and the pigment granules (Inaba et al., 1958). Where appropriate, information from these reports will be considered in this chapter.

By R. A. Jenkins, University of Wyoming. The work included in this chapter was supported by NSF Grant No. GB 6405.

Blepharismas are relatively large, highly vacuolated cells, and seem especially sensitive to osmotic shock. As a consequence, it has been difficult to preserve all aspects of cellular fine structure adequately with a single fixation procedure, even using newer techniques (e.g., glutaraldehyde applied in a variety of vehicles). Hence several different procedures must be used if one is to prepare the most accurate representation of all cellular details. The procedures used to prepare each of the electron micrographs included here are noted on pp. 54–55. The abbreviations given in the text are those used in the figures.

Cortical Structures

The pellicular complex. The surface of *Blepharisma* is bounded by a pellicle (P), whose structure is difficult to define. We believe it to consist of at least two membranes, each approximately 8 nm in width, which are separated by a less dense space about 10 nm wide (see Figs. 3.2, 3.3, and 3.12). The outermost membrane is often particularly dense, and occasionally seems to have a fine extraneous coat (Fig. 3.2, Ec). The structure of the pellicle is most evident in regions between the membranelles and in transverse sections of the cell. Kennedy (1966) has concluded that the pellicle is a single membrane serving as both pellicle and plasma membrane. It does happen on occasion that only a single limiting membrane is clearly resolved; however, at other times three component membranes seem to be present. A clear delineation of the pellicular structure is made difficult by problems in interpreting the orientation of sections, by the different preparative techniques employed, and by the vesicles and microtubules that lie just beneath the surface of the cell. Nevertheless, an examination of many cross sections of the organism indicates that the pellicle is a tripartite complex with a total thickness of some 25–30 nm.

Immediately beneath the inner membrane of the pellicle is a well-organized system of microtubules. In transverse sections this subpellicular microtubule (Spm) system is shown to be composed of microtubules about 22 nm in diameter, lying parallel to the long axis of the cell and spaced at intervals of about 25 nm (Fig. 3.3). The microtubules follow the surface contours but are absent directly beneath the lowest depressions of the cortical furrows (Fig. 3.3). Along the descending left side of each cortical ridge the microtubules join with the kinetodesmal fiber (Kf) in such a way that they appear to alternate with the distal microtubules in each vertical stack of the kinetodesmal fiber (Fig. 3.3). The rising right side of each ridge is devoid of Spm. As pointed out by Kennedy (1965), it is not clear whether the transverse fibers arising from the anterior kinetosome (K) of each pair become Spm or connect with the Spm system. Structurally, the elements of the system are apparently microtubules as generally described, although they may consist of two helical subfilaments (Kennedy, 1965). The Spm are most probably mechanical elements that help to maintain cell form; however, their possible involvement in irritability or motility should not be ruled out.

Pigment granules. The pinkish color of many blepharismas is due to a concentration of membrane-limited pigment granules (Pg), about 0.35 μm in diameter and lying just below the pellicle (Figs. 3.1, 3.2). The granules are concentrated under the ridges of the pellicle in longitudinal rows but are not uncommon much deeper in the cell (Fig. 3.1). Considerable variation in the appearance of the limiting membrane and general structure is found even in granules that are adjacent. As previously described by Inaba et al. (1958) and Kennedy (1965), there are two general types of granules: one is dense, homogeneous, and spherical; the other is less dense, granular, and irregular in outline. Inaba et al. (1958) attributed the color of living organisms to the granulated form and regarded the compact form as pigment-deficient. Kennedy (1966) has demonstrated that the cortical granules are readily extruded by the organism, leaving deep surface cups (Cu) formed by the fusion of the granular and pellicular membranes followed by an apparent dissolution of the outer membrane surface (Fig. 3.1). In some cases, partial extrusion apparently takes place (Figs. 3.2, 3.10); and in glutaraldehyde fixation intact granules are almost never found. The nature and function of the pigment within the granules are discussed in Chapter 11.

Somatic ciliature. The cilia of *Blepharisma* have a structure typical of that described for other ciliates. The body cilia occur only at the floor of the cortical furrows, with a single cilium (C) arising from the anterior member of each kinetosome pair (Figs. 3.1, 3.4). The ciliary shaft shows the classic filament pattern of nine doublet tubules (each doublet continuous with two of the three tubules of the kinetosome) arranged at the perimeter around two single, central tubules; the entire structure is bounded by a single unit membrane that is continuous with the pellicular membrane (Figs. 3.3, 3.4, and 3.14). The central pair of tubules terminates at a dense axosomal granule (Ag) located near the distal end of the kinetosome and just above the transverse septum that occurs roughly at the level of the cell surface (Fig. 3.4). Actually, the two central microtubules end at slightly different levels, and only one of the two extends into the axosomal granule (Fig. 3.14). The peripheral doublets terminate as the distal end of the cilium is approached, whereas the central pair extends very nearly to the tip.

The kinetosomes (K) are about 0.2 μm in diameter and 0.5 μm in length. Near the level of the cell surface, just beneath the slightly concave septum and the axosomal granule, the kinetosome appears as a cylinder of nine triplet tubules (Fig. 3.14). Cross sections nearer to the proximal end show the triplet tubules to be canted so that each makes an angle of 30–40 degrees with the tangent to the cylinder (Fig. 3.5). A cartwheellike structure with a single tubule at the center appears at the proximal end of the kinetosome (Fig. 3.5). The kinetosomes of a pair are not in line with one another parallel to the long axis of the cell; rather, the anterior member is offset to the left so that the pair is aligned at about 20 degrees to the long axis (Fig. 3.6).

Arising from the posterior kinetosome of each pair are 10–12 microtubules (Kmt) aligned in a stack or sheet (Figs. 3.3, 3.6) and running in a right-posterior direction. The component microtubules of each sheet are in contact or are joined by short bridges (Figs. 3.3, 3.5). Similar tubule sheets originate from more anterior kinetosomes, run posteriorly, and overlap the more posterior sheets to form a bundle (Figs. 3.3, 3.6) that corresponds to the kinetodesmal fiber of light microscopy. The way in which these microtubules are connected to the kinetosomes is not clear, although Kennedy (1965) has speculated that they are probably branches of the triplet tubules. Away from either end of the organism the kinetodesma consist of some 8–11 sheets of microtubules. Each single sheet arises at a kinetosome pair and the number of sheets is often 10, the microtubules from a pair extending posteriorly by about 10 kinetosome pairs (approximately 10 μm) and each sheet overlapping the preceding one (Fig. 3.3). In *Blepharisma*, as in other heterotrichs studied, the association of the kinetodesmos with the somatic kinetosomes and the overlapping pattern displayed by the compound fiber suggest that the system is designed for conduction-coordination, or perhaps contraction.

The space between the two kinetosomes of a pair appears to include fibrous and/or microtubular material (Fig. 3.5, Im) and seems to be the point of origin of an abbreviated sheet of tubules or fibers (Akf) that runs anteriorly toward the kinetodesmos (Figs. 3.5, 3.6). Our observations have revealed neither the structure nor the termination of this sheet. Kennedy (1965) refers to the structure as the anterior kinetodesmal fiber and believes that it may overlap or interwind with the kinetodesmos and thereby add stability to the system.

The anterior kinetosome of the somatic pair, near its proximal end and parallel with its triplet tubules, gives rise to a short sheet of about six microtubules, which curves gradually away from the kinetosome and extends upward into the ectoplasmic ridge (Fig. 3.6, Af). Its course beyond this point is not clear, but these sheets may splay apart to become the previously described subpellicular microtubules.

The fibrous lattice. Sections taken at the level of the proximal end of kinetosomes or slightly below pass through a rather poorly defined fibrous band (Figs. 3.7, 3.8, Fb). Examination of transverse sections indicates that the band is present at this location circumferentially, though somewhat discontinuously, and probably delineates an ecto-endoplasmic boundary, as has previously been suggested (Dembitzer and Hirshfield, 1966). The lattice is generally 80 nm in thickness but is slightly variable in structure and dimension. Its components are not tubular in appearance, but seem to be fine fibrils about 4 nm in diameter (Fig. 3.8). The fibrils are not aligned either longitudinally or circularly; rather, they exist in what Dembitzer and Hirshfield (1966) have called a branching network, which forms a fenestrated sheath around the endoplasm. Mitochondria (M) are heavily concentrated about the lattice and in many cases are embedded within fenestrations (Figs. 3.7, 3.8). At the present time, information about the fibrous lattice is so preliminary that no clear function can be ascribed to it. Perhaps the best possibilities are that it serves either as a structural framework or as a motile apparatus that allows the limited flexing of *Blepharisma*. We have found that the fibers are well preserved by osmium vapor and glutaraldehyde fixation.

Peroral and Oral Structures

The peristome in *Blepharisma* is a narrow groove usually limited to the anterior third or half of the cell. An undulating membrane (UM) borders the right peristomal edge, being most prominent toward the posterior half. The adoral zone membranelles (AZM), which lie on the other side, are each composed of three transverse rows of close-set cilia over most of the zone, but have only one or two rows in the anterior and posterior termini; they number 80–100 and are arranged in an antero-posterior band extending to the cytostome. This structure is often called the membranellar band.

The undulating membrane. The undulating membrane consists of three rows of cilia (Figs. 3.9, 3.11, Umk) whose kinetosomes run longitudinally along the margin of the peristome and seemingly follow a slightly elevated ridge in the cortex. The cilia are of the usual morphology except that the ciliary membrane bears numerous long filamentous projections, each ending in a spherical enlargement. This peculiarity is also found in the cilia of the AZM, and its significance will be discussed later. Ancillary kinetosomal fibers, which are typical of kinetosomes in the AZM and kineties, have not been seen associated with the kinetosomes of the undulating membrane. However, there are about 10 microtubules originating in the dense cap that closes the proximal end of each UM kinetosome (Fig. 3.11). These descend downward under the floor of the peristome and into the endoplasm, where they converge to form a rather large bundle of hexagonally packed tubules; and some of them are continuous with the kinetosomes of the AZM, thereby linking the two borders of the peristome (Fig. 3.9, Nf). These microtubules, together with those originating from the kinetosomes of the AZM, comprise the nemadesmal system of *Blepharisma,* which may function to coordinate motion or to give rigidity and support to the oral area.

Peristomal rods. Recent observations have disclosed the presence of peculiar, trichocyst-like rods (Pr) in the floor of the peristome of *B. japonicum* (Figs. 3.10, 3.12). These structures are present in groups, or perhaps rows, and may protrude into the peristomal groove. The entire structure appears to be membrane-limited and at the cell surface has its protruding tip covered by a distended pellicular membrane. Those measured were roughly 2 μm long and 0.25 μm in diameter. Distally, a peristomal rod is characterized by an extremely electron-dense tip; the median portion appears to consist of a fibrous cylinder, which apparently converts to a fibrous bundle at the proximal end (Fig. 3.12). Since cross sections of these rods have not been studied, details of their structure are lacking. Although there is no evidence that they are ejectile, it seems likely that they are trichocysts; this would be, to our knowledge, the first report of trichocysts in heterotrich ciliates.

Adoral zone membranelles. Each membranelle of the AZM is composed of many closely positioned cilia, and each is separated from the membranelles to either side by a small cortical ridge (Fig. 3.13, Cr). The cilia bear numerous projections (Cp), which are identical to those previously described for the undulating membrane but are more numerous and more conspicuous (Fig. 3.17). These projections are usually 0.5 μm in length and have a diameter near 20 nm, expanding to about 65 nm at the bulbous end. It is believed that the cilia are fused into the compound membranelles by an entanglement or zipping together of these protrusions. The AZM cilia of some blepharismas have electron-opaque granules (Dg) located in the cortex of the axoneme just inside the membrane (Fig. 3.15). However, the limited observations of these granules preclude further comment on their occurrence and significance.

At about the middle of the AZM in *B. americanum* each membranelle consists of three rows of cilia, the posterior two with about 14 cilia each and the anterior row somewhat shorter. The homologous region in a larger species, *B. japonicum*, shows at least 24 cilia per posterior row and also has fewer in the anterior row (Fig. 3.13). This pattern has been illustrated by light microscopy (Tuffrau, 1967). As Kennedy (1965) has reported, the kinetosomes of the AZM are arranged in rows such that each kinetosome of the middle row is surrounded by six equidistant kinetosomes.

The kinetosomes of the membranellar cilia are interconnected by fibrous strands (Fs) that are visible only in cross sections at precise levels, probably falling near the midlevel of the kinetosome (Fig. 3.13). Kennedy (1965) proposed that the fibers originate as branches of the peripheral microtubules of the kinetosome. It also seems probable that they might originate in the dense material bordering the triplets. Since the fibers are almost never clearly shown in longitudinal sections, this is a difficult question to resolve.

Below the level of the cartwheel, each kinetosome is closed at its proximal end by a dense fibrous cap (Pc) with a dimension larger than the kinetosomal diameter (Fig. 3.13). From the cap, or perhaps from the dense material alongside the kinetosome, there arise 10–25 nemadesmal microtubules (Nf in Figs. 3.9, 3.15), which extend deeper into the cell, those from each membranelle converging to form a broad, tapering fiber bundle. Successive fiber bundles curve toward the posterior and combine with other bundles to form a larger irregular bundle (Fig. 3.16, Lnb). As previously stated, some microtubules from the AZM fiber bundles appear to curve under the floor of the peristome and connect with the kinetosomes of the undulating membrane. Although the full course of the nemadesma has not been determined, the bundle is often encountered quite deep in the endoplasm and posterior to the cytopharyngeal region.

Originating from each kinetosome in the posterior row of every membranelle is a microtubule sheet (Pms) of 5–8 closely appressed microtubules (Fig. 3.13), which strongly resembles the somatic kinetodesmal sheets and, like them, curves posteriorly; according to Kennedy (1965), these sheets extend into the cortical ridges separating the membranelles. Pitelka (1969) has speculated that such sheets may extend in a posterior direction along the wall of the cytopharynx, thus forming the cytopharyngeal ribbons (to be described). Each kinetosome of the anterior row gives rise to a sheet of about six microtubules (Ams), which is aligned parallel to the kinetosomal rows and appears to curve to the anterior away from the kinetosome and toward the pellicle (Fig. 3.13).

Cytopharyngeal structures. The cytopharyngeal region of the buccal cavity is characterized by the absence of membranelles, the presence of cytopharyngeal ribbons (Cy) arranged perpendicular to the wall of the cytopharynx, and, at its base, a system of elongate vesicles (Ev) often separated by the cytopharyngeal ribbons (Fig. 3.18).

Dembitzer (1968) has shown that food vacuole formation involves a concentration of bacteria (*Blepharisma*'s normal food) at the terminus of the cytopharynx, with backflow prevented by a protruding lip or valvelike structure. From his micrograph (Dembitzer, 1968: Fig. 18) it would appear that a membrane then detaches from the cytopharyngeal wall to enclose the food organisms; however, actual ingestion is not described. He also treats the acid phosphatase activities of various stages of food vacuole function in detail. I have not observed or photographed the stages in food vacuole formation, but have encountered two seemingly distinctive vacuole forms worthy of note. One form has numerous fingerlike projections (Ve) extending into the vacuole content (Fig. 3.19); the other has numerous evaginating micropinocytotic vesicles (Mpv) at the vacuole membrane (Fig. 3.20).

The Internal Membranes

Vacuoles, channels, vesicles, and rough endoplasmic reticulum. The existence of a well-developed, interconnecting cytomembrane system has not been clearly demonstrated for *Blepharisma*. The cytoplasm of a fixed organism contains numerous vacuoles, but these are for the most part entirely electron-lucid, which would imply that they are perhaps osmotically produced by the shrinkage of the cell's ground substance and/or the dilation of smaller vesicles. A clear pattern of arrangement for the vesicles (Ve) or vacuoles (Va) has not been determined; neither have we been able to show that they interconnect to enclose a common space (Fig. 3.1). Recently, in glutaraldehyde-fixed specimens, some evidence has been found to support the proposition that at least some of the electron-lucid, membrane-limited spaces are part of an interconnecting system of channels (Dembitzer and Hirshfield, 1966). Dembitzer (1968) has interpreted the channels as an intracytoplasmic system wherein transport phenomena related to digestive processes are completed. The fact that newly produced posterior daughters (nonfeeders) have an essentially avacuolar cytoplasm may support this concept.

In addition to the extensive vacuolar structures, a great many small, membrane-bound vesicles (Ve) that contain small granules, vesicles, or fine material occur in the endoplasm (Figs. 3.1, 3.12, and 3.24). The more conspicuous oval or elongate vesicles have tiny, microvilluslike projections (Ov) extending inward from the membrane (Figs. 3.21, 3.23). Such vesicles often appear to contain granular material and are apparently identical to bodies previously described (Utsumi and Yoshizawa, 1957). Small saclike vesicles (Sv) with a moderately electron-dense content are present in some sections (Figs. 3.7, 3.12) and have been previously described (Dembitzer, 1968).

I have made only a very few observations of rough-surfaced endoplasmic reticulum (Er) in the vesicular form (Fig. 3.22). In no case have the nuclear envelopes and endoplasmic reticulum shown continuity.

Golgi bodies. Golgi bodies of the dictyosome form (G) are numerous throughout *Blepharisma*'s endoplasm. Each body consists of a curved stack of four or five flattened cisternae with dilated margins and a number of small spherical vesicles within their concave centers (Figs. 3.1, 3.21, 3.22, and 3.29). At least some of the cisternae are fenestrated (Fig. 3.21). Both Kennedy (1965) and Dembitzer (1968) found an association of granular membranes with the concave side of the Golgi bodies. Functionally, Dembitzer (1968) associates the Golgi bodies with acid phosphatase production and/or packaging; and I have some evidence associating them with the process of microtubule dissolution that follows cell division.

Contractile vacuole. The contractile vacuole system consists of a large terminal vacuole and anterior to it a collection of smaller vacuoles. It appears that the final collecting vacuole lies within a membrane-limited cavity, and, as Kennedy (1965) states, it is without radiating channels. Microtubules are not presently described as components of the system.

Other Organelles and Inclusions

Mitochondria. These vary considerably in size and shape but usually appear as rather dense, oval or rod-shaped bodies 0.5 to 0.75 μm in diameter (M in Figs. 3.1, 3.7, and 3.8). They are highly concentrated at the ecto-endoplasmic boundary, where they follow very closely the depth of the fibrous lattice but seldom lie immediately below the kineties (Fig. 3.3). Other mitochondria appear uniformly distributed throughout the endoplasm (Fig. 3.1). The ultrastructure of each mitochondrion is very similar to that found in other ciliates. Within the outer limiting membrane is a highly convoluted system of tubular cristae that essentially comprises the entire internal content (Figs. 3.21, 3.22). In some preparations small electron-opaque granules occur within the mitochondria.

Paraglycogen bodies. Kennedy (1964) succeeded in cytochemically identifying the oval, amorphous, mitochondrion-sized, non-membrane-limited granules (Pa) found throughout the cytoplasm as paraglycogen that provides a stored carbohydrate reserve for the organism (Figs. 3.1, 3.23). As he points out, these bodies have strikingly different appearances following different types of preparation for electron microscopy. In general, the paraglycogen bodies are best seen after OsO_4 vapor fixation, methacrylate embedding, and lead-citrate staining; they usually show as electron-lucid areas when the cells are in glutaraldehyde-epoxy preparations.

The cytoplasmic ground substance consists primarily of small granules (ribonucleoproteins?), extremely small vesicles, and perhaps a fine fibrous component.

Nuclei

Observations on nuclear structure can probably be applied generally to all blepharismas, since our studies have revealed no significant differences in ultrastructure for the species studied.

Micronuclei. The interphase micronucleus (Mi) is a nearly spherical body 1–2 µm in diameter (Figs. 3.1, 3.23), and is limited by a two-membrane envelope in which pores may (Kennedy, 1965; Inaba and Sotokawa, 1968) or may not (Seshachar, 1964; Jenkins, 1967) be present. The micronucleoplasm has a cortex consisting of a fine matrix surrounding an electron-dense, reticular central region that appears to be a densely packed fibrillar mass (Fig. 3.23). The several micronuclei may be located throughout the cytoplasm; however, most are found very near the macronucleus but not in contact with it. Neither ribosomes nor nucleolar material are present in the micronuclei.

Prophase micronuclei are enlarged to a diameter of about 3–4 µm and lack the dense central chromatin mass, which transforms to give rise to several small, dense chromosomes (Ch) distributed throughout the nucleoplasm (Fig. 3.1). At a slightly later stage, prometaphase, a few spindle microtubules (Smt) begin to appear in a random pattern (Fig. 3.24). Neither kinetochores nor centrioles are identifiable as sites of attachment or points of origin for spindle microtubules in this or any later stage.

In metaphase the chromosomes are aligned at the equatorial plate, and well-defined 22-nm spindle microtubules are present in large numbers (Fig. 3.25); some spindle microtubules appear to terminate at the chromosomes, and others pass between chromosomes, apparently extending from pole to pole. The matrix surrounding the microtubules is finely fibrous and evenly distributed throughout the micronucleus (Fig. 3.25). The nuclear envelope remains intact, as it does until division is completed; but its component membranes are sometimes difficult to distinguish. Metaphase chromosomes are masses 200–300 nm across with a poorly defined substructure except for a generally fibrous appearance (Fig. 3.25). All section orientations reveal the same morphology, which leads to the conclusion that the chromosome is a tightly folded spherical mass.

The early anaphase micronuclei provide a clear demonstration that both continuous and chromosomal spindle microtubules are present (Fig. 3.26). In mid-anaphase, when a chromosome separation of 4–5 µm has been effected, spindle microtubules are present at the poleward side in greatest numbers, but they are also present in the interzone (Fig. 3.27). Measurements of chromosome-to-pole distances in metaphase and anaphase indicate only a slight movement of the chromosomes toward the poles as division progresses, but the pole-to-pole distance increases greatly. Therefore, the separation of daughter chromosome sets must occur primarily by elongation of the continuous spindle microtubules. Since separations of daughter nuclei by more than 30 µm are common, the chromosome movement in *Blepharisma* must be regarded as one of the most extensive known. By late anaphase, the chromosomes of the daughter nuclei are fused as single masses (Cm) resembling the interphase form (Figs. 3.28, 3.29), and are located at opposite ends of the separation spindle (Ss).

When spindle elongation is completed, the two presumptive daughter nuclei are enclosed together within the intact nuclear envelope. As telophase progresses, a new nuclear envelope (Nne) is formed within the confines of the old (One) and closely juxtaposed to the chromatin mass (Figs. 3.29, 3.30), apparently forming from a coalescence of small vesicles and flattened cisternae. The new envelope thus separates and excludes essentially all of the spindle material from the chromatic substance of the daughter nucleus. Telophase is completed by the disruption of the original nuclear envelope, the release of the newly limited nucleus into the cytoplasm, and the dispersal of the separation spindle.

Meiotic micronuclei have been studied only in a very preliminary way. Figure 3.31 shows a portion of a prophase I micronucleus of *B. americanum* that includes a synaptinemal complex (Sc).

Fine-structure studies of the entire conjugation process are now in progress, emphasizing nuclear phenomena, cell attachment, and cytoplasmic bridge formation. Newly fused pairs show limited regions of cytoplasmic continuity but, for the most part, the pellicles (P) show only a close apposition, perhaps with increased membrane density (Fig. 3.32). Only the earliest stages of fusion have been studied.

The macronucleus. The vegetative macronucleus of *Blepharisma* is similar in structure to that described for other ciliates. Dense bodies of two general sizes are present within the macronucleus (Figs. 3.33, 3.34). The larger (Lb), above 0.5 µm in diameter, are regarded as nucleoli and have a diffuse granulo-fibrous appearance; they are fewer in number, and after lead staining often show numerous electron-opaque granules (E) about 10–20 nm in size. The smaller bodies (Sb), about 0.15 µm in diameter, are more numerous and present a more compact appearance. Some macronuclei show the margins of the small bodies, which are presumed to be chromatin, merged so that a broad reticulum results (Fig. 3.1, Ma). The balance of the nucleoplasm consists of a moderately dense matrix. In some macronuclei of interphase *B. americanum* and *B. undulans* dense spherical bodies 0.45 to 0.80 μm in diameter and consisting of a very compact reticulum are found (Fig. 3.35, Mb). Kennedy (1965) has identified these structures as a carbohydrate-protein complex perhaps stored for use in macronuclear division.

Jenkins and Giese (unpublished) encountered macronuclear inclusions of 4–6 μm in monoxenically grown *B. japonicum*. These consist of a ring of fine material very much like the nucleolar component, enclosing a moderately dense core resembling the nucleoplasm and often containing very dense ovoid inclusions (Fig. 3.37). Since nucleolar bodies are generally lacking in these macronuclei, it seems likely that they are formed by a coalescence of nucleoli like that occurring in the early division of *B. musculus* v. wardsi (Inaba and Sotokawa, 1968). It is also possible that this configuration relates to the formation or utilization of the carbohydrate-protein bodies described earlier.

The macronucleus is limited by an envelope consisting of two membranes separated by a less dense space 8–10 nm in width. Many pores (Np) about 80 nm in diameter with associated annuli are clearly evident (Fig. 3.36).

The details of ultrastructural changes in dividing macronuclei are presented in two reports (Inaba and Sotokawa, 1968; Jenkins, unpublished). Organisms studied in this laboratory have either filiform or moniliform vegetative macronuclei. When cell division begins, these nuclear morphologies first convert to a condensed spherical mass, then reelongate as rods and subsequently divide (see Chapter 4). During condensation the macronuclear content changes from its interphase morphology, and by the time condensation is completed the large and small bodies are not easily distinguished and the nucleoplasm is generally homogeneous (Fig. 3.25). Work with *B. musculus* v. wardsi (Inaba and Sotokawa, 1968) shows the sequence to involve first an enlargement of nucleoli, later a diminution but not a dissolution; meanwhile the chromatin material becomes diffuse and later reorganizes as small bodies.

Coincident with the onset of elongation from the condensed macronuclear form is the appearance of numerous microtubules (Mt) closely applied to the cytoplasmic side of the macronuclear envelope (Figs. 3.38, 3.39). They are aligned parallel with the direction of elongation (corresponding to the long axis of the cell) and are arranged circumferentially about the macronucleus. These microtubules are present throughout elongation and disperse at its completion (Inaba and Sotokawa, 1968; Jenkins, 1968 and unpublished). It has been shown (Jenkins, 1969 and unpublished) that colchicine blocks the elongation of the macronucleus. Electron microscopy reveals that the microtubules (the division sheath) surrounding the macronucleus during normal elongation are absent or diminished in number (and perhaps disoriented) after this treatment. We can tentatively conclude that the block of elongation is caused by the dissolution and/or dysfunction of the microtubule sheath that normally provides its control and/or motive force.

As the elongation of the macronucleus continues, the large and small bodies reappear and resume their interphase morphology. Division of the macronucleus apparently occurs by a progressive thinning at the site of the fission furrow and results when cytokinesis is completed.

It is evident that the ciliate protozoan is a marvelously complex cell. Although we are now beginning to assemble a reasonably complete description of ciliate morphology, the functions of many components are unknown, and the known functions of others lack explanations at the molecular level. However, knowledge of the fine structure of *Blepharisma* is a prerequisite for the interpretation of many subjects to be considered in subsequent chapters of this book.

LITERATURE CITED

Borysko, E., and H. Dembitzer. 1958. The fine structure of the cortical region of a pigmented ciliate, *Blepharisma undulans*. J. Appl. Phys. **29**: 19–21.

Dembitzer, H. M. 1968. Digestion and the distribution of acid phosphatase in *Blepharisma*. J. Cell Biol. **37**: 329–44.

Dembitzer, H. M., and H. I. Hirshfield. 1966. Some new cytological observations in the heterotrichous ciliate, *Blepharisma*. J. Cell Biol. **30**: 201–7.

Inaba, F., R. Nakamura, and S. Yamaguchi. 1958. An electron microscope study on the pigment granules of *Blepharisma*. Cytol. **23**: 72–79.

Inaba, F., and Y. Sotokawa. 1968. Electron-microscope observation on nuclear events during binary fission in *Blepharisma wardsi* (Ciliata: Heterotrichida). Jap. J. Genet. **43**: 335–48.

Jenkins, R. A. 1967. Fine structure of division in ciliate protozoa, 1: Micronuclear mitosis in *Blepharisma*. J. Cell Biol. **34**: 463–81.

——— 1968. Observations on the fine structure of nuclear divisions in *Blepharisma* and *Didinium*. J. Protozool. **15** (suppl.): 10a.

——— 1969. The role of microtubules in macronuclear division in *Blepharisma*. J. Protozool. **16** (suppl.): 10a.

———— Unpublished. Fine structure of division in ciliate protozoa, II: Macronuclear division in *Blepharisma*.

Kennedy, J. R. 1965. The morphology of *Blepharisma undulans* Stein. J. Protozool. **12**: 542–61.

———— 1966. The effect of strychnine and light on pigmentation in *Blepharisma undulans* Stein. J. Cell. Biol. **28**: 145–53.

Kurita, M. 1969. Electron microscopy of the pigment granules in *Blepharisma*. Biol. J. Nara Women's Univ. **18**: 50–52.

Pitelka, D. R. 1969. Fibrillar systems in Protozoa. *In* Research in Protozoology (T. T. Chen, ed.), III, 280–388, New York.

Repak, A. J., and R. M. Pfister. 1967. Electron-microscopical observations on the extracellular structures of the resting cyst of *Blepharisma stoltei*. Trans. Amer. Microsc. Soc. **86**: 417–21.

Seshachar, B. R. 1964. The fine structure of the nuclear apparatus of *Blepharisma intermedium* Bhandary (Ciliata: Spirotricha). J. Protozool. **11**: 402–9.

Shigematsu, N. 1967. Electron-microscopic observations on the macronucleus of the Niigata 1 strain of *Blepharisma*. Biol. J. Nara Women's Univ. **17**: 41–43.

Tuffrau, N. 1968. Les structures fibrillaires somatiques et buccales chez les cilies heterotriches. Protistol. **3**: 369–94.

Utsumi, K., and K. Yoshizawa. 1957a. Fibrous organelles in *Blepharisma*. Saibokagaka-Symposium **5**: 143–50.

———— 1957b. Intracellular structure of *Blepharisma* as revealed by electron microscope. Zool. Mag. (Dobut. Zasshi) **66**: 234–39.

The organisms studied and included in the following portfolio of electron micrographs were: *B. americanum; Blepharisma* sp., Turtox strain; *B. japonicum,* Suzuki #3 strain; *B. japonicum* v. intermedium; and *B. japonicum* v. intermedium, albino. Polyxenic mass cultures of these stocks were maintained under reduced light at 25–30° C in a 0.1% Cerophyl-lettuce infusion buffered with a 5-mM phosphate buffer solution (pH 6.8) and inoculated with *Bacillus subtilis* 12 to 24 hours before the ciliates were introduced. Monoxenic cultures were reared under similar conditions of light and temperature in a lettuce infusion inoculated with *Pseudomonas ovalis.*

The selection of a particular species for study naturally depends on the structural aspect under consideration, as well as on the ease of culturing that species in the laboratory. The predominance of *B. japonicum* both in our stock cultures and in the following micrographs is in large part due to the hardiness, large size, and prominent structures of that species.

In order to examine and illustrate various aspects of *Blepharisma's* structure by electron microscopy one must use a wide variety of preparation techniques. These procedures are steadily improving, as are the comparable techniques used in light microscopy.

The following fixation procedures were employed in preparing specimens for examination:

A. Osmium tetraoxide vapor. A small drop of culture fluid containing the ciliates was placed at the center of a coverslip, which was then inverted over the mouth of a container of aqueous 2% osmium tetraoxide. The usual fixation time was 4 minutes at 23° C.

B. Immersion in 2% osmium tetraoxide plus 0.5% calcium dichromate for 30 minutes at room temperature.

C. A 4% solution of glutaraldehyde in .05 M phosphate buffer (pH 7.2) for 20 minutes, followed by 1% osmium tetraoxide in the same buffer for one hour.

D. Treatment with 2.5% glutaraldehyde and 3% acrolein in .05 M phosphate buffer (pH 7.2) for 20 minutes, followed by 1% osmium tetraoxide in the same buffer for one hour.

E. Treatment with 0.5% osmium tetraoxide in a .05 M phosphate buffer for 10 minutes. Glutaraldehyde was then added to produce a final concentration of 4%, in which the cells were treated for a further 30 minutes. Finally, 1% osmium tetraoxide in the same buffer solution was applied for one hour.

The embedding media employed to hold cells for sectioning were the following:

1. A cross-linked methacrylate mixture consisting of 57 ml n-butyl methacrylate, 43 ml ethyl methacrylate, 1.5 ml divinylbenzene, and 1 g benzoyl peroxide.

2. An Epon-Araldite mixture consisting of 20 ml Araldite 502, 25 ml Epon 812, 60 ml DDSA, 10 ml D.E.R. 732, and 4 ml DMP-30. DDSA is dodecenylsuccinic anhydride, a hardener included in epoxy embedding mixtures; D.E.R. is Dow epoxy resin, a flexible resin designed for embedding; DMP is 2,4,6-tri(dimethyl-aminomethyl)-phenol, a catalyst for hardening epoxy mixtures.

3. An Epon-D.E.R. mixture consisting of 2 ml Epon 812, 8 ml D.E.R. 736, 9 ml nadic methyl anhydride, and 0.35 ml DMP-30.

The cells were dehydrated in graded acetone or ethanol solutions, with acetone always used in transition.

In all cases the cells were embedded singly, either in capsules or, with the epoxies, in a flat matrix so that specific orientations could be achieved. Thin sections were cut with an LKB or Reichert ultramicrotome, mounted on grids with thin Parlodion or Formvar supporting films, and either stained with calcium permanganate or doubly stained with uranyl acetate and lead citrate. The micrographs were taken with an RCA EMU 3F or 3G electron microscope operated at 50 or 100 Kv.

Using A–E to identify the fixation procedure and 1–3 to identify the embedding medium, the captions in the following series list the species and preparation techniques employed for each micrograph. Unless otherwise noted all figures are unpublished electron micrographs taken at the University of Wyoming by the author.

Fig. 3.1. Survey micrograph of the midregion of a longitudinal section of *B. americanum* (preps. A and 1). One lobe of the moniliform macro-nucleus (Ma) is centrally located and is surrounded by five micronuclei (Mi), two of which show the chromosomes (Ch) of prophase. Mito-chondria (M), paraglycogen granules (Pa), pigment granules (Pg), Golgi bodies (G), and a variety of vesicles (Ve) and vacuoles (Va) are visible. The gullet (Gu) is cut in approximate cross section, and the distinctive vacuoles associated with the gullet terminus are obvious. At the bottom of the figure a somatic cilium (C) arises from the anterior kinetosome of a pair, and cups in the pellicle (Cu) mark the sites of pigment loss. × 6,000. From Jenkins, 1967.

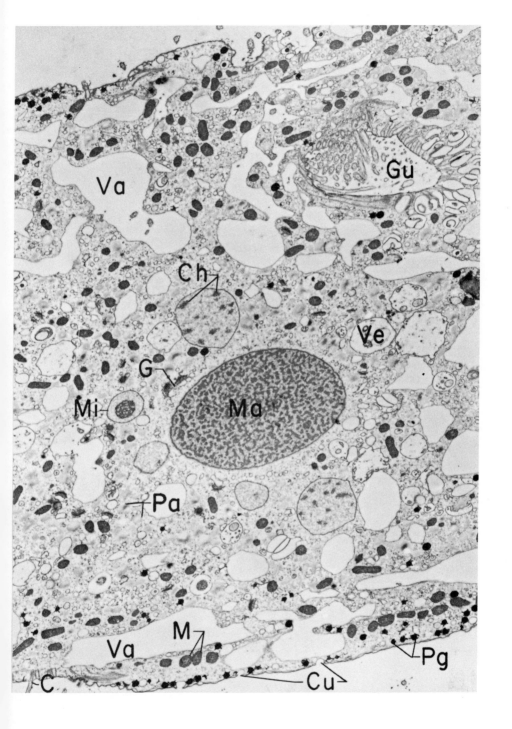

Fig. 3.2 (*above*). A portion of one cortical ridge, produced by a skimming longitudinal section. Three full rows of pigment granules (Pg) are present, some (arrows) showing a partial voiding of pigment. Pigment granule membranes are easily discerned. The pellicle (P) gives some evidence of an extraneous coat (Ec), with an array of microtubules (Spm) immediately beneath it. *B. japonicum*, preps. B and 1, × 67,000.

Fig. 3.3 (*below*). Cross sections of the organism show the best definition of the pellicle (P) and the arrangement of microtubules that lie beneath the pellicle (Spm) and those (Kmt) constituting the kinetodesmal fiber (Kf). Although no kinetosomes are visible in this section, one somatic cilium (C) is present in a cortical furrow. *B. japonicum*, preps. B and 1, × 50,000.

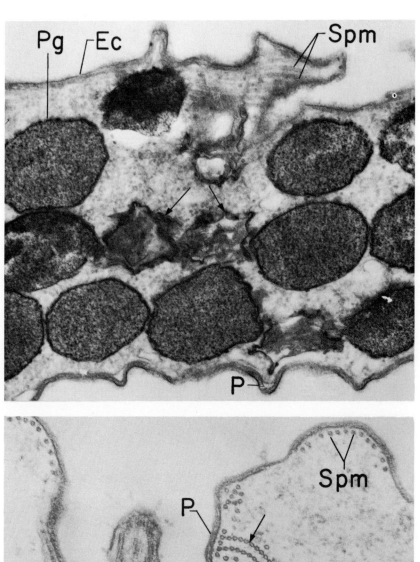

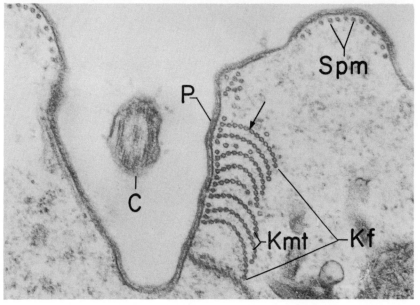

Fig. 3.4 (*above, left*). Only the anterior member (K) of the kinetosome pair develops a cilium (C). Continuities of the pellicular membrane (P) and ciliary membrane and of axoneme peripheral doublets and kinetosome tubules are shown. The central pair of microtubules terminates in the axosomal granule (Ag). *B. japonicum* v. intermedium albino, preps. C and 3, × 63,000.

Fig. 3.5 (*above, right*). This longitudinal section was taken at a level just below the floor of a cortical furrow. Two somatic kinetosome (K) pairs have associated microtubule sheets which compose the anterior fiber (Af) and the kinetodesmal fiber (Kf); the small arrows show regions of bridging between the Kf microtubules. The poorly defined anterior kinetodesmal fiber (Akf) appears to arise from the dense material (Im) between the kinetosomes. The cartwheel pattern of the proximal region of kinetosomes is indicated at the long arrow. *B. japonicum*, preps. D and 3, × 65,000.

Fig. 3.6 (*below*). Part of a somatic row of kinetosomes sectioned longitudinally at the appropriate level reveals the compounding of the kinetodesmal fiber (Kf) from kinetodesmal microtubules (Kmt) arising at the posterior kinetosome of each pair. Both the anterior fiber (Af) and the anterior kinetodesmal fiber (Akf) are clearly shown. A typical pigment granule (Pg) is present in the region of the furrow. *B. americanum*, preps. A and 1, × 40,000.

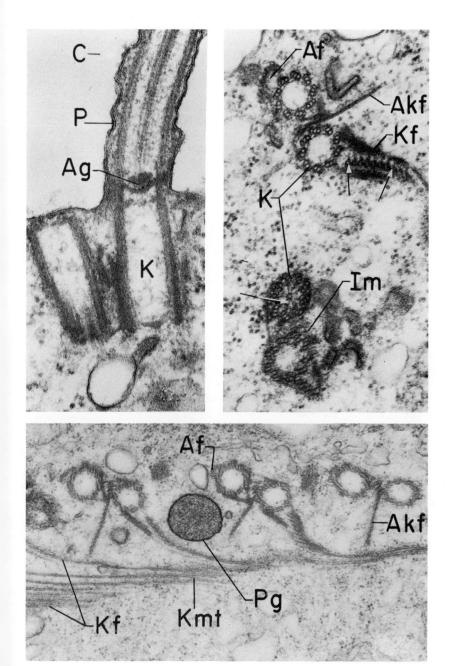

Fig. 3.7 (*above*). Since the fibrous lattice (Fb) is relatively thin, any skimming section of the curved cell surface will include only a small region in which the fibrous material is present. Mitochondria (M) are often enclosed within fenestrations of the lattice material. Vesicles (Sv and Ve) and vacuoles (Va) are characteristic of the cytoplasm. The kinetosomes (K) are cut at a level that does not include the kineto-desmos. *B. japonicum*, preps. D and 3, × 24,000.

Fig. 3.8 (*below*). The thickness of the fibrous band (Fb) is shown clearly when the cell is cross-sectioned. Mitochondria (M) are usually closely concentrated along the band. The 4-nm fibers (F) are apparently embedded in a fine, fibrous matrix. *B. japonicum* v. intermedium albino, preps. C and 3, × 42,000.

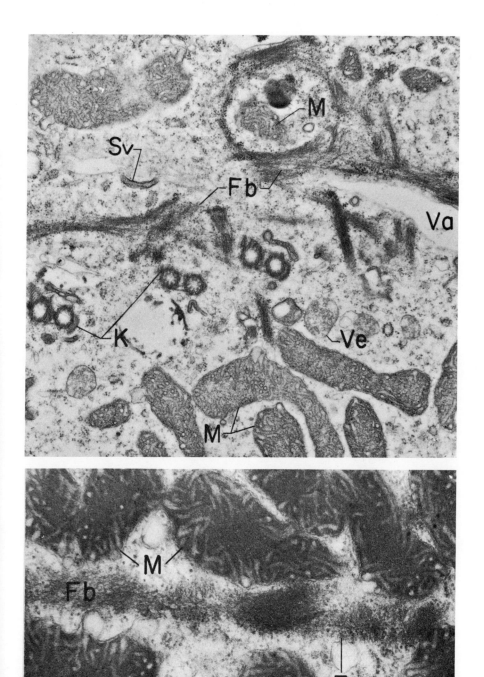

Fig. 3.9 (*above*). When the organism is cross-sectioned at the level of the peristome (Figs. 3.9–3.12 are so sectioned), the ciliary rows of the AZM are visible (center to upper right). The nemadesmal fiber (Nf) has continuity under the peristomal floor with the kinetosomes (Umk) of the undulating membrane, but the bundle leaves the plane of section in this micrograph. *B. japonicum*, preps. C and 3, × 8,000.

Fig. 3.10 (*below*). At higher magnification a region of the peristomal floor shows a regular pattern of what are thought to be posterior microtubule sheets (Pms) and the less regularly placed trichocyst-like peristomal rods (Pr). A reasonably intact pigment granule (Pg) and one essentially voided (arrow) are also shown. The AZM is out of the micrograph to the right, and a single kinetosome (Umk) of the UM is at the left. *B. americanum*, preps. A and 1, × 32,000.

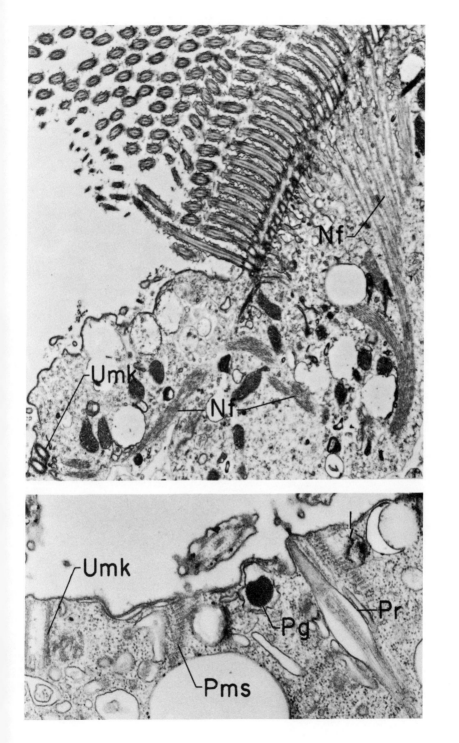

Fig. 3.11 (*above*). All three kinetosomal rows of the undulating membrane are included in this micrograph (Umk). It is typical that the innermost kinetosome (leftmost here) is canted toward the AZM, so that its cilium lies over the peristomal floor. Microtubules of the nemadesmal fiber (Nf) arise from the dense proximal cap (Pc) of the kinetosomes. *B. japonicum*, preps. E and 3, × 27,000.

Fig. 3.12 (*below*). In some regions of the peristomal floor the peristomal rods (Pr) are sectioned longitudinally and show a complex internal structure. Some details in the structure of the pellicle (P) and the arrangement of microtubules in the posterior microtubule sheets (Pms) are apparent. Vesicles typical of the cytoplasm but especially of the region of the Pr are present (Sv and Ve). *B. japonicum*, preps. E and 3, × 38,000.

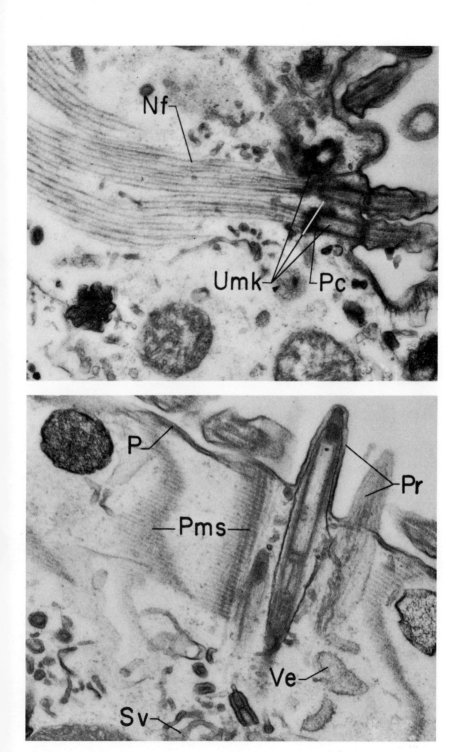

Fig. 3.13. Each component membranelle of the AZM is separated from those anterior and posterior to it by a thin cortical ridge (Cr). In this section along the AZM (anterior toward the bottom of the figure), anterior microtubule sheets (Ams) arising from each kinetosome in the anterior row, posterior microtubule sheets (Pms) originating at the kinetosomes of the posterior row, and interconnecting strands between kinetosomes (Fs) are clearly evident. Cross sections of cilia near the distal end of the kinetosome include the axosomal granule (Ag), and sections at the proximal end of kinetosomes show the extremely dense fibrous cap (Pc) from which nemadesmal microtubules originate. Pigment granules (Pg) are not common within the AZM. *B. japonicum*, preps. B and 1, × 39,000.

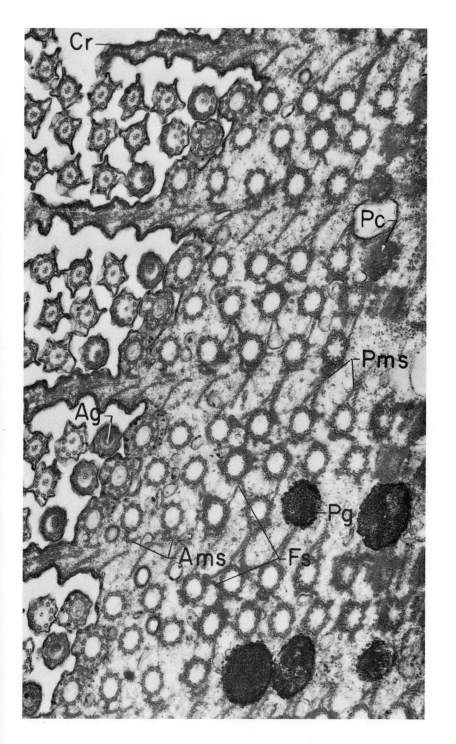

Fig. 3.14 (*above*). This micrograph, a very small portion of one membranelle, reveals the typical pattern of microtubules in the cilium (C), the continuation of one microtubule of the central pair beyond the other (arrows), and the pattern of triplets in the distal end of the kinetosome (K). *B. japonicum*, preps. B and 1, × 70,000.

Fig. 3.15 (*below*). Occasionally cilia will include very dense granules just exterior to the peripheral doublets. These cross sections of AZM cilia show numerous granules (Dg) near their proximal ends. Posterior microtubule sheets (Pms) and microtubules of the nemadesma (Nf) are also visible. *B. japonicum* v. intermedium albino, preps. C and 3, × 48,000.

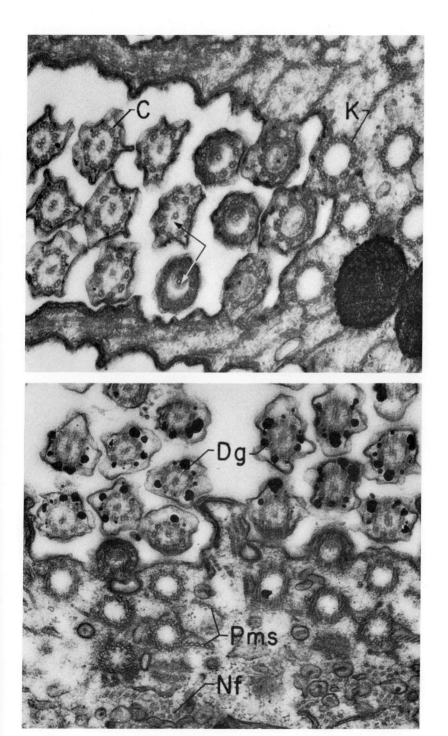

Fig. 3.16 (*left*). A survey micrograph of a section along the AZM reveals the course of the nemadesmal fibers (Nf) from each membranelle downward and posteriorly to form the large nemadesmal bundle (Lnb). Rarely, as in this case, paraglycogen granules (Pa) are preserved by glutaraldehyde-epoxy procedures. *B. japonicum*, preps. D and 3, × 8,700.

Fig. 3.17 (*right*). The component cilia of both the AZM and the UM bear distinctive projections (Cp) that loosely join the cilia as a unit. Nemadesmal fibers (Nf) and pigment granules (Pg) are also shown. *Blepharisma* sp., preps. A and 1, × 41,000.

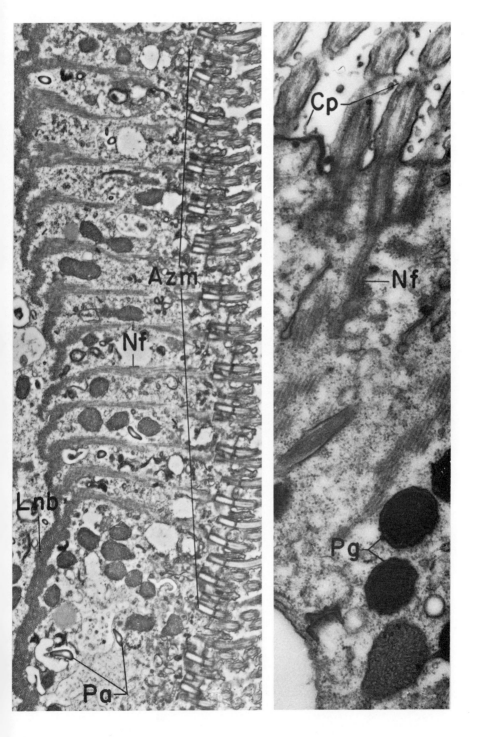

Fig. 3.18 (*left*). This longitudinal section reveals the termination of the AZM within the gullet (Gu) and the appearance of cytopharyngeal ribbons (Cy) at that level. The heavy-walled elongate vesicles (Ev) are typical of the terminus of the cytopharynx. *B. americanum*, preps. A and 1, × 10,000.

Fig. 3.19 (*above, right*). The food vacuoles (Fv), here containing a partially digested bacterium (B), very often have fingerlike projections (Vp) into the vacuole content. *B. americanum*, preps. A and 1, × 40,000.

Fig. 3.20 (*below, right*). The micropinocytotic vesicles (Mpv) formed into the cytoplasm most likely carry hydrolysate from the food (B) being digested within the food vacuole (Fv) into the cytoplasm. *B. japonicum*, preps. D and 3, × 15,000.

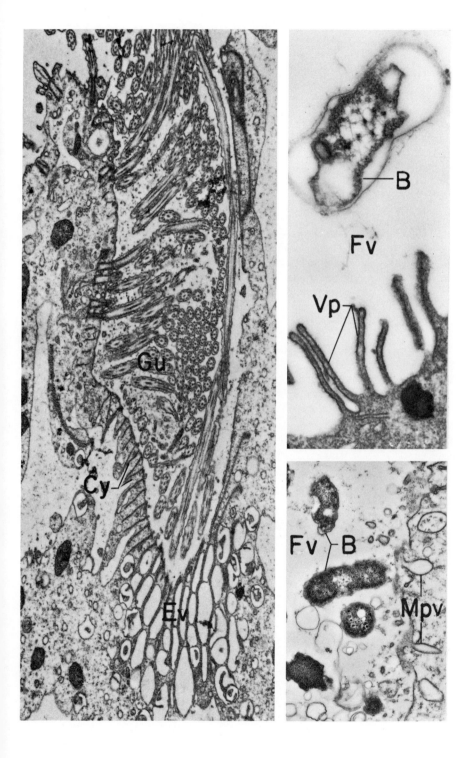

Fig. 3.21 (*above*). Dictyosomelike Golgi (G) are typically abundant in *Blepharisma*. The two Golgi bodies that are cross-sectioned here reveal the stacked lamellae and the vesicles within the concave face. The arrows indicate fenestrations within a lamella that is sectioned face-on. The typically dense-membraned oval vesicle (Ov) and one region of a mitochondrion (M) are included. *B. japonicum*, preps. A and 1, × 65,000.

Fig. 3.22 (*below*). Endoplasmic reticulum in a lamellar array has not been encountered in *Blepharisma*, but several procedures have revealed areas that include great amounts of vesicular, rough-surfaced endoplasmic reticulum (Er). Such regions often have Golgi bodies (G) nearby. A mitochondrion (M) is also present. *B. japonicum*, preps. D and 3, × 27,000.

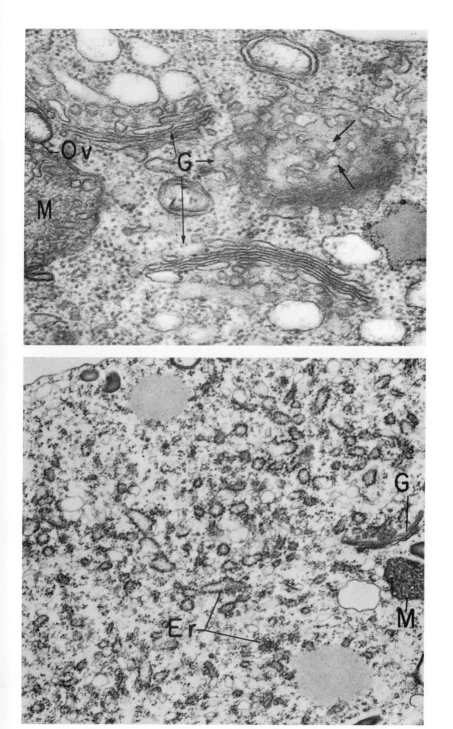

Fig. 3.23 (*above*). The interphase micronucleus (Mi) is limited by a two-membrane envelope in which pores seem to be lacking or greatly reduced. The chromatin material appears as a dense central mass. Near this micronucleus are typical mitochondria (M), paraglycogen granules (Pa), and a distinctive oval vesicle (Ov). *Blepharisma* sp., preps. A and 1, × 45,000.

Fig. 3.24 (*below*). The prometaphase micronucleus (Mi) reveals rather well-defined chromosomes (Ch) scattered throughout and a few poorly oriented spindle microtubules (Smt). The micronucleus has increased in dimension and maintained the nuclear envelope intact. A vesicle with a variety of internal contents (Ve) and a paraglycogen granule (Pa) are included. *Blepharisma* sp., preps. A and 1, × 40,000. From Jenkins, 1967.

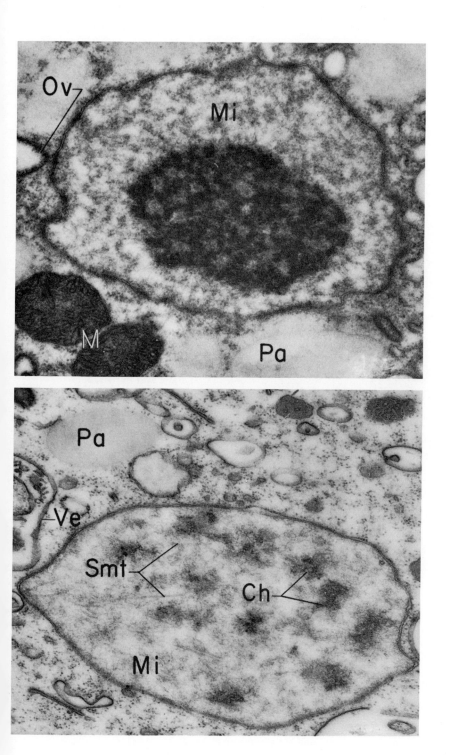

Fig. 3.25 (*above*). The late metaphase micronucleus (Mi) is fusiform and roughly 5 μm in length. At this stage the tightly coiled chromosomes (Ch) lie very near the equator and are attached to some of the spindle microtubules; other microtubules (Smt) appear to extend from pole to pole and do not attach to chromosomes. A small portion of the condensed macronucleus (Ma), with its homogeneous nucleoplasm, is included at the top of the figure. *Blepharisma* sp., preps. A and 1, × 37,000. From Jenkins, 1967.

Fig. 3.26 (*below*). Sister chromosomes (Ch) show very early separation in this micrograph. Note the apparent termination of some spindle microtubules in chromosomes (upper arrows, left and right) and the continuity of others through the equator (top center and bottom right arrows). *Blepharisma* sp., preps. A and 1, × 46,000. From Jenkins, 1967.

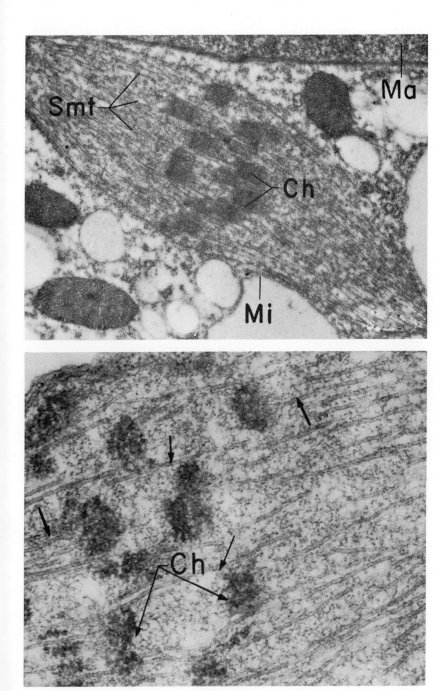

Fig. 3.27 (*left*). In this longitudinal section of a mid-anaphase micronucleus, chromosomes (Ch) are separated by about 5 μm. Many spindle microtubules (Smt) are present both on the poleward side of the chromosomes and within the interzone (I). The nuclear envelope (Ne) remains intact, although the intermembrane spacing is somewhat irregular. A small portion of the macronucleus (Ma) is present at the lower right. *B. americanum*, preps. A and 1, × 22,000. From Jenkins, 1967.

Fig. 3.28 (*right*). By late anaphase the elongation of the spindle microtubules (Smt) in the separation spindles (Ss) is completed, and individual chromosomes are no longer distinguishable but are now combined as the dense chromatin mass (Cm). The macronucleus (Ma) is completing elongation parallel with the long direction of the separation spindles. *B. japonicum* v. intermedium, preps. A and 1, × 20,000. From Jenkins, 1967.

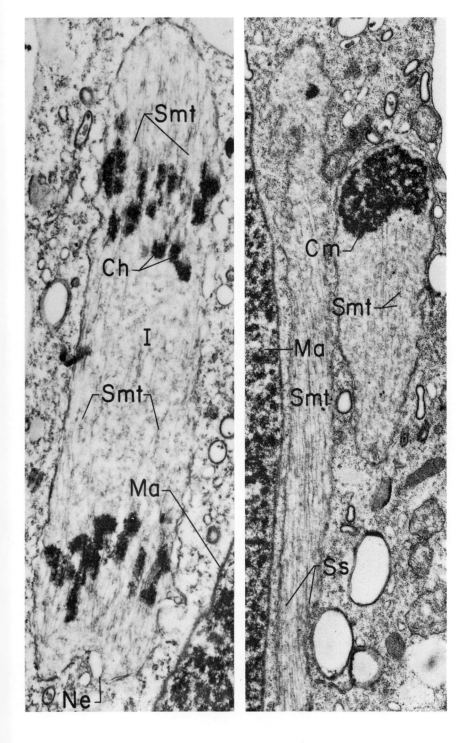

Fig. 3.29 (*above*). Shortly after chromosome movement is completed, the spindle microtubules of the separation spindle (Ss) undergo degradation to a fine fibrous material. Interior to the old, intact nuclear envelope (One) flattened cisternae form, closely appressed to the chromatin mass (Cm), and apparently fuse to form the new nuclear envelope (Nne). Face-on and cross-sectioned Golgi bodies (G) are present. *B. americanum*, preps. A and 1, × 36,000. From Jenkins, 1967.

Fig. 3.30 (*below*). The telophase daughter micronucleus (Mi) shows the new nuclear envelope (Nne) closely applied. This envelope has formed within the confines of the old nuclear envelope (One), which now fragments to release the new nucleus. *B. japonicum* v. intermedium, preps. A and 1, × 65,000. From Jenkins, 1967.

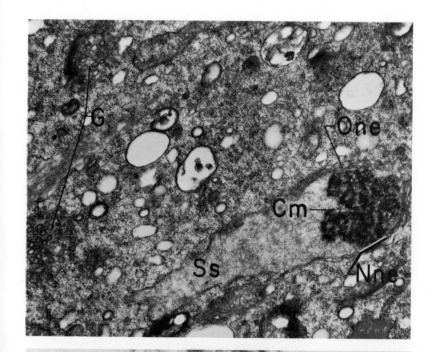

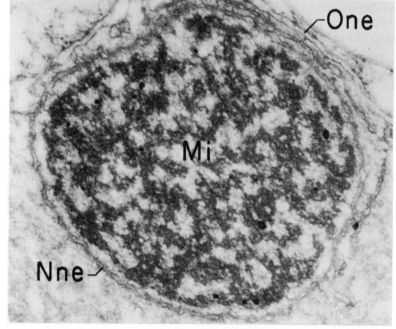

Fig. 3.31 (*above*). The synaptinemal complex (Sc) is found within meiotic nuclei at prophase I. During conjugation micronuclei undergo meiosis, and in this micrograph portions of two synaptinemal complexes of prophase I can be identified. Meiotic prophase micronuclei are larger than those in mitotic prophase; but they are similar in that the nuclear envelope (Ne) remains intact. *B. americanum*, preps. A and 1, × 72,000.

Fig. 3.32 (*below*). A small region along the zone of attachment of two conjugants (1 and 2). The contiguity of the pellicles (P) of the two cells is evident in this micrograph. Pigment granules and mitochondria are present as in vegetative cells. *B. americanum*, preps. A and 1, × 42,000.

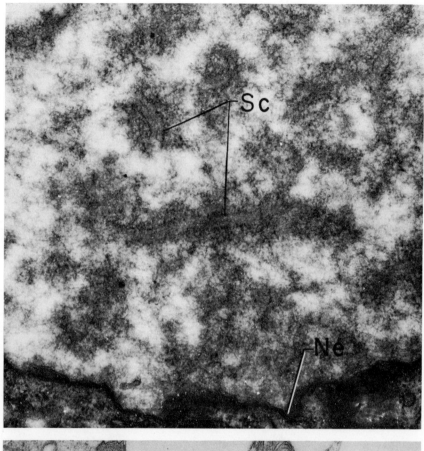

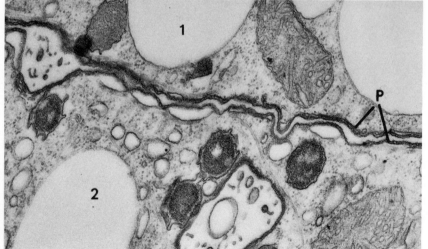

Fig. 3.33 (*left*). Survey micrograph including a small part of an inter-phase macronucleus (Ma) and showing the numerous small bodies (Sb) and large bodies (Lb). The nuclear envelope (Ne) is typical. *B. japoni-cum*, preps. D and 3, × 15,000.

Fig. 3.34 (*right, above*). In some preparations the large bodies (Lb) are marked by electron-dense granules (E), whereas the small bodies (Sb) never are. *B. japonicum*, preps. B and 1, × 50,000.

Fig. 3.35 (*right, below*). Some organisms have within their interphase macronuclei very dense spherical inclusions (Mb) that are clearly visible. *B. americanum*, preps. A and 1, × 44,000.

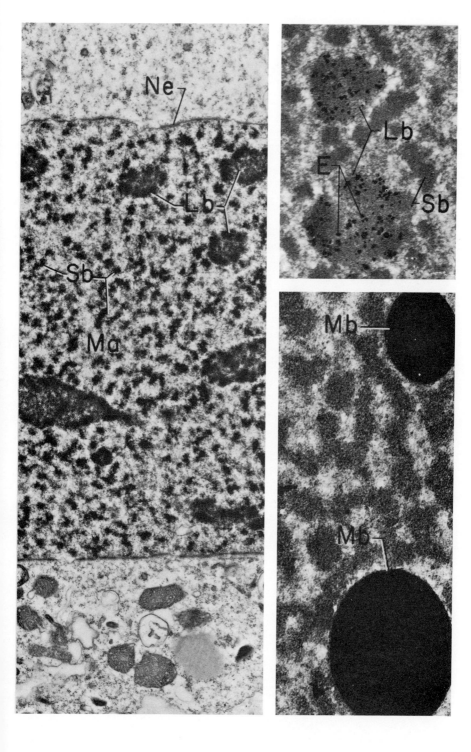

Fig. 3.36 (*above*). This grazing section of the macronucleus (Ma) presents the best orientation for demonstrating the structure, size, and numbers of nuclear pores (Np). *B. japonicum*, preps. D and 3, × 45,000.

Fig. 3.37 (*below*). Extremely large and distinctive macronuclear inclusions like the one depicted here (occupying most of the figure) have occasionally been encountered. Large bodies are generally lacking in such nuclei, but small bodies (Sb) seem unchanged. Nucleoplasm is separated from cytoplasm by the nuclear envelope (Ne). *B. japonicum*, preps. A and 1, × 23,000.

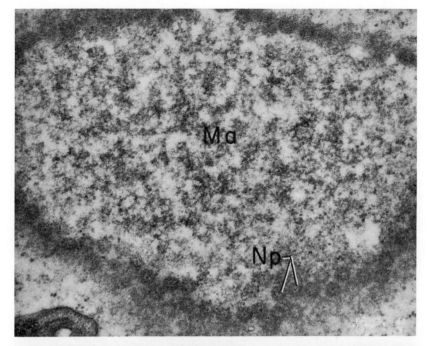

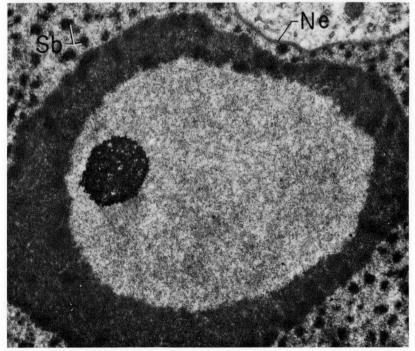

Fig. 3.38 (*above*). This micrograph was produced from a section cut transversely across an elongating macronucleus (Ma). During the elongation of the macronucleus in division, microtubules (Mt) appear just external to the nuclear envelope (Ne) and parallel with the direction of elongation. These form a sheath around the elongating macronucleus. The cross-bridged spindle microtubules (Smt) of two micronuclear separation spindles (Ss) are also shown. *Blepharisma* sp., preps. A and 2, × 55,000.

Fig. 3.39 (*below*). The microtubule sheath surrounding the macronucleus (Ma) can also be shown if the elongating macronucleus is sectioned at a slight angle to its surface. The orientation and number of the microtubules (Mt) is evident. There is no connection between the microtubules and the nuclear pores (Np). The highly convoluted, tubular cristae of the mitochondria appear at M. *B. americanum*, preps. A and 1, × 30,000.

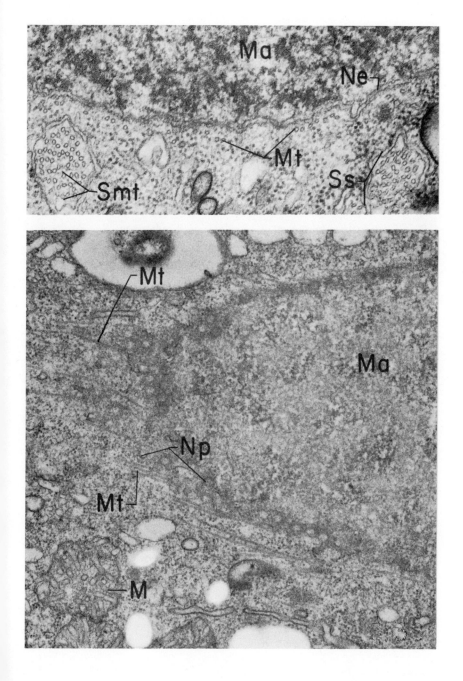

CHAPTER FOUR

Ecology and Culture

Relatively little is known of the ecology of *Blepharisma*. Species of the genus have been found in fresh, brackish, and sea water; and one, *B. halophilum*, has been reported from brine pools. Most investigators do not mention whether they collected the organisms from the surface, sides, or bottom of pools or streams (e.g., see Table 12.2). A systematic search in most localities is discouraging, inasmuch as so few pools appear to contain blepharismas. For example, Noland (1925) found *B. lateritium* in only six out of 78 collections. Our experience, and that of R. A. Jenkins (personal communication), has been similar. Wang (1928), in an extensive survey of one pond through a seasonal cycle, did not encounter *Blepharisma* at any time, although he found many other protozoans (including six species of *Stentor* and two of *Spirostomum*), some of them repeatedly.

In India *Blepharisma* is commonly found in pools throughout the country during the season between the monsoons and the drying out of the ponds (B. R. Seshachar, unpublished). In Japan it is easily obtained in a culture containing decomposing stubble from rice paddies, and was once seen in runoff from a rice paddy in such large numbers as to color the water red (S. Suzuki, unpublished). Except for these scattered observations, the ecology of the Asiatic strains of *Blepharisma* does not seem to have been studied either.

In spite of these difficulties, laboratory experience in culturing *Blepharisma* has given considerable data on the organism's limits of resistance to various environmental conditions, some of them pertinent to its ecological parameters in nature.

Food and Culture

Blepharisma is considered a bacterial feeder in nature (Stolte, 1926; Sandon, 1932; Dawson, 1928, 1953). Most cultures used by investigators are polyxenic: that is, they may contain other organisms besides *Blepharisma*, sometimes other protozoans and usually many species of bacteria. Pure cultures of *Blepharisma* in a polybacterial infusion are probably most common, but cultures with only one species of bacteria as food are also used. Less frequently, the cells are raised by axenic culture—growth on a synthetic medium of inorganic and organic material with no bacteria present.

Polyxenic cultures are most like the natural environment, since *Blepharisma* normally lives in waters containing many other protozoans and bacteria. Under these conditions, it seems to compete successfully with other ciliates (Vandermeer, 1969). But, although blepharismas may be most vigorous in wild cultures, they cannot be observed accurately when so many variables are present. For experimental purposes one must have repeatable cultures, and these can be obtained only when the nutrient is controlled—that is, when the culture is monobacterial or axenic. Table 4.1 gives comparative data on *Blepharisma*'s growth (measured by rate of division) in polybacterial, monobacterial, and axenic cultures. It will be seen that the time between generations is shortest when many species of bacteria are available as food, next best when one species is present (provided it is edible), and significantly longer when an axenic medium is used.

Blepharisma may be regarded as a microphagous filter feeder, and it usually subsists on the bacteria found in decomposing vegetation. The vibrating membranelles of the peristome set up a vortex that draws in nearby bacteria, and the undulating membrane helps scoop them down the oral groove to the cytostome and gullet, where they are enclosed in a food vacuole. Many food vacuoles can be seen in actively feeding

TABLE 4.1

Generation Time of *B. japonicum* v. intermedium at 25° C

Medium	Generation time (hr)	Conditions	Source
Cerophyl[a] 0.05%	15.2 ± 3.2	Monoxenic, polybacterial	Smith, 1965
Cerophyl 0.05%	17.0 ± 3.7	Monoxenic, monobacterial	Smith, 1965
Yeast extract, lyophilized bacteria, vitamins, etc.	30–40[b]	Axenic	Smith and Giese, 1967

[a] Dehydrated and powdered cereal grass greens.
[b] See Table 4.2.

blepharismas, and they often distend the posterior end of the body (Fig. 4.1). Even a small species of *Blepharisma* (e.g., *B. americanum*) may feed on such other small protozoans as *Khawkinea*, *Colpidium* (Giese, 1938), and *Tetrahymena* (Landon, 1959). In this case, the blepharismas enlarge, especially in their mouth parts, and can eventually engulf prey larger than themselves. Stolte (1924) says that large specimens will even eat paramecia and rotifers. When some members of a pure culture of *Blepharisma* become smaller during a period of starvation, they are eaten by larger ones, which then become cannibal giants (see Chapter 5). Cannibalism should always be considered a possibility when culturing *Blepharisma*.

Many experimental studies of *Blepharisma* have been performed with monobacterial cultures. In our laboratory the bacterium *Pseudomonas ovalis*, which was isolated from lettuce infusion, proved satisfactory both for *Blepharisma* and for other ciliates (Giese and Taylor, 1935). Blepha-

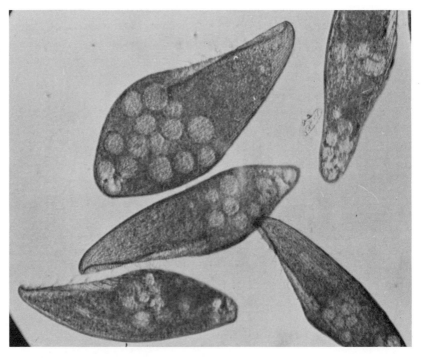

Fig. 4.1. A group of actively feeding blepharismas (*B. japonicum* v. intermedium) in a monoxenic polybacterial culture medium.

rismas were freed of bacteria by a series of baths (after Parpart, 1928) in a sterile balanced salt solution (modified from Taylor and Strickland, 1935) held in small watchglasses, sterile micropipettes being used for bathing. Single blepharismas were then placed in individual growth tubes, each containing an autoclaved infusion that had been inoculated with *Ps. ovalis* several hours earlier. Counts were made every 12 hours to determine the rate of division in each tube (Giese, 1945), and the culture that showed the most rapid division was chosen as a stock for later cultures.

Division rate may or may not be synchronous in a series of culture tubes taken at random from a single stock culture (Fig. 4.2). For this reason, each symbol plotted on the figures in this chapter and others represents the average number of divisions per tube in a group of 10–12 culture tubes. Usually, three series of experiments were performed, but only one set is represented in figures. When the same sequence of events was not found in each of the three series, additional experiments were performed.

Satisfactory cultures of *Blepharisma* on *Ps. ovalis* have been grown in my own laboratory for 40 years without clear evidence of deterioration (Giese and McCaw, 1963a). I have found, however, that different species, as well as different stocks of the same species, sometimes divide at different rates under seemingly identical conditions (see Table 4.4). It is not certain whether these differences could be eliminated by using other species of bacteria as food. Other investigators have in fact had equal success using other bacterial species; for example, Suzuki (1957) used *Bacillus subtilis* and *Pseudomonas fluorescens*.

Completely defined axenic media are available for several ciliates (Hall, 1965, 1967), but these media, when tested, failed to support the growth of *Blepharisma* (Smith, 1965). Axenic culture media for ciliates contain nucleic acid factors, B vitamins, a mixture of amino acids, and sometimes other factors (Hall, 1965). Seshachar and Saxena (1968), by testing hydrolytic activity on various substrates, found that *B. japonicum* v. intermedium secreted carbohydrases and proteinases, but no evidence of lipases was obtained. (Among the carbohydrases, identified by their action, were amylase, an unknown invertase with transglucosidase activity, β-glucosidase, and α-glucosidase; there was no evidence of a β-galactosidase.) Since lipases are common in free-living organisms, including protozoans, further study on *Blepharisma* is called for. If lipase

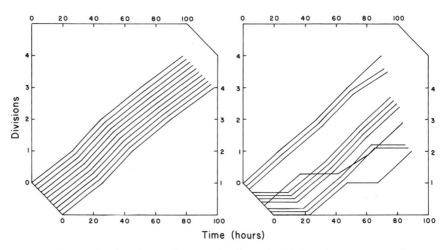

Fig. 4.2. Synchrony and asynchrony in the division of *B. japonicum* v. intermedium. *Left*: plot of 11 isolated cells descended from a single ancestor four generations back; the four succeeding generations traced in the graph maintain perfect synchrony. *Right*: the relatively asynchronous division of 11 other cells of the same strain that were taken at random from a stock culture many generations removed from a common ancestor. The time and division axes in both graphs are staggered to emphasize synchrony and asynchrony. From Giese, 1968; originally from data of B. McCaw.

is truly absent in *Blepharisma*, lipids or lipid precursors may be a critical component of successful axenic media.

When an autoclaved (or lyophilized) *Ps. ovalis* suspension was supplemented by yeast extract (to supply amino acids and nucleic acid factors), lettuce extract (probably to supply stigmasterol), and various B vitamins (see Tables 4.2 and 4.3), the medium was found to support the growth of *Blepharisma japonicum* v. intermedium with a generation time of 32 hours (Smith, 1965). Although this is not a rapid rate, the growth appeared normal; at least, no abnormal forms appeared, as they often do in less suitable media, and *Blepharisma* grew in the medium with unabated vigor for approximately five years. Nevertheless, a completely defined axenic medium for *Blepharisma* has not yet been achieved (Smith and Giese, 1967).

Christie and Hirshfield (1968) found that even if yeast extract, protease peptone, and vitamins were included in the axenic medium (Lilly and Farina, 1967), *B. americanum* developed abnormalities in its macronucleus, failed to encyst, and rarely conjugated, whereas the bacteria-fed controls encysted and conjugated freely. Division rate was not measured.

In 1948 a brief report described a *Blepharisma* (dark pink in color and resembling *B. lateritium* in size, shape, and macronuclear type) that appeared to possess green chlorellae (*Chlorella conductrix*) in its cytoplasm. The relationship resembles that of *Chlorella* with *Stentor polymorphus*, except that *Stentor* is not known to occur without the chlorellae (Tartar, 1961). It was found in Marble Lake, northwest Iowa. The blepharismas ingested bacteria, small flagellates, ciliates, and algae; but ingestion of food organisms was lowest in the blepharismas that had the largest numbers of chlorellae. The green color of the chlorellae was lost after two weeks in darkness, but the blepharismas survived in darkness by ingesting bacteria; and the chlorellae regained their color on exposure to light. The chlorellae remained in the blepharismas for at least four months, at which time observations were terminated (Johnson, 1948). There are no studies of the division rates in blepharismas possessing chlorellae but deprived of bacterial food, which might determine whether they could utilize the nutrients produced by the chlorellae; and no other reports of such a relationship between chlorellae and *Blepharisma* have appeared.

TABLE 4.2

Permutations of the Basic Media for Axenic Culture of *Blepharisma*

Ingredient	Medium[a]				
	1[b]	2[b]	3[c]	4[c]	5[c]
Yeast extract (ml/liter)	40.0	50.0		50.0	
Yeast autolysate (g/liter)			5.0		5.0
Bacteria (slant cultures/liter)[d]	33.3	33.3	33.3		
Vitamin mix I (ml/liter)[e]	1.0	1.0			
Vitamin mix II (ml/liter)			10.0	10.0	10.0
Glucose (ml/liter)	1.0	1.0			
Lyophilized bacteria (g/liter)				0.75	0.75
Generation time (hr)	40	30	40	30	35

SOURCE: Smith and Giese, 1967.

[a] Basal mixture used in all media: 0.1% (w/v) lettuce; 0.1 M Na$_2$HPO$_4$ at 18.8 ml/l; 0.1 M NaH$_2$PO$_4$, at 1.2 ml/l.

[b] Lettuce, buffer, and bacteria were autoclaved together. Vitamins, glucose, and yeast extract were each prepared separately and added aseptically.

[c] All constituents were autoclaved together.

[d] The 33.3 slant cultures/liter of bacteria are approximately equivalent to the 0.75 g of lyophilized bacteria used in media 4 and 5.

[e] See Table 4.3 for vitamin mixtures.

TABLE 4.3

Vitamin Mixtures for Axenic Culture of *Blepharisma*

Ingredient	Mixture I[a]	Mixture II[b]
Water (ml)	10.0	100.0
Thiamine-HCl (g)	0.006	0.006
Calcium pantothenate (g)	0.002	0.002
Pyridoxal HCl (g)	0.002	0.002
Nicotinamide (g)	0.002	0.002
Riboflavin (g)	0.002	0.002
Folic acid (g)	0.001	0.001

SOURCE: Smith and Giese, 1967; both mixtures modified from the work of Miller and van Wagtendonk, 1956.

[a] This mixture was sterilized by filtration and added aseptically to media; it was stored at 5° C.

[b] This mixture was not sterilized before being added to media; therefore, freshly mixed solutions were added to media that were subsequently autoclaved.

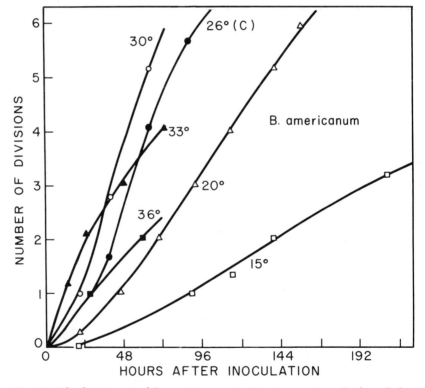

Fig. 4.3. The division rate of *B. americanum* at various temperatures. Each symbol represents a test group of 10–12 culture tubes. From Giese and McCaw, 1963a.

Temperature as a Factor in Growth

Blepharismas can actually withstand a wider range of temperature than that allowing their growth. For example, the larger species (e.g., *B. japonicum* and *B. japonicum* v. intermedium) can be kept in a refrigerator for prolonged periods at 5° to 7.5° C. At this temperature range they drop to the bottom of the culture tube and remain in the detritus; but even after two weeks they swim in normal fashion if warmed to room temperature. A smaller species (*B. americanum*) was found to swim even at 7.5°. Blepharismas kept at 7.5° without feeding remained alive up to five weeks. They can therefore withstand the periods of low temperature typical of wintertime in California. Blepharismas are less resistant to low temperature if taken from a culture in the logarithmic state. Therefore, if stocks are to be kept in reserve in the refrigerator, they should be put there just after peak population has been reached.

When blepharismas are placed in ice water at 0° C they shed pigment (see Chapter 8). If quickly warmed up to room temperature after 90 seconds they survive and multiply at the same rate as controls, but if kept at such low temperatures for more than two minutes they almost invariably die. *Blepharisma* is thus unable to withstanding freezing except in the encysted state (Giese, unpublished). No one has yet attempted to preserve blepharismas by the freezing procedure employed for some other protozoans (Diamond, 1964).

Blepharisma japonicum v. intermedium cultures do remarkably well at 13° C. They do not usually grow, but remain in a healthy state for two months. Some cultures I have observed lasted for even a month more, and these, after first being acclimated, were able to grow slowly. Cultures in nature probably exist chiefly at temperatures lower than 30°. Kasturi Bai et al. (1969) suggest 28° as best for the growth of *B. japonicum* v. intermedium, since at this temperature the cells store optimal amounts of glycogen, basic protein, lipids, and acid phosphatase.

Growth occurs over the entire range of 15–33° C, the division rate increasing with temperature up to 30°. At 33° the rate is slower than at 30° (Fig. 4.3); and above this it is progressively still slower, ceasing entirely at about 38°. At this temperature various nutrient reserves in the cells decrease markedly (Kasturi Bai et al., 1969). However, blepharismas kept at 38° for several hours and then placed back at 25° divide normally, with a slight lag that perhaps indicates a small degree of injury. Exposure to 40°, when it does not kill the blepharismas, also has little effect on division after they are replaced at 25°, except for a similar lag before division begins. Temperature affects growth rates in *B. japonicum* v. intermedium and *B. americanum* in a similar manner, resulting in temperature coefficients (for increase in rate of division calculated for a 10° temperature interval) of approximately 3.84, 2.92, and 1.59 over the ranges 13–18°, 18–25°, and 25–30°, respectively. Another measure of growth, the rate of regeneration, has a similar relation to temperature, the curves for division and regeneration rates being almost parallel (Fig. 4.4).

Growth and cell division do not always occur at the same rate in different species of *Blepharisma* grown under the same culture conditions and at the same temperature. In the observations shown in Table 4.4 two stocks of *B. americanum*, and three stocks of *B. japonicum* all had a generation time of approximately 15 hours at 25° C; other stocks had about 20 hours, and the one stock of *B. undulans* had a generation time of 40 hours. Similar differences prevailed at 30°, except that the generation time was shorter owing to the higher temperature. At 13° some of the stocks died; others showed differences exaggerating those present at higher temperatures, and in the same relative order for different stocks.

TABLE 4.4

Generation Time for Various Stocks of *Blepharisma*

Species	Stock	Size[a] (in μm)	Generation time (hr)[b] at 13° C	25° C	30° C
B. americanum	Stanford(G)	149 × 43	93.6 ± 48.6	15.9 ± 4.2	10.1 ± 0.4
	Rao B	147 × 56	112.0 ± 29.5	21.8 ± 2.8	17.9 ± 4.5
	Balamuth	148 × 46	84.7 ± 13.1	15.2 ± 2.1	10.6 ± 1.0
B. stoltei	Nara	224 × 78	died	22.3 ± 2.8	14.5 ± 1.3
B. japonicum	Niigata	293 × 95	250.0 ± 31.1	25.4 ± 2.3	15.6 ± 2.8
	Suzuki #3	318 × 96	172.0 ± 58.6	13.9 ± 1.0	9.8 ± 2.8
	Intermedium	294 × 76	175.5 ± 31.2	17.5 ± 6.9	10.9 ± 0.9
	Suzuki #5	315 × 95	146.0 ± 65.4	15.2 ± 1.9	10.7 ± 1.8
B. undulans	Suzuki #3	176 × 27	died	39.8 ± 3.0	27.3 ± 5.2

SOURCE: Giese and McCaw, 1963a.

[a] All measurements were made on log-phase cells (grown under the standard conditions described in the text) that had just completed division and had not yet begun feeding again. Each specimen was placed in a drop of 3% methyl cellulose and measured by ocular micrometer. Averages of 20 specimens.

[b] Measured on log-phase blepharismas grown in the standard manner described, 10–12 of each species, placed individually in 4-mm tubes and maintained at the temperature under study. All specimens used had just divided, and all were therefore in the same interdivisional stage. Data are averages of three series. Generation time given is the average of the first three divisions after inoculation; the first division almost always takes longer than subsequent divisions.

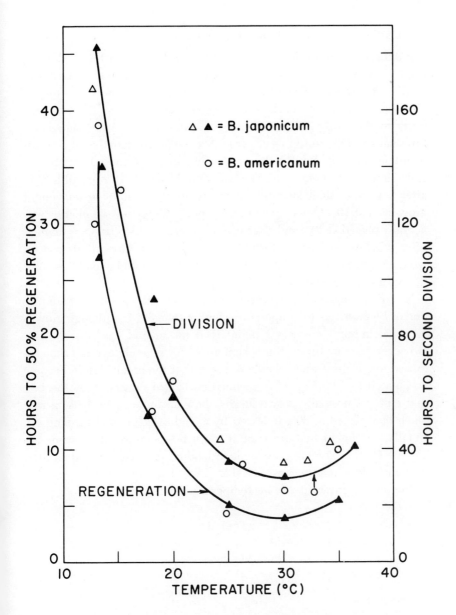

Fig. 4.4. Regeneration and division at various temperatures in three *Blepharisma* stocks from two different species. From Giese and McCaw, 1963a.

Acclimation to Lower or Higher Temperatures

Blepharisma, as a rule, does not grow after being transferred directly from 25° C to 13°, although some specimens (about one in ten) will divide after several days of acclimation (Fig. 4.5). However, after acclimation at 13° for a month growth is consistent, and after three months fairly good cultures can be obtained. Transferring these acclimated cultures back to 25° results in a growth rate even better than that of controls maintained at 25°, but the difference, though suggestive, is not statistically significant (Giese and McCaw, unpublished). It is possible that after a very gradual lowering of the temperature *Blepharisma* might grow even at 10°. One culture I had kept at 13° for several months was actually placed at 10°, and after several weeks the blepharismas divided (Fig. 4.5, lowest line). Unfortunately, both this culture and its control were discarded by accident before observations could be made, as were the others long acclimated to 13°

No convincing evidence has been obtained for the permanent adaptation of *Blepharisma* to temperatures higher than 30° C, although growth occurred in some cultures I maintained for several weeks at 33–35° However, the fact that cultures kept at 30° for several days and then returned to 25° grow more slowly suggests that the organisms do become acclimated to 30° (Fig. 4.5). Acclimation is also suggested by the fact that cultures normally grown at 25° show an increase in division rate when first placed at 30°, followed by a slight decline and leveling off. Finally, specimens that are kept at lower temperatures do become acclimated to the extent of growing in individual size even when their division rate does not increase (Table 4.5). This agrees with data on *Tetrahymena* grown at various temperatures (Thormar, 1962).

TABLE 4.5

Size of *B. japonicum* v. intermedium after Acclimation to
Different Temperatures

Temperature	Number of generations observed	Generation time (hr)	Dimensions (in μm)
30° C	66	12	182 × 58
25°	stock culture[a]	18	249 × 76
13°	25	96	327 × 105

SOURCE: Unpublished experiments of Barbara McCaw. Data are averages for 20 cells.
    [a] Number of generations not recorded.

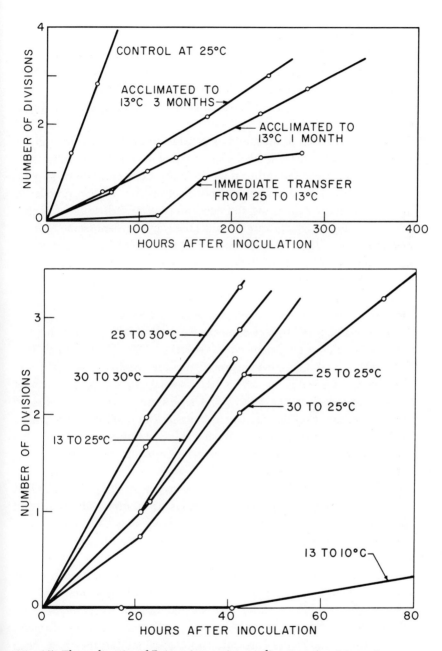

Fig. 4.5. The acclimation of *B. japonicum* v. intermedium to various temperatures, as measured by division rate. *Above*: acclimation to 13°C. *Below*: the results of transferring blepharismas to other temperatures to determine whether they are acclimated. From data of B. McCaw.

Osmotic Tolerance

Since most of the species of *Blepharisma* that have been studied occur in fresh water, the balanced salt solution (modified from Taylor and Strickland, 1935) used in our Stanford laboratory is an approximation to pond water (Table 4.6).

The concentration of all solutions considered in this chapter is given in osmoles: that is, in terms of the sum total of dissolved molecules and / or ions per unit volume rather than the molar concentration of specific ions of electrolytes or molecules of nonelectrolytes. The first practice is more meaningful than citing the concentration of individual salts, because in biological media various salts are always present (some in trace amounts), as well as various nonelectrolytes. Osmolal concentration is here determined by one of the colligative properties of a solution (e.g., depression of freezing point or change in vapor pressure); that is, by properties dependent on the number of particles free to act. A 1.0 osmolal solution depresses the freezing point by $1.86°$ C.

Unit osmolality (UO), as used in the figures and tables in this chapter, is the osmolality of our balanced salt solution: 4.35×10^{-3} osmolal (Hilden, 1969). The standard axenic growth medium (Smith, 1965) is approximately ten times this, or 4.35×10^{-2} osmolal ($10 \times$ UO). For convenience, most data on the figures and tables are given in multiples of unit osmolality; from this the true osmolality can readily be calculated.

Despite the fact that it lives in fresh water containing a variety of salts, *Blepharisma*, like many other freshwater protozoans, can be washed essentially free of salts without visible ill effects by a series of baths in glass-distilled water. The cells appear to swell very little, if at all. Conversely, as they are subjected to solutions of progressively increasing osmolality the blepharismas shrink; and above $40. \times$ UO they become completely flattened and fail to grow unless soon transferred to a lower osmolality.

Determining the water content and osmolality of a protozoan cell is usually difficult, and *Blepharisma* offers no special advantage in this respect. The studies of water content and osmotic pressure in other ciliates, mostly from fresh water, have been summarized by Kitching (1967). The values he cites are only approximations, but they have been obtained through a variety of methods and lines of approach and are similar to the values reported for other types of living cells. The water

TABLE 4.6
Standard Balanced Salt Solution

Salt	Concentration
NaCl	1.78×10^{-3} M
KCl[a]	3.08×10^{-4} M
$MgCl_2$	4.16×10^{-4} M
$MgSO_4$	1.62×10^{-6} M
$CaCl_2$	6.80×10^{-6} M
Approximate total osmolality	4.35×10^{-3} osm.

NOTE: Modified from Taylor and Strickland, 1935. The solution here described was designated the unit standard balanced salt solution (USBSS) in several earlier papers from this laboratory (Giese et al., 1965; Hilden and Giese, 1969; Giese and Benedetti, 1971). It is designated unit osmolality (UO) in this chapter.
   [a] The original medium of Taylor and Strickland had 3.08×10^{-5} KCl.

content of *Tetrahymena* has been estimated (from a densely packed pellet of cells) to be about 80.6% (Dunham and Child, 1960); and the osmotic pressure of a freshwater peritrich was estimated (from the osmolality required to just prevent water uptake in a cyanide-treated cell) at 0.05 osmoles. The value of $10 \times$ UO (.0435 osmolal) obtained for the osmotic pressure of *Blepharisma* (Hilden, 1969) is of the same order of magnitude.

Freshwater ciliates are less permeable to water than many other kinds of cells (Kitching, 1967); however, the permeability constant of *Blepharisma* to water has not been measured. Blepharismas transferred from Cerophyl medium to distilled water scarcely swell, whereas those placed in $41 \times$ UO quickly shrink, suggesting that water passes outward through their cell membranes more rapidly than inward. The osmotic gradient for a *Blepharisma* in distilled water is approximately 0.97 atmospheres, considering the osmolality of *Blepharisma* itself to be $10 \times$ UO. In a $41 \times$ UO medium the osmotic pressure is 3.9 atmospheres; therefore, the difference in osmotic pressure between the outside and inside of the cell under these conditions is $3.9 - 0.97$, or 2.93 atmospheres.

The osmotic pressure of *Blepharisma*'s cytoplasm depends in part on the osmolality of the medium in which the cells have been grown. Many cells take up ions, and perhaps accumulate organic metabolites, when placed in media of high osmolality. When they are thus acclimated and are then returned to a lower osmolality, they swell and sometimes burst, indicating that they are taking up water in response to the osmotic gradient but are unable to void the osmotically active material inside them as rapidly as they take up water. Reacclimation to a lower osmolality may take several days (Giese and Benedetti, 1971).

Possibly, water entry into blepharismas transferred from 1 × UO to distilled water is reduced by the elastic properties of the cell membrane, which to some extent negate the tendency for water to enter the cell. However, when a *Blepharisma* loaded with salts by gradual acclimation to 41 × UO is subsequently placed into distilled water, it swells until it bursts, the membrane not being strong enough to withstand the larger osmotic pressure gradient.

In axenic media little if any growth can be detected in blepharismas transferred from unit osmolality to 30 × UO, and it is slow at 20 × UO. However, cultures maintained by serial transfers acclimate and grow at 20 × UO. When cultures acclimated at this level are transferred to media of still higher osmolality, they grow slowly, and after many serial transfers some cultures will reproduce at 30 or 40 × UO. In all these cases, however, growth is very slow, and the cells remain somewhat shrunken. It has proved impossible to obtain any growth in axenic media of osmolality higher than 40 × UO, even after three years of acclimation to levels just below this. No determinations of the division interval in axenic cultures at different UO values have been made (Hilden, 1969).

Since *Blepharisma* grows well on the bacterium *Pseudomonas ovalis*, which survives and grows even at osmolalities above 41 × UO, the division rate of our blepharismas was determined immediately after their transfer to media at different osmolalities in infusions of Cerophyl inoculated with *Ps. ovalis*. Surprisingly, the division rate in a medium of 11 × UO was more rapid than in unit osmolality; in 21 × UO, division was almost as rapid as in 11 × UO; and in 31 × UO, some cells died, and others divided slowly after a long lag (see Fig. 4.6, *C*). This was true for both *B. japonicum* v. intermedium and *B. japonicum* (Suzuki #3 strain), suggesting that growth is improved when the external osmolality is close to the internal, perhaps because less effort is required for maintaining the internal environment.

Acclimation to High Osmolality

As measured by division rate. Although blepharismas fed on *Ps. ovalis* grew poorly when first transferred to media with an osmolality

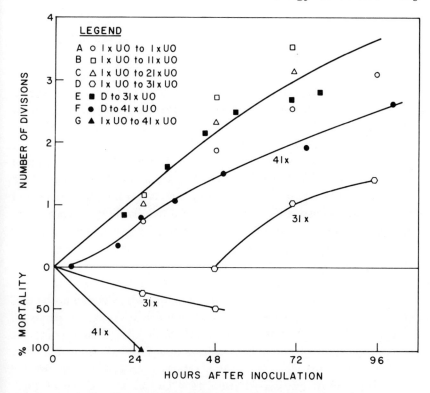

Fig. 4.6. Growth and mortality of *B. japonicum* v. intermedium on Cerophyl infusion inoculated with *Ps. ovalis* at various salt concentrations. Note the rapid acclimation to 31 and 41 × UO of cells that survive the first transfer.

greater than 21 × UO (Fig. 4.6, *D* and *G*), the cells that did not die acclimated rapidly. Thus blepharismas that grew slowly when first transferred from 1 × UO to 31 × UO (Fig. 4.5, *D*) grew almost as well as those in 11 × UO after a second transfer to new 31 × UO medium (Fig. 4.6, *E*). When blepharismas were transferred from a healthy culture in 31 × UO to 41 × UO, they grew, but not quite as rapidly as at 11 × UO, 21 × UO, or 31 × UO (Fig. 4.6, *F*). Furthermore, it proved difficult to maintain cultures at this osmolality because growth was slower with each successive transfer.

Blepharismas not only grow very slowly on *Ps. ovalis* at high osmolality, but are altered in other ways. The cells are smaller in volume and with sparser pigment than in media with lower osmolalities, and they are brownish in color rather than red. They also swim much more slowly than controls at unit osmolality, possibly because of the increased viscosity of the medium.

That blepharismas had acclimated to media of higher osmolality in one experimental case was indicated by injury and a slower division rate when they were returned to media of lower osmolality (Fig. 4.7). Almost all the cells transferred from $41 \times$ UO to $1 \times$ UO died (curve G); the few that survived started dividing only after a lag of 36 hours, and then divided a little more slowly than controls (curve A). When transferred from $41 \times$ UO to $11 \times$ UO, few blepharismas were killed, but the long lag (about 30 hours) preceding division suggests a necessary period of recovery and adjustment; once the cells started dividing, however, they did so at the rate of controls (curve B). The lag preceding division in blepharismas transferred from 41 to $21 \times$ UO was shorter (curve C). When the blepharismas that had survived the transfer from 41 to $1 \times$ UO were allowed to adjust for a week before being returned to $11 \times$ UO, they not only started dividing without a lag but also divided at the rate of controls kept at $11 \times$ UO, indicating complete acclimation (curve E).

Apparently, the blepharismas had truly acclimated themselves to the higher osmolality, presumably by raising their internal osmolality. They swelled to the bursting point after a transfer from $41 \times$ UO to distilled water; and when transferred from $41 \times$ UO to $1 \times$ UO all of them swelled and most died without bursting. Yet when blepharismas are transferred directly from UO to distilled water they scarcely swell. Judging from the experimental data, acclimation to $41 \times$ UO from $1 \times$ UO takes over a week, and reacclimation downward takes about the same amount of time.

Perhaps growth and cell division are best at $11 \times$ UO because this approximates the internal osmolality of *Blepharisma*, as already mentioned (Hilden, 1969). Presumably, less water would enter at $11 \times$ UO than at $1 \times$ UO; and less effort would be expended on maintaining a gradient on salt transport, which would presumably be required in $1 \times$ UO owing to leakage from the cell.

Acclimation as measured by regeneration rate. It is also possible to use the rate of regeneration of a peristome on a postperistomal fragment of *Blepharisma* as a measure of acclimation to high osmolality, and we have tested this for osmolalities from 1 to $75 \times$ UO. Regeneration at unit osmolality takes about five hours at $25°$ C. Although *Blepha-*

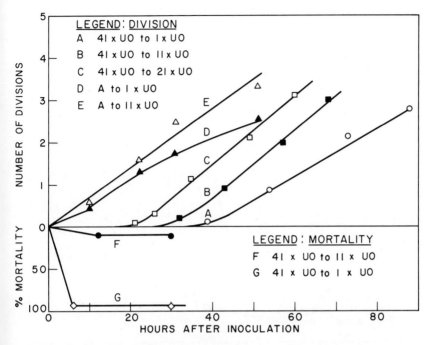

Fig. 4.7. Growth and mortality of *B. japonicum* v. intermedium on Cerophyl infusion after transfer from high osmolality to low.

risma will not grow or regenerate at $75 \times$ UO, it will tolerate such osmolalities for several hours. The regeneration of blepharismas acclimated to lower osmolalities was slow when they were placed at high osmolalities for a test; but the rate for those grown at a high osmolality (in axenic media) and then placed at a high osmolality to regenerate was equal to that of controls at unit osmolality (Fig. 4.8). For example, those grown for two years in an axenic medium of $40 \times$ UO, when placed in a medium of this osmolality, regenerated at approximately the rate of controls at unit osmolality and were only slightly retarded by $50 \times$ UO. At higher osmolalities regeneration was progressively retarded. When blepharismas grown at high osmolalities were placed in media of lower osmolality, regeneration was also retarded, slowing down in proportion to the disparity between the osmolality of the growth medium and the osmolality of the test medium (Hilden and Giese, 1969).

As I have mentioned, blepharismas acclimated to high osmolalities do not reacclimate to low osmolalities at once. When cells grown at

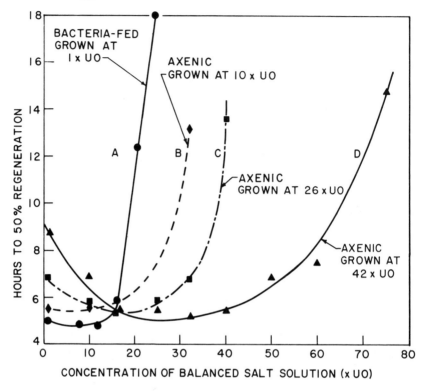

Fig. 4.8. Regeneration rate of *B. japonicum* v. intermedium in axenic medium at various osmolalities (from Hilden and Giese, 1969). Each symbol represents the average rate of 24 postperistomal fragments, handled as described in Chapter 9.

$42 \times$ UO are placed in an axenic medium of $10 \times$ UO, they swell (Fig. 4.9); and it is almost impossible to transect them for regeneration studies, since the protoplasmic contents generally flow out without healing when the pellicle is cut. It is necessary to acclimate the blepharismas gradually, in periodic steps of about one-third dilution with standard axenic medium over a month or so. After seven days at a reduced osmolality it is possible to cut the cells for regeneration tests. However, little real acclimation occurs even after 14 days. After 21 days the cells will regenerate at approximately the normal rate of somewhat over five hours to 50% regeneration. But even after 28 days, reacclimation is still incomplete, and the cells require somewhat longer to regenerate than controls maintained at the lower osmolality (Giese and Benedetti, 1971).

When sucrose is substituted for the balanced salts, regeneration is delayed in much the same manner as with salts but on an osmolal basis

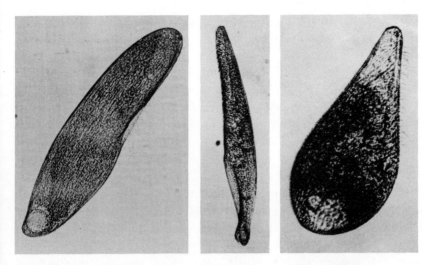

Fig. 4.9. *Left, B. japonicum* v. intermedium growing in an axenic medium at
10 × UO. *Center,* the same cell transferred to 42 × UO. *Right,* a cell grown at
42 × UO after one hour at 10 × UO. From Giese and Benedetti, 1971.

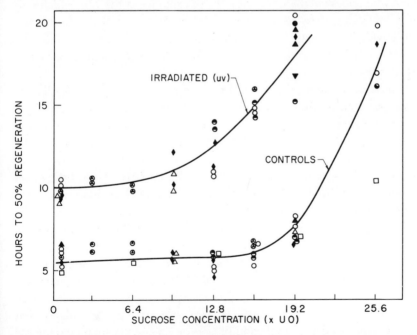

Fig. 4.10. Sucrose concentration and the regeneration of *B. japonicum* v. intermedium. The fragments plotted on the upper curve received 3,200 ergs/mm² of
UV radiation (265 nm) before they were placed in the test solution. The various
symbols indicate experiments done on different days.

to a somewhat greater degree. Thus there is a slight retarding effect in 19.2 × UO and a marked delay in 25.6 × UO (Fig. 4.10). When the cell is injured, however, as by UV irradiation, even a 12.8 × UO sucrose concentration is somewhat damaging, and regeneration is considerably retarded. Sucrose, it is true, is not likely to be found in the natural environment of blepharismas except in minute traces. However, the experiment points up the difference in action between salts and nonelectrolytes (Giese et al., 1965).

Effect of pH

It is difficult to determine the effect of pH on growth and cell division because *Blepharisma* does not tolerate buffer concentrations that effectively maintain the pH. A Sørensen phosphate buffer of 0.1 M with respect to phosphate is almost immediately toxic to *Blepharisma*; one-tenth this concentration is usually satisfactory, provided that sodium salts are used, potassium being especially unfavorable. Although the best results have been obtained with 0.005 M phosphate buffer, this concentration does not maintain the pH (for example, at pH 7.0), which falls to a low value after the growth of bacteria in a Cerophyl infusion and rises with the growth of the protozoans. The oscillations are naturally greater when the original pH is poised further from neutrality (Giese et al., 1965).

I have also tested Tris buffer (hydroxymethyl aminomethane), but in nontoxic concentrations it is no more effective in maintaining the pH than Sørensen phosphate buffer. And like the phosphate buffer it is toxic at a concentration of 0.1 M, probably because it has a similar effect on the osmosis of protozoans.

Initial buffering over the range from pH 5.0 to pH 8.0 has little effect on the rate of division of *Blepharisma* in a Cerophyl medium. However, a pH of 9.0 is usually quite unfavorable, and pH 8.5 may be also. At the other end of the scale, an initial pH of less than 5.0 is also unfavorable for growth (Giese et al., 1965). Essentially the same may be said of the effect of pH on rate of regeneration, there being no meaningful difference in rate over the same pH range of 5.0 to 8.0. Since the blepharismas are tested over a short period of time, the pH remains close to the value initially set (Giese et al., 1965). In any case, it is quite unlikely that *Blepharisma* under natural conditions ever encounters such extreme pH values at either end of the scale (Noland, 1925).

Oxygen Requirements

Little information is available on the oxygen requirements of various species of *Blepharisma*. Noland (1925) did record the oxygen content of ponds in which he found *Blepharisma*. And *B. japonicum* has been collected from papyrus swamps in Uganda where the water is completely anaerobic within an inch of the surface (Beadle and Nilsson, 1959). Periodic sampling of the oxygen content of the water with the Winkler method showed that whereas the ciliate *Bursaria* died soon after the water became anaerobic, *B. japonicum* lived for three days under anaerobic conditions. Emerson (1929) measured the oxygen consumption of *Blepharisma* with the Warburg method and found that the endogenous respiration had a respiratory quotient of 1.0, suggesting the use of carbohydrate as an energy source. In a nitrogen atmosphere the blepharismas produced gas (probably CO_2) by glycolysis. On returning to air, they recovered and respired much as before, and the respiratory quotient returned to unity. This suggests that no oxygen debt had been incurred.

The survival of *Blepharisma* for three days under anaerobic conditions implies that it can rely on glycolysis or some other anaerobic mode of respiration (fermentation) when necessary. This ability is valuable, since it allows *Blepharisma* to enter mucky pond water and obtain bacteria as food. However, because it cannot divide in the absence of oxygen (although it will regenerate; Giese and McCaw, 1963b) the organism must return to aerated water after feeding.

In a medium lacking nutrients, stationary-phase blepharismas are even more resistant to lack of oxygen than in a medium rich in nutrients and bacteria. In my recent investigations I reduced the oxygen partial pressure in such a culture to about 0.1% of that initially present by exhausting the culture to a vacuum of about 2 mm Hg in a Thunberg tube; nevertheless, the blepharismas continued to swim about. When a low-oxygen culture of *B. americanum* was placed at 13° C encystment occurred. In another culture kept at room temperature cannibal giants appeared, and within a week practically all the smaller cells had been eaten. When the exhaustion procedure was repeated twice more, reducing the oxygen partial pressure to little more than one-billionth, the blepharismas lived for shorter periods. The large African stock of *B. japonicum* survived for only 12–18 hours, the smaller *B. japonicum* about 37 hours; *B. americanum* lasted for several days at room temperature and for a week or more at 13°.

The response of *Blepharisma* to graded changes in oxygen partial pressure has not been tested, and no studies appear to have been made of its anaerobic and aerobic metabolic pathways. Nothing further seems to have been done on respiration, either.

Responses to Electromagnetic Radiation

When blepharismas in culture tubes are exposed to the light of early dawn, they do not appear to be highly responsive; but later in the day they are found in the debris at the bottom of the culture tube. If small stones are substituted for the usual organic debris, the blepharismas are found among and under the stones. The reaction is not quick, and if the cells are suddenly exposed to bright light they are usually killed. This reaction is apparently a photooxidation, since *Blepharisma*'s pink pigment is a photosensitizer (see Chapter 11). Light is thus an important factor in the ecology of *Blepharisma*. Perhaps species of this genus are not found as often as some other common protozoans because they are more likely to be hidden in bottom detritus, especially since collections are usually made by day. This may account for one collector's failure to find any members of this genus in an extensive search over the seasons of one year (Wang, 1928).

Like all cells, blepharismas are also sensitive to far UV radiation and X-rays. These radiations have therefore been used to analyze some problems in the physiology of the genus. Most of this information is considered in Chapters 9 and 11.

Predation

One of the most important ecological factors for the survival of any species is avoidance of predators by prey. In some way enough members of a species, whether predator or prey, must survive to reproduce and propagate their kind.

In developing a plan to seed natural ponds with *Blepharisma*, I took samples from open ponds and added blepharismas to them. Whenever small, filter-feeding crustaceans were already present in the pond samples, the introduced blepharismas soon disappeared; and whenever such predacious crustaceans become prominent in the ecological succession of a natural pond, it is unlikely that blepharismas will be found there.

No studies of blepharismas living in natural ponds have yet been made.

In laboratory cultures containing the rhizopod protozoan *Actinosphaerium* blepharismas were seen trapped on that organism's filopodia and were later engulfed in telltale red food vacuoles. *Actinosphaerium* does not thrive on *Blepharisma* alone, but it can eat large numbers of them. Interestingly, if an *Actinosphaerium* that has engulfed numerous blepharismas is suddenly exposed to bright light, the red vacuoles are quickly evacuated regardless of their stage of digestion. The photo-oxidation of *Blepharisma's* red pigment probably acts as a stimulant to this voiding (Giese and Pappas, unpublished). The pigment is toxic to other organisms not only in light but in darkness, if present in high concentrations; lower concentrations in darkness seem to be nontoxic. Furthermore, the pigment does not appear to leave the uninjured cells without bright light. Blepharismas can be kept in culture tubes with *Paramecium* under dim or moderate light, and each genus will divide at its characteristic rate, just as it would divide in an isolated culture (Giese, 1949).

Apparently many other protozoans will feed on *Blepharisma*, especially those with relatively nonselective feeding habits. Selective feeders like *Didinium nasutum*, however, will starve to death or encyst in thriving cultures of *Blepharisma*, even the albino strain. Since *Blepharisma* divides more slowly than *Paramecium* but serves equally well as food for various carnivorous protozoans and metazoan filter feeders, it is likely to be consistently less prominent than *Paramecium* when the two are found in the same ponds.

Note on Experimental Methods

Though of minor interest theoretically, a brief discussion of experimental methods for determining *Blepharisma's* division rate might help those attempting such measurements for class or research purposes. The stock cultures used are most conveniently grown in fairly large test tubes. For individual experiments, small culture tubes 6 cm long and 5 mm in outer diameter have proved satisfactory, since observations can be made on them for several days to a week with no danger that the culture medium will suffer excessive loss by evaporation. These containers can be made of soft glass tubing by fusing one end of a 6-cm section in the hot tip of a Bunsen flame and flaring the other end with a small, tapered carbon rod twirled in the red-hot opening (Fig. 4.11,

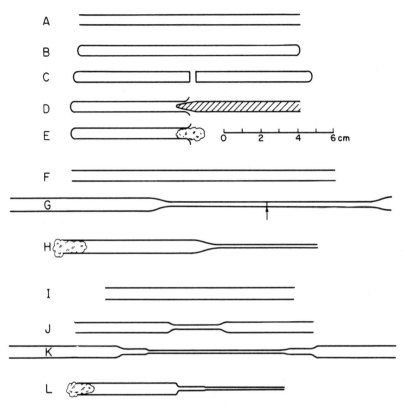

Fig. 4.11. Equipment for cell-division experiments. *Culture tube* (*A–E*): Soft 5-mm glass tubing 10–12 cm long is sealed at both ends and cut; the cut ends are heated and flared with a tapered carbon rod. *Pipette for culture medium* (*F–H*): A piece of 6-mm tubing 15–16 cm long is heated and gently pulled to a diameter of about 1 mm, and the middle of the narrow section is scratched and broken. *Pipette for blepharismas* (*I–L*): A 10-cm length of 6-mm tubing is heated and pulled very gently to half its diameter; when it has become rigid again, the center of the narrow segment is carefully reheated and rapidly drawn out to a very fine diameter. Both culture tubes and pipettes should be plugged at the wide end with rolled cotton to prevent contamination.

A–D). A small cotton plug serves to close the open end. The tubes are most easily held in a 50- or 100-ml beaker, supported by a rack made of 1-mm rigid plastic sheeting 5 cm square and drilled with a dozen numbered holes of appropriate size. The plugged culture tubes should be sterilized before use in an experiment.

Mouth-operated transfer pipettes are used to introduce culture medium and blepharismas into the culture tubes. It is best to have two kinds of pipettes: one of relatively large tip diameter (somewhat less than 1 mm) for transferring the culture medium, and several much finer ones (about 200 μm tip diameter) for transferring the blepharismas. The pipettes for culture medium are made by heating a 12–14-cm piece of 6-mm outer diameter soft glass tubing in a flame, making a pull when the glass is soft, and cutting at the middle of the thin section (Fig. 4.11, *G*). The wide ends can be plugged with cotton and the pipettes sterilized in a large test tube (about 20 × 2.5 cm), the narrow ends resting on a cotton wad at the bottom of the test tube.

The pipettes for transferring blepharismas are made from 10–12-cm pieces of soft glass tubing 5 or 6 mm in diameter. An initial draw is made to narrow the tube to about one-third its original diameter; and a second rapid draw, made after heating a small central section of the narrowed portion, produces a very fine tip (Fig. 4.11, *I–L*). The tip can be broken cleanly by scratching it with a carborundum crystal (or diamond tip) and pressing gently; its final diameter should be about 200 μm (several times the size of a *Blepharisma*). These small pipettes can be sterilized in the same manner as the larger ones.

To use either kind of transfer pipette, one fits a three-foot piece of rubber tubing snugly over the wide end of the pipette; the other end of the tubing is tipped with a medicine dropper, wide end outwards, for holding in the mouth. By sucking or blowing gently on the mouthpiece one can take up or expel fluid and culture medium with organisms and at the same time watch the pipette tip under a dissecting microscope.

The larger pipettes are used to transfer culture medium inoculated several hours to a day earlier with some bacteria suitable as food for *Blepharisma* (e.g., *Pseudomonas ovalis*). The smaller pipettes are used to transfer blepharismas, generally taken from a Columbia watch glass holding a sample of the stock culture (the watch glass should be held in a Petri dish and should be sterilized before use). With a fine tip, the blepharismas can be released one at a time into the small culture tubes. The number of blepharismas in a small culture tube can easily be counted under low power of a dissecting microscope while the tube is lying on the microscope stage, since the culture fluid is held in the tube by capillarity. From such counts the division rate can be determined.[*]

[*] These methods have been described before (Giese, 1945); more detail can be obtained from Mertens (1966), who describes an experiment for the study of "population explosion in a test tube."

Division rate may or may not be synchronous in a series of culture tubes taken at random from a single stock culture. For this reason, each symbol plotted on the statistical charts given in this chapter represents the average number of divisions per tube in a group of 10–12 small culture tubes, each inoculated at the start with a single cell. It is not possible to count accurately if there are more than about 64 blepharismas in a single tube, so the data are limited to the six divisions after transfer.

LITERATURE CITED

Beadle, L. C., and J. R. Nilsson. 1959. The effect of anaerobic conditions on two heterotrich ciliate Protozoa from papyrus swamps. J. Exp. Biol. **36**: 583–89.
Bhandary, S. V., and H. I. Hirshfield. 1964. Comparative studies of RNA synthesis in cannibal giant *Blepharisma*. J. Cell. Comp. Physiol. **63**: 217–24.
Bragg, A. N. 1937. Protozoan ecology. Science **86**: 307–8.
Christie, S. L., and H. I. Hirshfield. 1969. Morphological variations between axenic and bacteria-fed *Blepharisma*. J. Protozool. **16** (Suppl.): 20 (Abstr.).
Dawson, J. A. 1928. A comparison of the life-"cycles" of certain ciliates (*Blepharisma undulans*). J. Exp. Zool. **51**: 199–208.
—— 1953. The culture of *Blepharisma undulans* and *Stentor coeruleus*. Biol. Rev., City College of New York **15**: 13–15.
Dembitzer, H. M. 1958. Digestion and distribution of acid phosphatase in *Blepharisma*. J. Cell Biol. **37**: 329–44.
Diamond, L. S. 1964. Freeze-preservation of Protozoa (Method). Cryobiology **1**: 95–102.
Emerson, R. 1930. Measurements of the metabolism of two protozoans. J. Gen. Physiol. **13**: 153–58.
Farina, J. P. 1967. Axenic culture of *Blepharisma undulans*. Doctoral dissertation, St. Johns University.
Farina, J. P., and D. M. Lilly. 1965. Axenic culture of *Blepharisma undulans*. Amer. Zool. **5**: 735 (Abstr.).
Giese, A. C. 1938. Cannibalism and gigantism in *Blepharisma*. Trans. Amer. Micr. Soc. **57**: 245–55.
—— 1945. A simple method for division rate determination in *Paramecium*. Physiol. Zool. **18**: 158–61.
—— 1949. A cytotoxin from *Blepharisma*. Biol. Bull. **97**: 145–49.
—— 1968. Cell physiology. 3d ed. Philadelphia, 671 pp.
Giese, A. C., and T. Benedetti. 1971. Reacclimation of salt-acclimated *Blepharisma* to low salt concentration as measured by regeneration rate. Physiol. Zool. **44**: 1–8.
Giese, A. C., and B. K. McCaw. 1963a. Regeneration rate of *Blepharisma* with special reference to the effect of temperature. J. Protozool. **10**: 173–82.

—— 1963b. Effect of metabolic and other inhibitors on regeneration in *Blepharisma undulans* (*B. undulans japonicum*). Exp. Cell Res. 32: 130–46.

Giese, A. C., S. G. Smith, and B. J. Berry Dau. 1965. Effect of osmotic pressure, ionic imbalance, and pH upon the regeneration rate in *Blepharisma* (*B. intermedium*). Exp. Cell Res. 39: 145–60.

Giese, A. C., and C. V. Taylor. 1935. Paramecia for experimental purposes in controlled mass cultures on a single strain of bacteria. Arch. Protistenk. 84: 225–31.

Hall, R. P. 1965. Protozoan nutrition. New York, 90 pp.

—— 1967. Nutrition and growth of Protozoa. *In* Research in protozoology (T. T. Chen, ed.), I, 337–404. New York.

Hilden, S. A. 1969. Sodium and potassium levels in *Blepharisma intermedium*. Doctoral dissertation, Stanford University. 129 pp.

Hilden, S. A., and A. C. Giese. 1969. Effect of salt concentration on regeneration rate in *Blepharisma* acclimated to high salt levels. J. Protozool. 16: 419–22.

Johnson, L. P. 1948. A symbiotic *Blepharisma*. Proc. Iowa Acad. Sci. 55: 391–93.

Kasturi Bai, A. R., K. Srihari, M. Shadaksharaswamy, and P. S. Jyothy. 1969. The effects of temperature on *Blepharisma intermedium*. J. Protozool. 16: 738–42.

Kattar, M. B. 1940. Observaçãoes sobre a reprodução de *Blepharisma sinuosum* Sawaya. Fac. Fil. Cienc. Letras Univ. São Paulo Bol. Zool. 25: 417–24.

Kitching, J. A. 1967. Contractile vacuoles, ionic regulation, and excretion. *In* Research in protozoology (T. T. Chen, ed.), I, 307–36. New York.

Landon, S. 1959. *Blepharisma undulans* in bacteria-free culture. Master's thesis, Stanford University. 51 pp.

Lazo, A. W. 1953. Acción de terramicina sobre algunos protozoos. Invest. Zool. Chilenas 2: 9–10.

Lilly, D. M., and J. P. Farina. 1967. The axenic culture of *Blepharisma undulans* in conditioned, supplemented, and unconditioned medium. J. Protozool. 14 (Suppl.): 36 (Abstr.).

McManus, M. A., and M. S. Geraghty. 1962. The effect of kinetin on the multiplication rate of *Blepharisma undulans*. Proc. Iowa Acad. Sci. 69: 610–15.

Mertens, T. R. 1966. Population explosion in a test tube. Amer. Biol. Teacher 28: 103–7.

Miller, C. A., and W. J. van Wagtendonk. 1956. The essential metabolites of a strain of *Paramecium aurelia* and a comparison of the growth rate of different strains of *P. aurelia* in axenic culture. J. Gen. Microbiol. 15: 280–91.

Noland, L. E. 1925. Factors influencing the distribution of fresh-water ciliates. Ecology 6: 437–52.

Parpart, A. K. 1928. The bacteriological sterilization of *Paramecium*. Biol. Bull. 55: 113–20.

Richards, O. W., and J. A. Dawson. 1927. The analysis of the division rates of ciliates. J. Gen. Physiol. 10: 853–58.

Sandon, H. 1932. The food of Protozoa. Egypt. Univ. Publ. Fac. Sci. #1. 187 pp.

Sani, B. P., and P. L. Narasimha Rao. 1966. Antibiotic principles of *Garcinia morella*, 8: Antiprotozoal activity of morellin, neomorellin, and other insoluble neutral phenols of the seed coat of *Garcinia morella*. Ind. J. Exp. Biol. **4**: 27–28.

Saxena, D. M. 1970. Enzyme systems in the ciliates *Blepharisma intermedium* and *Spirostomum ambiguum*: Phosphatases, urease, and dehydrogenases. Acta Protozool. **7**: 81–86.

Seshachar, B. R., and D. M. Saxena. 1968. Digestive enzymes of *Blepharisma intermedium* Bhandary. Acta Protozool. **6**: 291–96.

Seshachar, B. R., and K. N. Saxena. 1963. Free amino acids and related compounds in different species of *Blepharisma* Perty (Ciliata: Spirostomatidae). Physiol. Zool. **36**: 174–83.

Seshachar, B. R., K. N. Saxena, and H. Girgla. 1971. Some factors governing the feeding behavior of *Homalozoon vermiculare* (Ciliophora: Holotricha). J. Protozool. **18**: 90–95.

Smith, S. G. 1965. Nutrition and axenic culture of *Blepharisma intermedium*. Doctoral dissertation, Stanford University. 73 pp.

Smith, S. G., and A. C. Giese. 1967. Axenic media for *Blepharisma intermedium*. J. Protozool. **14**: 649–54.

Stolte, H. A. 1924. Morphologische und physiologische Untersuchungen auf *Blepharisma undulans* Stein. Arch. Prot. **48**: 245–301.

Stolte, H. A. 1926. Die Kultur von *Blepharisma undulans* Stein und seine Verwendung im zoologischen Kursen. Zool. Anzeiger **65**: 213–16.

Suzuki, S. 1957. Morphogenesis in the regeneration of *Blepharisma undulans japonicus* Suzuki. Bull. Yamagata Univ. Natur. Sci. **4**: 85–192.

Tartar, V. 1961. The biology of *Stentor*. New York, 413 pp.

Taylor, C. V., and A. G .R. Strickland. 1935. Some factors in the excystment of dried cysts of *Colpoda cucullus*. Arch. Protistenk. **86**: 181–90.

Thormar, H. 1962. Cell size of *Tetrahymena pyriformis* in culture at various temperatures. Exp. Cell Res. **28**: 269–79.

Utsumi, K. 1955. Cytochemical studies on Ciliata, II: Phosphatases in *Paramecium aurelia* and *Blepharisma undulans japonicus*. Igaku to Seibutsugaku **34**: 245–48.

Vandermeer, J. H. 1969. The competitive structure of communities: An experimental approach with Protozoa. Ecology **50**: 362–71.

Wang, C. C. 1928. Ecological studies on the seasonal distribution of Protozoa in a fresh-water pond. J. Morph. and Phys. **46**: 431–78.

CHAPTER FIVE

Cannibalism

Cannibalism among the Protozoa was first reported by Haime in 1853, and has since been found in many species of protozoans. It appears to be especially common among the ciliates. Cannibalism in *Blepharisma*, first observed by Penard in 1922, occurs in many species of the genus, in some much more frequently than in others. Cannibal blepharismas usually become giants, growing to several times their normal size and greatly enlarging their mouthparts.

Possible Causes of Cannibalism

Blepharisma is primarily a bacterial feeder, but it also ingests particulate detritus, small protozoans, and even algae (Sandon, 1932). In a healthy culture in logarithmic phase the cells are dividing regularly, and the size of individuals at any stage between divisions is approximately the same. But when the food supply dwindles, some cells divide but fail to grow thereafter for lack of food, while others remain considerably larger, perhaps because they cannot get sufficient food to complete division. Whatever the reason, the larger cells often tend to engulf the smaller ones; and upon doing so they grow larger, still without dividing, and become true cannibal giants. Cannibalism also occurs when large and small species of *Blepharisma* are mixed, the larger species engulfing the smaller and developing into giants (e.g., *B. japonicum* eats *B. americanum*).

Cannibalism presents several questions: Is it a racial or genetic character? Is it an adaptation to larger prey, to meals that are highly assimilable because of possessing the same type of protoplasm, or both? Is hypertrophy a result of growth accompanied by an inhibition of division? Is cannibalism an adaptation to starvation by which some individuals will survive even though no normal food is to be had?

Nilsson (1967), studying an African race of *B. japonicum*, found that cannibalism occurred among all stocks of the species. She cloned cannibal giants and found that cannibals occurred with no greater frequency in their progeny than in clones fed bacteria, and only under similar conditions. I have obtained the same results with *B. americanum*. Tartar (1961) found that cannibalism occurred in nine stocks of *Stentor coeruleus* isolated from widely different sources. Apparently, cannibalism is not a restricted genetic trait.

Steinberg (1959) reasoned that since *Blepharisma* cannibals appeared in old cultures in which division was inhibited, the accumulated excretions may have inhibited division and thus induced large forms that were able to engulf small ones. He filtered the blepharismas from an old culture and boiled one aliquot of the infusion, keeping another aliquot as control; then he returned a few cells to each portion. Cannibals appeared and remained large even after exhausting the food, but only in the unboiled infusion. Steinberg interpreted this to mean that some thermolabile inhibitor of division was effective, and probably required, in the induction of cannibalism.

When I first approached this problem (Giese, 1938) I considered cannibalism a result of the chance variation in size of individuals and their mouthparts in a declining bacteria-fed culture. If so, it should be possible to produce cannibals at will by feeding blepharismas with more nutritious food to increase their size and develop larger mouthparts (Table 5.1). This approach was most successful when *B. americanum* was fed with the small ciliate *Tetrahymena*. It was necessary to wash the tetrahymenas free of food and then starve them for a day; otherwise, very few blepharismas could have engulfed them. Most of the vigorous blepharismas from a logarithmic bacteria-fed culture could eat the treated *Tetrahymena*; and those who did grew considerably, developed larger mouthparts, and were then able to capture smaller, bacteria-fed blepharismas when these were added to the culture. Thus in this species cannibalism can be induced at will and is not solely due to starvation conditions. A similar procedure has been used to induce cannibalism in *B. japonicum* (Nilsson, 1967), in *B. americanum* (Bhandary and Hirshfield, 1964), in *B. japonicum* v. intermedium albino (Giese, unpublished), and in an unspecified large species of *Blepharisma* (Padmavathi, 1961).

In many stock cultures minute blepharismas can sometimes be ob-

TABLE 5.1

Size of *B. americanum* Fed Various Foods

Food organism	Average size of food organism	Average size of *Blepharisma* so fed
Bacteria:		
Pseudomonas ovalis	1.5×0.5 µm	$149 \pm 22 \times 58 \pm 9.8$ µm
Fed *Ps. ovalis*, then starved	—	$143 \pm 20.2 \times 42.9 \pm 6.7$
Flagellate:		
Khawkinea halli	$42 \pm 8 \times 8 \pm 1.5$	$150 \pm 18.1 \times 67 \pm 13.6$
Ciliates:		
Tetrahymena pyriformis	$30 \pm 3.3 \times 15 \pm 4.1$	$206 \pm 28.7 \times 89 \pm 9.9$
Blepharisma americanum	$132 \pm 29.5 \times 27 \pm 4.7$	$217 \pm 24.7 \times 109 \pm 20.3$
Colpidium colpoda	$58 \pm 8.6 \times 33 \pm 4.4$	$240 \pm 25 \times 114 \pm 18.9$
Stylonychia curvata[a]	$71 \pm 12 \times 31 \pm 4.5$	290×160

SOURCE: Giese, 1938.

[a] *Blepharisma* ingests this organism so rarely that the figure given for a *Stylonychia*-fed cell is far too incomplete to determine standard deviations.

served. When isolated, these grow to normal size and divide to produce normal-sized individuals. The origin of these dwarfs was finally resolved when blepharismas trapped in the bacterial slime that often covers glass culture surfaces were observed for prolonged periods. In attempting to withdraw from the slime a *Blepharisma* would occasionally pull itself in two, one part being much smaller than the other. Presumably, as long as the small piece contained a portion of the macronucleus it could regenerate, forming thereby a dwarf otherwise perfect in shape. It is possible (but not likely) that such dwarfs could induce cannibalism in the other cells of a culture, since they usually appear in the early stages of a culture cycle.

It may be stated that any condition causing an increase in the size of individual blepharismas may induce cannibalism. Chemical inhibitors of division or low temperatures might also help to maintain cannibalism by preventing the rapid division of the enlarged cells. When cannibal giants are placed in a fresh medium containing bacteria, however, they rapidly divide to form the smaller cells characteristic of bacteria-fed blepharismas, and cannibalism ceases. It would be interesting to use division inhibitors or low temperatures (cf. Table 4.5) to see if the resulting enlarged cells would become cannibals when mixed with normal-sized bacteria-fed cells in a fresh medium maintained under the inhibiting conditions.

Cannibalism can be maintained for extended periods in a *Blepharisma* culture that also contains other small ciliates—for example, I have used *Colpidium colpoda*. Under these conditions, the cannibal giants of *B. japonicum* (African strain) on occasion ingested blepharismas when available, but fed on *Colpidium* between meals on their own kind. Apparently, feeding on *Colpidium*, a relatively small ciliate with a rapid division rate, nevertheless kept the cannibals and their mouthparts large enough to ingest a small *Blepharisma* whenever one was encountered. In fact, giants were often seen to have food vacuoles containing *Colpidium* side by side with those containing *Blepharisma*, the proportions of the two kinds depending largely on the relative numbers of *Colpidium* and small blepharismas in the culture. In a wild culture this strain often shows cannibals more or less continuously—probably for the same reason, since other small ciliates and rotifers are usually present in nature (Nilsson, unpublished).*

It would be interesting to determine whether extracts from small blepharismas—or from *Colpidium*, etc.—can induce an enlargement of mouthparts in other normal cells. This is known to occur following the application of stomatin extracted from *Tetrahymena pyriformis* to microstomatous *Tetrahymena vorax*. About 70 to 90% of these microstomatous filter feeders were transformed to macrostomatous carnivorous forms by this extract in eight hours (Buhse, 1967).

Ingestion in Cannibal Giants

We have already described ingestion in normal bacteria-fed blepharismas (Chapter 4). Ingestion in cannibal giants is quite dramatic, and has been described in detail by Nilsson (1967) for *B. japonicum* (African strain), a species especially favorable for observation because of its large size (Fig. 5.1). The potential prey that encounters a cannibal "is caught by the oral membranelles, by means of which it is oriented so that the anterior pole of the prey points toward the cytostome of the cannibal and the oral areas of the two organisms are in close contact. As soon as the prey is oriented and well lodged by the membranelles, a large vacuole is formed at the cytostome of the cannibal prior to the engulfing process. The cannibal rotates around its own axis, and when

---

* I have not seen *Blepharisma*, even giants, feed on *Paramecium aurelia*, although Padmavathi (1961) misquotes me to that effect. I have seen *Blepharisma* giants struggle with paramecia, never successfully. However, Dawson (1929) mentions that *Blepharisma* (presumably *B. americanum*) may on occasion eat a *Paramecium*.

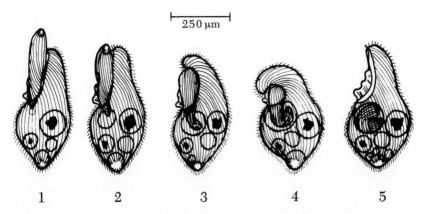

250 µm

Fig. 5.1. The engulfment of a *Blepharisma* by a cannibal giant of *B. japonicum* (African stock). From Nilsson, 1967; by permission of the Danish Science Press.

the engulfing starts, the anterior end of the cannibal bends over the posterior end of the prey, thus helping the oral membranelles to push the prey through the cytostome. In the completed food vacuole the prey is U-shaped, and movements of the prey can be detected for some time. . . . The whole engulfing process lasted 3–6 minutes when the prey was half the size of the cannibal, a shorter time if the prey was smaller." (Nilsson, 1967: 9–10.)

In species with a large undulating membrane, such as *B. americanum*, the membrane appears to take part in engulfment, acting as a scoop. The first steps in engulfment by this species are slower than the final ones, which may sometimes occur in less than a minute (Giese, 1938). This was also true of a stock of *B. japonicum** studied by Ibara (1939).

Sometimes the prey struggles vigorously, and occasionally manages to escape engulfment. Even if engulfed, a trapped *Blepharisma* continues to swim vigorously for a time within the cannibal's food vacuole. If assisted to escape, it may revive and appear completely normal (Dawson, 1929). A second *Blepharisma* may sometimes be engulfed while the first is still swimming actively in a food vacuole; and as many as six red vacuoles have been observed in a cannibal (Giese, 1938; Nilsson, 1967).

Digestion of the ingested prey often begins rapidly. In a *B. ameri-*

---

* Ibara described his culture as *B. undulans;* but from his camera lucida sketches of the macronucleus it appears to be *B. japonicum.*

canum cannibal the prey ceases swimming in about an hour and becomes opaque. Digestion is usually complete within a day, and cannibals fed in the morning will eliminate the indigestible residue, including the concentrated red pigment of the engulfed blepharismas, by nightfall. In some strains, however, digestion appears to be much slower, taking more than a day; in these cases the prey will swim within the food vacuole for many hours (Dawson, 1929).

Tests were made with dyes specific to DNA and RNA during the digestion of a *Blepharisma* by a cannibal giant. During the first three hours the macronucleus of the prey and all DNA present disappear from the food vacuole; during the last six hours the RNA also disappears. Presumably, the digested nucleic acids are absorbed by the cannibal (Tulchin and Hirshfield, 1962).

As long as the appropriate food is available, cannibal giants continue to divide and form other giants, which also ingest the smaller blepharismas; and eventually a culture may consist almost entirely of giants. When starved, the giants dwindle in size slowly, and will not divide unless they are placed in a fresh, bacterized nutrient medium.

Morphology and Behavior of Cannibal Giants

The enormous increase of mass in *Blepharisma* cannibals has been noted by all who have observed them (Fig. 5.2). The three-dimensional increase in bulk is even more striking than the enlargement evident in a two-dimensional figure. Measurements show that the giants are proportionately enlarged in all organelles (Giese, 1938). Thus the membranellar band and undulating membrane are greatly increased (Bhandary and Hirshfield, 1964). The number of kineties increases from 60 to 100 in cannibal giants of *B. japonicum* (Nilsson, 1967), in part owing to the larger number of kineties in the V-zone; counts of kineties have not been made on other species.

The number of micronuclei in *B. japonicum* cannibals was found to be 21 ± 3, which is essentially the number (21 ± 5) found in bacteria-fed cells (Nilsson, 1967). In *B. americanum*, however, the depth of Feulgen staining suggests that the micronucleus becomes polyploid in cannibal giants (Hirshfield and Pecora, 1955). It would be interesting to make chromosome counts on the dividing micronuclei of a cannibal giant, but this has not been done for any species.

The cannibal giants of *B. japonicum* sometimes develop two macro-

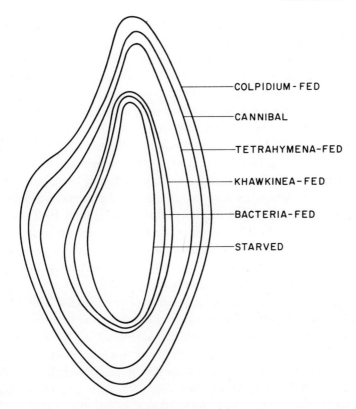

COLPIDIUM-FED

CANNIBAL

TETRAHYMENA-FED

KHAWKINEA-FED

BACTERIA-FED

STARVED

Fig. 5.2. Relative sizes of *B. americanum* cells starved or fed on various diets. From camera lucida sketches (Giese, unpublished).

nuclei instead of the usual single filament, and their macronuclear behavior is abnormal in several other respects. The macronucleus may be fragmented at right angles to its long axis into two or more pieces; rarely, it may become Y-shaped (Nilsson, 1967). In *B. americanum* giants the nodes of the beaded macronucleus increase in size (Giese, 1938; Bhandary and Hirshfield, 1964). In *B. musculus* v. wardsi, also a multinodal strain, the macronuclear nodes increase in size and number, appear to lose their connecting strands, and move closer to one another. Sometimes several macronuclear strands appear. Large Feulgen-negative bodies that accept RNA-specific stains appear in the nodes, and evidence indicates that there is a copious synthesis of protein in these bodies, much as there is in nucleoli. Moreover, these structures persist in the macronuclei of the giants' small-sized progeny after the resumption of bacterial feeding (Bhandary and Hirshfield, 1964).

Not all cannibal giants show macronuclear aberrations; and conversely, aberrations are sometimes found in healthy, noncannibal blepharismas. The number of macronuclear aberrations in the cannibal giants of *B. japonicum* (African strain) increases proportionally with the increasing size of the cells, being about 10% for those approximately 275 μm long and almost 60% for those 450 μm long (Nilsson, 1967). The giants produced by feeding blepharismas with other protozoans also showed macronuclear aberrations (Hirshfield, Chunosoff, and Bhandary, 1963). Although a correlation between cannibalism and aberrant macronuclei was suggested in one study (Tulchin and Hirshfield, 1960, 1962), it does not seem probable. In this respect it would be of interest to study the macronuclei of noncannibal giant *Blepharisma* fed on other protozoans; the aberrant macronuclei are perhaps a result of mechanical factors inherent in giantism, and not of cannibalism as such.

Cannibal giants divide at about the rate of bacteria-fed cells (Table 5.2). Since the volume of protoplasm formed per unit time is much larger in cannibals than in normal *Blepharisma*, the diet is evidently effective. However, *Blepharisma* protoplasm is not necessarily the most assimilable for *B. americanum*: the largest giants obtained were noncannibal giants fed *Colpidium* (see Fig. 5.2). Although the division-rate data for these giants were not obtained in isolation cultures, they indicate that the rate of division was about the same as that of bacteria-fed cells (Giese, 1938).

TABLE 5.2

Division Rate of *B. americanum* on Different Diets

Accustomed diet	Experimental diet	Average divisions per day[a]
Ps. ovalis	bacteria	1.40
Tetrahymena	*Tetrahymena*	1.34
Cannibal	*Blepharisma*	1.40
Tetrahymena	starved	1.58
Cannibal	starved	1.95
Tetrahymena	bacteria	2.44
Cannibal	bacteria	2.47

[a] Considerable variability in division rate was obtained, especially with cannibal giants. Data from Giese, 1938.

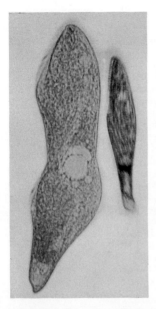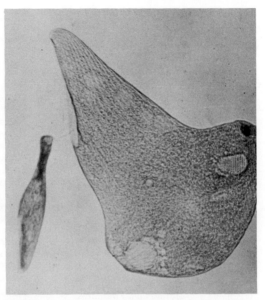

Fig. 5.3. *Left*: normal division of a cannibal giant (*B. americanum*); the smaller specimen is a bacteria-fed cell of the same species, somewhat compressed by starvation. *Right*: an abnormal monster cell (resulting from the failure of normal division in a cannibal giant), compared to a bacteria-fed cell. By courtesy *Journal of the American Microscopical Society*.

Not all cannibal giants of *B. americanum* divide normally. At times L- or T-shaped monsters are formed, as though the oversize food vacuoles have deranged the division line (Fig. 5.3). These usually reorganize themselves after a time and divide to form normal cells.

Blepharisma cannibal giants are definitely an unstable state of the species. Kept in an old culture medium they usually remain large, shrinking only gradually when starved. However, when placed in fresh culture medium with bacteria or in balanced salt solutions without food, they undergo a series of divisions, each giant producing 4–11 offspring of normal size. This would appear to be a natural regulation back to normal size (Giese, 1938).

Conclusions

Cannibalism is widespread among the Protozoa, and giantism following cannibalism is also not restricted to *Blepharisma* (Table 5.3). For

TABLE 5.3
Observed Cases of Cannibalism in Protozoa

Class	Genus/Species	Sources
Ciliata	*Oxytricha* sp.	Haime, 1853
	Oxytricha hymenostoma	Dawson, 1919
	Onychodromus grandis	Maupas, 1888
	Fabrea salina	Henneguy, 1890
	Balantidium coli	Hegner et al., 1924
	Pleurotricha lanceolata	Joukowsky, 1898; Penn, 1934
	Blepharisma undulans[a]	Penard, 1922
	Stentor coeruleus	Johnson, 1893; Gelei, 1925; Tartar, 1961
	Stentor roeseli	Gales, 1925
	Tintinnidium	Hofeneder, 1930
	Gastrostyla steini	Meyer, 1930
	Lembadion magnum	Kahl, 1930–31
	Stylonychia curvata	Giese and Alden, 1938
	Bursaria truncatella	Giese, 1937
	Woodruffia metabolica	Johnson, 1937
	Holosticha flavorolina	Schaeffer, 1937
Flagellata	*Actinomonas mirabilis*	Griessmann, 1913
	Ochromonas granularis	Doflein, 1921
	Gymnodium heterostriatum	Kofoid and Swezy, 1921
	Trichonympha campanula	Cleveland, 1925
Rhizopoda	*Trichosphaerium siebaldi*	Schaudinn, 1899
	Amoeba (*proteus?*)	Jennings, 1915
	Valkampfia magnum	Oehler, 1916
	Chlamydophrys, all sp., esp. *C. schaudini*	Belař, 1921
	Amoeba vespertilio	Lapage, 1922
	Hartmanella aquarum	Oehler, 1924
	Amoeba terricola	Mattes, 1924; Ivanič, 1927
	Amoeba sphaeronucleola	Mattes, 1924; Ivanič, 1927
	Amoeba verrucosa	Ivanič, 1927
	Entamoeba histolytica	Cleveland and Sanders, 1930

SOURCE: Summarized mostly from Sandon, 1932; citations to the original papers may be obtained from Sandon.
[a] Subsequent studies on cannibalism in *Blepharisma* are cited in the text.

example, cannibal giants have been observed in *Stylonychia* (Giese and Alden, 1938) and *Amoeba* (Lapage, 1922; Ivanič, 1927). On the other hand, cannibalism is not always accompanied by giantism. Thus in *Stentor coeruleus* a cannibal may remain the same size as its prey (Tartar, 1961).

The engulfing of some cells by others during development in the laboratory has also been seen in many invertebrates. For example, the phagocytic nutritive cells in the gonads of sea urchins engulf relict sperm or eggs and store the nutrients for another reproductive cycle. Again, in some invertebrates one egg grows at the expense of other eggs (Giese and Pearse, in press). Perhaps these events are somehow related to cannibalism in protozoans.

Cannibalism indicates that to a primitive organism with relatively nonselective feeding habits any other organism with which it collides is "food" if it can be engulfed, whether or not it is of the same species. Although the literature abounds with statements that cannibalism may be racial (genetic), or simply habitual, in some species of protozoans, there is really no proof for these contentions in *Blepharisma*.

Cannibalism appears to be just one aspect of feeding, but it may be a useful aspect. Routine surveys of stocks of *Blepharisma* grown as described in Chapter 4 have shown that in those cultures in which cannibals were recorded about three weeks after subculture a small number of healthy, pink blepharismas of about normal size were always to be found a month later. Conversely, cultures in which cannibals did not develop contained numerous, minute, starving cells three weeks after subculture, and only sickly minute ones after another month, if any were present at all. Cannibalism therefore appears to serve a useful purpose, maintaining the few at the expense of the many. This lends support to what has been called the "lifeboat theory" of cannibalism.

A question arises here. Is cannibalism in *Blepharisma* a phenomenon occurring in nature, or is it only a laboratory curiosity? It might be argued that a natural population would rarely contain enough blepharismas in one place to produce cannibals. However, cannibalizing ciliates of even the species with large populations have yet to be collected in nature, and the question thus remains open.

LITERATURE CITED

Bhandary, A. V., and H. I. Hirshfield. 1964. Comparative studies of RNA synthesis in two strains of cannibal giant *Blepharisma*. J. Cell. Comp. Physiol. **63**: 217–24.

Buhse, H. E., Jr. 1967. Microstome-macrostome transformation in *Tetrahymena vorax* strain V_2 type S induced by a transforming principle, stomatin. J. Protozool. **14**: 608–13.

Dawson, J. A. 1929. Cannibalism in a ciliate, *Blepharisma*. Proc. Soc. Exp. Biol. and Med. **26**: 335.

Giese, A. C. 1938. Cannibalism and gigantism in *Blepharisma*. Trans. Amer. Microsc. Soc. **57**: 245–55.

Giese, A. C., and R. H. Alden. 1938. Cannibalism and giant formation in *Stylonychia*. J. Exp. Zool. **78**: 117–34.

Giese, A. C., and J. S. Pearse. In press. Introduction: General principles. *In* Reproduction of marine invertebrates (Giese and Pearse, eds.). 7 vols. New York.

Haime, J. 1853. Observations sur les métamorphoses et sur l'organisation de la *Trichoda lynceus*. Ann. Sci. Nat. Zool. **19**: 109–34.

Hirshfield, H. I., and P. Pecora. 1955. Reconstitutive events in *Blepharisma undulans* as affected by colchicine. Exp. Cell Res. **9**: 414–27.

Hirshfield, H. I., L. Chunosoff, and A. V. Bhandary. 1963. Macronuclear variability of *Blepharisma* associated with growth. *In* Cell growth and cell division (Symp. Int. Soc. Cell Biology, R. J. C. Harris, ed.), II, 27–56. New York.

Ibara, Y. 1939. An observation on *Blepharisma undulans* with special reference to cannibalism and giantism. Annot. Zool. Jap. **18**: 21–28.

Ivanič, M. 1927. Über den Kannibalismus bei *Amoeba verrucosa* (Ehrbg.) nebst: Bemerkungen über den Kannibalismus bei Protozoan im allgemeinen. Zool. Anz. **74**: 313–21.

Lapage, G. 1922. Cannibalism in *Amoeba vespertilia* (Penard). Quart. J. Micr. Sci. **66**: 669–701

Nilsson, J. R. 1967. An African strain of *Blepharisma japonicum* (Suzuki): A study of the morphology, giantism and cannibalism, and macronuclear aberration. Compt. Rend. Trav. Lab. Carlsberg **36**: 1–24.

Padmavathi, P. B. 1961. Giant cannibals in *Blepharisma undulans* (Protozoa: Ciliata). Arch. Protistenk. **105**: 341–44.

Penard, E. 1922. Etudes sur les Infusoires d'eau douce. Geneva, 331 pp.

Sandon, H. 1932. The food of Protozoa. Cairo, 187 pp.

Steinberg, P. 1959. The cause of giantism and cannibalism in *Blepharisma undulans*. Biol. Rev., City College of New York **21**: 4–10.

Tartar, V. 1961. The biology of *Stentor*. New York, 413 pp.

Tulchin, N., and H. I. Hirshfield. 1960. Studies of cannibal giant *Blepharisma*. Biol. Bull. **19**: 345 (Abstr.).

——— 1962. Nucleic acid digestion and macronuclear form in cannibal *Blepharisma*, N.Y.U. strain. J. Protozool. **9**: 200–203.

CHAPTER SIX

Surface Properties and Salt Relations

The surface of *Blepharisma*, like that of any ciliate, differs from that of an amoeba. The surface of amoeboid cells is naked except for a coating of mucilaginous polysaccharides; but the surface of ciliates is bounded by a stiff, elastic, proteinaceous pellicle, which gives the organisms their characteristic shapes. Also, no ciliate has yet shown signs of the pinocytosis found in amoeboid cells, although it may possibly occur on the freshly cut surface of a ciliate, through which some enzymes (e.g. RNAase) appear to pass (Giese and McCaw, 1963).

The presence of a pellicle in *Blepharisma* does not prevent its moving through very small interstices in culture medium or pond muck. In fact, blepharismas are able to perform some remarkable contortions in squeezing through narrow cracks and passages. When free of unequal pressure, however, a cell will maintain its shape. The ectoplasm of the cell body itself probably lends additional support to the pellicle; only the endoplasm in the more rounded posterior of the cell is truly fluid, and food vacuoles circulate freely within it. The elasticity of the pellicle is evident during *Blepharisma*'s changes of shape under various conditions—slender when starved, pyriform when well fed, flattened almost to the shape of a leaf when put in hypertonic media, and bloated to a teardrop when transferred from a solution of higher osmolality to one of lower osmolality. During encystment the cells are able to double themselves up completely just before the thin cyst wall forms.

It has been shown that the surface rigidity of *Blepharisma* may be affected by a number of conditions: hydrostatic pressure, enzyme action, the extrusion of protein and pigment, sound waves, far UV radiation, and changes in osmotic pressure. Each of these factors will change the surface properties of the cell.

Changes in Shape Under Hydrostatic Pressure

The application of hydrostatic pressure, up to 6,000 pounds per square inch (psi), has little effect on the shape of *Blepharisma*. Since pressure of this magnitude generally causes a solation of protein and protoplasm, as measured by decreased viscosity (Marsland, 1958), it appears that the surface of *Blepharisma* can maintain its structure remarkably well. Higher pressures induce a characteristic shortening of the cell, the first stage of breakdown in the surface structure. The pressure at which this occurs varies with the temperature: 8,000 psi at 12° C, 8,700 at 15°, 9,200 at 20°, and 9,300 at 25°. Thus higher temperatures can counteract the effect of pressure to some extent (Auclair and Marsland, 1958). But pressures above 9,300 psi invariably cause cytolysis, that is, a rupturing of the cell surface and an extrusion of protoplasm. The actual rate of cytolysis depends on the pressure applied: at 15,000 psi (over 1,000 atmospheres) the process is rapid, and every cell in a culture cytolyzes within five minutes; at 12,000 psi complete cytolysis takes over 20 minutes. (Figs. 6.1 and 6.2.)

Interestingly, the postperistomal fragments of transected blepharismas cytolyze about as rapidly as whole cells at a given pressure, even though one might expect the cell surface at the cut end to be weakened. Perhaps cytolysis depends not only on the structure of the pellicle at the surface but also on the structure of the cell's ectoplasm (Giese, 1968b). However, we do not know how rapidly a new pellicle develops on the cut surface, and the 15 minutes that commonly elapse in the laboratory between cutting and the application of pressure may suffice.

If the cells are irradiated with UV, much lower pressures will induce cytolysis. After irradiation with 6,000 ergs/mm² at wavelengths of 230, 265, and 280 nm, the pressures required to cytolyze 50% of the blepharismas were 5,000, 6,500, and 7,000 psi, respectively. Wavelengths less readily absorbed by protoplasm (254 or 302 nm) had no noticeable effect (Hirshfield et al., 1957). Tschakotine (1936) found that microbeam irradiation of *Blepharisma* at 280 nm caused first a contraction

Fig. 6.1 (*above*). Equipment for applying hydrostatic pressure. The pump, constructed from a truck jack, applies pressure to the bomb chamber. The effect on cells in a culture tube within the bomb may be observed through a microscope.

Fig. 6.2 (*below*). The cytolysis of *B. japonicum* v. intermedium at various pressures (temperature 25° C).

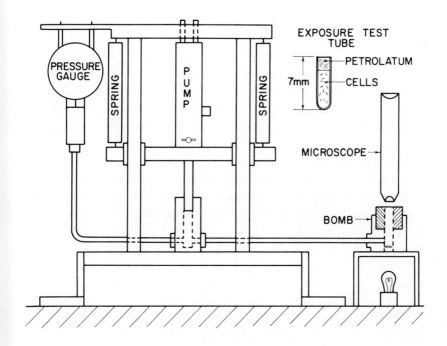

EXPOSURE TEST
TUBE

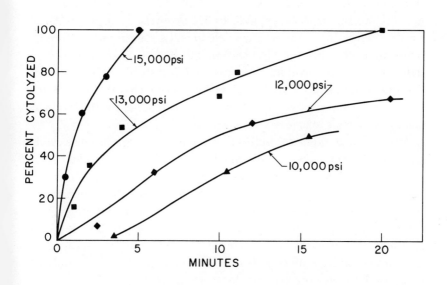

and then a bulge at the target spot, indicating a weakening of the injured surface.

The surface of a cell treated with proteases is also cytolyzed by lower hydrostatic pressures. For example, whereas 50% of an untreated control group cytolyze at 9,000 psi, a group treated with a very dilute solution of trypsin or chymotrypsin will cytolyze to the same extent at 7,000 psi. Presumably, some protein is present at the surface of *Blepharisma*, and its removal by the enzyme weakens the surface structure and leads to quicker cytolysis when pressure is applied. Neither α nor β amylase had any action alone, even at relatively high concentrations; but after a preliminary treatment with protease, α amylase lowered the pressure required for cytolysis. This suggests the presence of carbohydrates. Finally, β-hyalyuronidase had the same effect as protease in reducing resistance to pressure, indicating that mucopolysaccharides are also present. This has been confirmed by recent work with dyes (Nilsson, unpublished); and it is not too surprising, since mucopolysaccharides are known to occur at the surface of many cells.

When the surface of a *Blepharisma* is treated with a strychnine sulfate solution (Nadler, 1929), the cell extrudes a capsule consisting of protein and pigment (see Chapter 7). In this case, too, the surface of the cell is weakened, and to the same extent as after protease treatment; again, a pressure of 7,000 psi induces 52% cytolysis, as against 9,000 psi for the control. It has not been possible to find a concentration of strychnine sulfate that measurably weakens the surface of the cell without inducing capsule shedding (Asterita and Marsland, 1961). And the capsule shedding itself probably removes so much structural protein from the cell surface that any other effect of treatment with strychnine sulfate is difficult to assess.

Although high pressure applied for a minute or more will cause cytolysis in blepharismas, an exposure of a few seconds has no residual effect, and neither the rate of regeneration nor the rate of division is altered. Presumably, the bonds weakened by high pressure of brief duration reform normally on its release. However, the same bonds cannot reform after prolonged pressure, and cytolysis results (Giese, 1968b). It is clear that any kind of injury to the integrity and structural strength of the cell surface, perhaps affecting both pellicle and ectoplasm, causes *Blepharisma* to become more susceptible to pressure.

Effect of Sound Waves

Intense sonic waves passed through a fluid induce the formation of gas bubbles, which can cause mechanical damage in any living cells present in the fluid (Smith, 1935). Sonication, as this treatment is called, is now a routine laboratory method for disrupting cells before the cell components are fractionated by centrifuge. When sonication is applied to a suspension of cells, an anomalously greater effect is observed at what are considered the resonance frequencies of the cell structure. Each species of protozoan appears to have its own frequency, and the frequency of a particular *Blepharisma* will differ from that of all other ciliates.

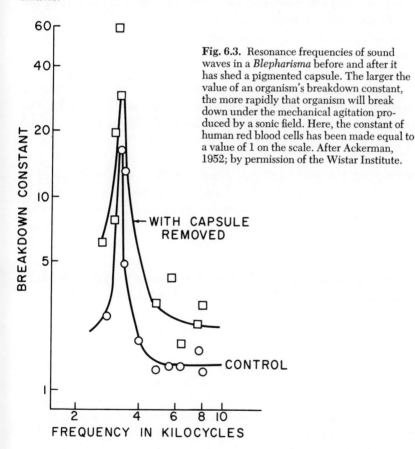

Fig. 6.3. Resonance frequencies of sound waves in a *Blepharisma* before and after it has shed a pigmented capsule. The larger the value of an organism's breakdown constant, the more rapidly that organism will break down under the mechanical agitation produced by a sonic field. Here, the constant of human red blood cells has been made equal to a value of 1 on the scale. After Ackerman, 1952; by permission of the Wistar Institute.

Blepharisma offers an especially good opportunity to test whether resonance frequency and cell fragility change when a cell surface is altered. When a capsule is removed from *B. undulans* by strychnine sulfate, the resonance frequency is the same as before removal. This may mean that the resonance effect depends on the entire cell cortex, which is not markedly affected by the removal of the capsule (Fig. 6.3). But after capsule shedding the mechanical strength of the cell surface is reduced to half its previous value, and only half the amount of energy is needed to disrupt the cell by sonication—a quantitative verification of Nadler's qualitative observation that cells with pigmented capsules removed are much more fragile and difficult to handle (Ackerman, 1952).

Regulation of potassium and sodium in the cell. A major part of the osmotically active material in any cell is electrolyte, and it can be quantified by testing the cell's conductivity with microelectrodes. The electrolyte content of *Blepharisma*, so determined, is 0.04 N, which is similar to that of a variety of ciliates (Table 6.1) but much higher than that of *Amoeba proteus* and very much less than that of a marine cell like the oocyte of the sea star *Pisaster ochraceus* (Gelfan, 1927, 1928). The osmolality of the KCl solution in which the osmotic pressure is expressed in Table 6.1 is approximately twice the molality.

The two major cations in *Blepharisma* are K^+ and Na^+, with K^+ predominating. The changes in concentration of these cations in the cell as external concentrations change are a measure of the capacity of the cell surface to regulate the ionic composition of the cell. The potassium concentration inside cells is higher than the sodium concentration, whereas in axenic media and balanced salt solutions the sodium concentration is much higher than potassium (Table 6.2); both ions are easily measured by flame photometry. The ratio of potassium to sodium in *Blepharisma* is comparable to that in most cells (Hilden, 1970).

When *Blepharisma* is grown in media containing more than 47 milliosmolar (mM) balanced salt, some of the cells continue swimming while others become nonmotile and fall to the bottom of the culture. The proportion of nonmotile cells increases as the osmolality of the culture medium increases (Hilden, 1970). Motile and immotile cells respond differently to increased salt concentrations. When the balanced salt concentration in the suspending medium is increased, the sodium inside motile cells begins to increase at a lower level of external concentration than does that in nonmotile cells (Fig. 6.4). Since sodium is

TABLE 6.1

Electrolyte Content of Various Cells, Determined by Conductivity

Organism	Normality (KCl equivalent)	Specific conductance in mho/cm^2 (all $\times$ 10^{-3})
Amoeba proteus	0.01	1.225
Euplotes sp.	0.035	4.1
Spirostomum teres	0.0385	4.4
Blepharisma sp.	0.04	4.7
Oxytricha sp.	0.05	5.8
Frontonia sp.	0.053	6.1
Paramecium sp.	0.06	6.9
Nitella protoplasm	0.04	4.7
Nitella central sap vacuole	0.07	7.9
Pisaster ochraceus oocyte[a]	0.25	26.2

SOURCE: Gelfan, 1928.

[a] This is a seastar egg that normally exists in the electrolyte concentration of seawater. Other cells are freshwater organisms.

TABLE 6.2

Sodium and Potassium Levels in *Blepharisma* When the Salt Concentration of the Medium Is Varied

Salt varied	Concentration (mM/liter)[a]	μM per gram of cellular protein	
		Sodium ions	Potassium ions
NaCl	17.8	39 $\pm$ 18	292 $\pm$ 30
	35.6	65 $\pm$ 27	346 $\pm$ 72
	71.2	242 $\pm$ 67	242 $\pm$ 67
KCl	3.1	42 $\pm$ 19	336 $\pm$ 81
	6.2	51 $\pm$ 20	298 $\pm$ 72
	12.4	61 $\pm$ 6	366 $\pm$ 27
CaCl$_2$	0.068	47 $\pm$ 24	354 $\pm$ 60
	0.136	44 $\pm$ 10	328 $\pm$ 30
	0.272	28 $\pm$ 10	330 $\pm$ 30
MgCl$_2$	0.42	47 $\pm$ 24	354 $\pm$ 60
	0.84	50 $\pm$ 24	362 $\pm$ 36
	1.68	55 $\pm$ 28	351 $\pm$ 28
MgSO$_4$	0.16	47 $\pm$ 24	354 $\pm$ 60
	0.32	70 $\pm$ 25	370 $\pm$ 24
	0.64	56 $\pm$ 10	341 $\pm$ 43
Sucrose	0.0	59 $\pm$ 15	315 $\pm$ 10
	28.0	82 $\pm$ 44	306 $\pm$ 14
	56.0	91 $\pm$ 51	382 $\pm$ 111

SOURCE: Hilden, 1970.

[a] In each case, the concentration of salts other than the one listed is the same as in a solution of 10 $\times$ UO: that is, 17.8 mM NaCl, 3.1 mM KCl, 0.068 mM CaCl$_2$, 0.42 mM MgCl$_2$, and 0.16 mM MgSO$_4$. All figures are for motile cells. With NaCl at 71.2 mM/liter and other salts at 10 $\times$ UO, the concentrations in immotile cells are: sodium ions, 110 $\pm$ 5 μM; potassium ions, 266 $\pm$ 11 μM. (UO, unit osmolality, is defined on p. 106.)

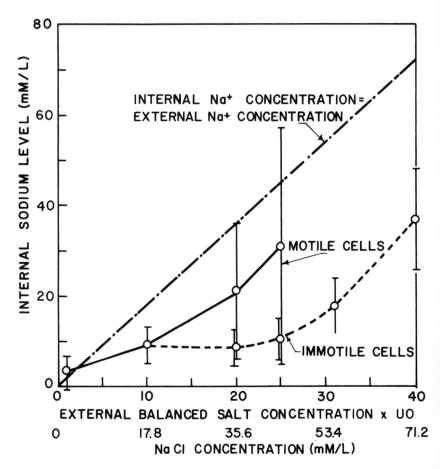

Fig. 6.4. Internal sodium levels in motile and immotile *B. japonicum* v. intermedium at various external balanced salt concentrations. The lines through points are standard deviations. After Hilden, 1969.

probably entering the cell continuously, it is now thought that *Blepharisma* possesses a "sodium pump" to extrude any excess. This regulation fails when the external sodium concentration is above 44 mM for non-motile cells, and at a much lower level in motile cells. Possibly, motile cells are not able to expend the same effort on sodium regulation. The internal potassium level of both motile and nonmotile cells does not change much over the entire range of external concentration levels tested (Fig. 6.5); however, the probable errors for these determinations are large.

When the concentration of each salt in the suspension medium is varied separately, the internal potassium concentration is maintained even when the external NaCl, KCl, $CaCl_2$, $MgCl_2$, or $MgSO_4$ concentration is increased fourfold over that in a 10 × UO solution. The sodium concentration is also maintained, except in two instances: when the ex-

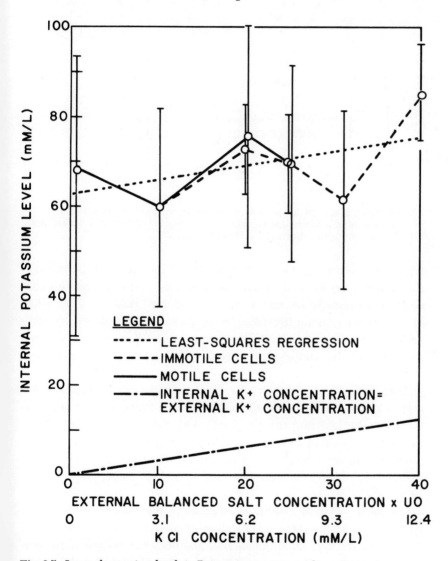

Fig. 6.5. Internal potassium levels in *B. japonicum* v. intermedium at various external salt concentrations. After Hilden, 1969.

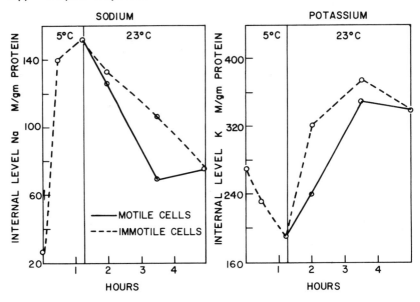

Fig. 6.6. Internal sodium and potassium levels in B. *japonicum* v. intermedium when cells suspended in a balanced medium are placed at 5° C for one hour and then returned to room temperature (23°). After Hilden, 1969.

ternal sodium reaches a value 40 times that found in unit balanced salt, the sodium level inside the cells rises markedly; and even half this concentration causes a 33% rise in internal sodium (Hilden, 1970). Thus in spite of the osmotic stress exerted on its surface membrane by these variations in external salt, *Blepharisma* is able to regulate its internal sodium and potassium levels remarkably well—at least as effectively as most other protozoans.

That the regulation of internal sodium and potassium levels in *Blepharisma* is dependent on metabolically coupled transport functions can be shown by lowering the temperature to reduce metabolism. When the cells are chilled to 5° C, the internal sodium level rises and the internal potassium level falls. Conversely, when the chilled cells are warmed up to 23°, sodium is extruded and potassium accumulates (Fig. 6.6).

Chemical metabolic inhibitors also affect the ionic composition of *Blepharisma*. In the presence of sodium cyanide, which reduces aerobic respiration, the internal sodium almost doubles while potassium remains about the same. In the presence of sodium fluoride, which reduces glycolysis, the sodium level rises by over 50% and the potassium by about 20%. The most striking effect is that of ouabain, which selectively affects the cell's sodium pump: in a 10^{-5} M ouabain solution the internal sodium doubles and the internal potassium rises by about 20%. Some inconsistencies have been found in the action of other metabolic inhibitors (see Hilden, 1969, 1970). However, the positive results obtained support the idea that the movement of sodium and potassium through the surface membranes of *Blepharisma* occurs by active transport. It is possible that potassium may be accumulated by a potassium pump coupled to the sodium pump, as happens in some other cells (see Giese, 1968a), but no convincing evidence for this has appeared in experiments with *Blepharisma.*

Osmotic Effect of Electrolytes and Nonelectrolytes

If charges on the ions in a solution have no effect on osmotic activity and the cell surface, nonelectrolytes and electrolytes at the same osmotic pressure should have the same effect. For *Blepharisma* this can be tested by using a balanced salt medium (in multiples of UO) as the electrolyte and sucrose as the nonelectrolyte. The regeneration of postperistomal cell fragments is a good measure of the effects induced by different solutions because the experiments can be completed within a few hours, require only small numbers of cells, are easily observed, and can be terminated at a relatively objective point in time—namely, the first ingestion of bacteria by the regenerated mouth (see Chapter 9), an act signaled by the appearance of food vacuoles.

The balanced salt concentration in a $1 \times$ UO medium can be increased twelvefold (to 5.2×10^{-2} osmolal) without affecting the cells' rate of regeneration (Fig. 6.7). However, regeneration is delayed when the salt concentration is $16 \times$ UO, and markedly so at $20 \times$ UO (6.9×10^{-2} osmolal). Since ionic balance is maintained and only the total salt concentration has been increased, the delay of regeneration appears to be due to osmotic change. Using sucrose, a concentration of 5.6×10^{-2} osmolal has no effect, but 6.7×10^{-2} osmolal or more decidedly retards regeneration (Fig. 6.8). Regeneration, it seems, is retarded to about the same degree by the osmotic effects of both electrolytes and nonelectrolytes (Giese et al., 1965). Similar results have been obtained for two other stocks of *Blepharisma* tested: *B. americanum* and *B. japonicum* (African strain).

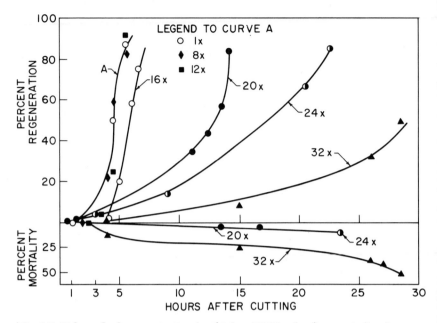

Fig. 6.7. Balanced salt concentration (multiples of UO) related to survival and regeneration rate in *B. japonicum* v. intermedium. After Giese et al., 1965.

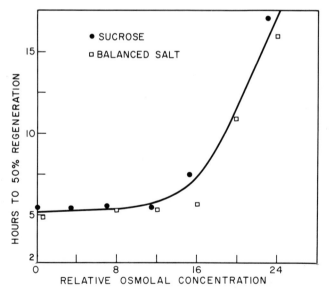

Fig. 6.8. The relation between concentrations (in UO) of balanced salt or sucrose solutions and regeneration in *B. japonicum* v. intermedium.

The Effect of Individual Ions on Surface Properties

Some experiments have been performed to see how *Blepharisma* responds when only a single kind of electrolyte is active at its surface—in other words, when the suspending solution is unbalanced. Regeneration of postperistomal fragments is again used as the criterion. Regeneration is as fast at unit osmolality (UO) in NaCl alone as in a balanced salt solution, but it is much slower at 8 × UO NaCl than at 8 × UO of balanced salts (Fig. 6.9).

Sodium chloride at a concentration of 16 × UO kills most of the cells; the addition of calcium chloride counteracts this fairly effectively, but regeneration is still retarded. The addition of magnesium salts also counteracts the killing action of sodium, though less effectively. Surprisingly, potassium chloride at 1 × UO is not very toxic to *Blepharisma* (Fig. 6.10), even though an 8 × UO concentration kills most of the cells. Again, the lethal action can be counteracted by adding calcium chloride. Unit concentrations of calcium or magnesium salts in the medium do not retard regeneration; but at higher osmolalities regeneration is retarded significantly, and part of the population is killed by osmotic pressure (Giese et al., 1965).

Calcium and the Integrity of the Cell Surface

Calcium ions have long been recognized as necessary for maintaining the normal permeability of cell membranes. Although the common statement that calcium tightens the pores of the cell membrane and lowers its permeability to water and other molecules is an oversimplification, the removal of calcium from the environment does alter the permeability markedly (Finean, 1966). It is of interest, therefore, to consider the effect of varying quantities of calcium on the surface properties of *Blepharisma*.

The effects of ethylene diamine tetraacetic acid (EDTA), a chelating agent that binds calcium, would be of great interest in studying permeability, but it has not been tested. However, it has been found (Prabhakara Rao, 1963) that EDTA will induce the shedding of pigment (about 34%) and protein, much as NaCl does, and that this effect is negated by the addition of $CaCl_2$. Similarly, the shedding of pigment and protein induced by sodium chloride, ammonium oxalate, or sodium tungstate can be annulled by appropriate amounts of $CaCl_2$. It is now believed

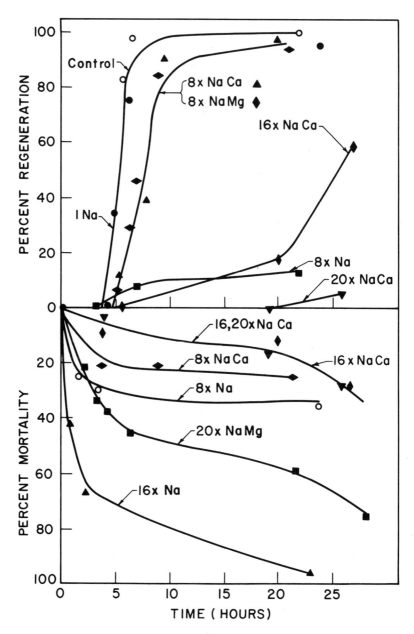

Fig. 6.9. The effects of NaCl and mixed ionic solutions of varying UO on regeneration in *B. japonicum* v. intermedium. From Giese et al., 1965; by permission of the Academic Press.

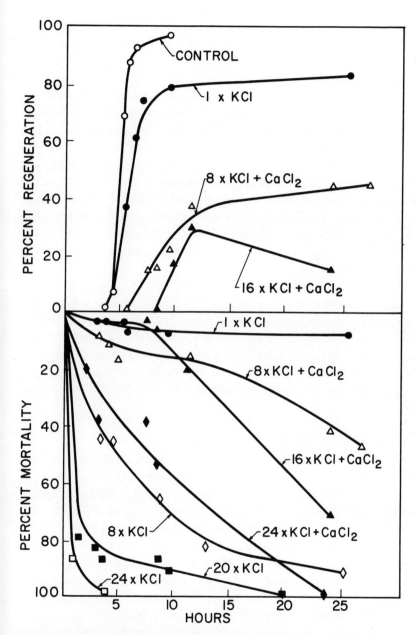

Fig. 6.10. Effects of KCl and mixed ionic solutions of varying UO on regeneration in *B. japonicum* v. intermedium. From Giese et al., 1965; by permission of the Academic Press.

that sodium salts induce the shedding of pigment by replacing calcium ions in the cell surface with sodium, thereby removing calcium as effectively as EDTA does; but the addition of new calcium ions reverses the effect (Prabhakara Rao, 1963).

EDTA at 1 × UO has very little effect on the rate of regeneration of *B. japonicum* v. intermedium, although some of the cut pieces do not heal and eventually die. When the EDTA concentration is increased by half, 31% of the fragments die; when it is doubled to 2 × UO about half the fragments die, and the survivors are somewhat slow to regenerate. Thus it requires EDTA at about twice the osmolality of the calcium in the medium—i.e., twice the amount needed to chelate all the calcium in the medium—to affect *Blepharisma*'s viability and rate of regeneration. The extra EDTA probably chelates the calcium in the cell membranes, which would certainly upset the cells' stability (Giese et al., 1965).

The damaging effects of single-salt solutions (KCl, NaCl, etc.) used to suspend blepharismas, described earlier, might also be explained as the result of calcium loss in the membrane. It is interesting that magnesium ions, which sometimes simulate the general effects of calcium, will do so in this case by reversing the damaging effect of sodium chloride on regeneration (Giese et al., 1965) but will not prevent the pigment and protein extrusion stimulated by NaCl, as calcium will (Prabhakara Rao, 1963).

The Contractile Vacuole

The contractile vacuole was first seen in a protozoan (probably *Paramecium*) by Spallanzani in 1776, but its function was not understood for some time. It was at first considered by many to be a kind of heart, circulating fluid within the cell. In 1849 Schmidt suggested that the contractile vacuole might open to the outside (quoted from Moore, 1934); but he thought that fluid entered and left freely through the vacuolar pore, perhaps as a breathing process. Conclusive proof that the contractile vacuole was an organelle for voiding fluids came only when Jennings (1904) showed that the outward movement of fluid from a *Paramecium* could be stopped completely by placing a glass needle across the pore. The actual expulsion could be demonstrated by adding opaque dyes or particles, such as India ink, to the fluid surrounding the cell.

The contractile vacuoles in protozoans are of two kinds: those with canals emptying into them, as in *Paramecium*; and those formed by the coalescence of smaller vacuoles into a large, definitive vacuole that discharges the fluid, as in *Blepharisma* (Wrzesniowski, 1869). Stein made the first observation of contractile vacuoles in *Blepharisma* in 1849; and Moore (1934) reviewed both this work and the later observations of Maupas, Wrzesniowski, Stolte, and Haye, most of whom worked with *B. lateritium*. Moore herself went on to describe the formation of contractile vacuoles in *B. undulans* (possibly *B. americanum*). Her observations were made both on whole blepharismas and on regenerates from which the posterior tip had been removed by transection.

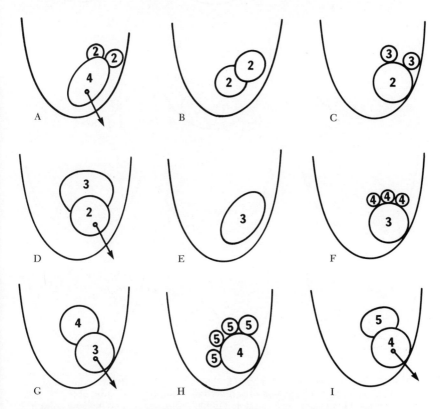

Fig. 6.11. Stages in the development of contractile vacuoles in *Blepharisma*. The vacuoles are numbered in the order of their appearance, and those appearing simultaneously have the same number. The arrows indicate systoles. From Moore, 1934; by permission of the Wistar Institute.

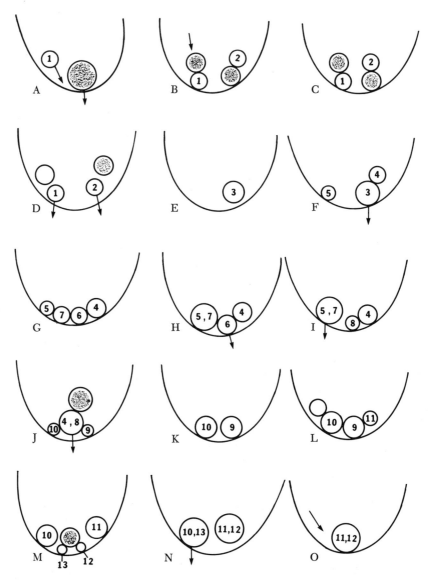

Fig. 6.12. Stages of vacuolar formation in the regenerating posterior fragment of a *Blepharisma*. The fluid vacuoles sometimes fail to empty in the order of their formation; and food vacuoles (containing indigestible matter) and fluid vacuoles may empty at different points. From Moore, 1934; by permission of the Wistar Institute.

These experiments indicated that the contractile vacuole is a temporary structure, formed within the granule-free and cilia-free posterior end of a *Blepharisma* but not necessarily appearing in exactly the same spot during successive evacuations (Fig. 6.11). Usually, two kinds of vacuoles are present: a primary vacuole formed by the coalescence of a number of smaller ones, and secondary vacuoles ("feeder vacuoles") that may be enlarging at the very time the primary one is undergoing systole. In addition, the cytopyge region (see Chapter 1) along the posterior border serves for both the discharge of the contractile vacuole and the evacuation of indigestible residue from the food vacuoles, which also form a composite vacuole; both are emptied by the contraction of the entire posterior end of the body. Sometimes, as in regenerating cells, there is competition between the two kinds of vacuole (Fig. 6.12), and the contractile vacuole may be temporarily deformed as a result.

Although the contractile vacuole was once claimed to be a derivative of the Golgi apparatus, Moore (1934) could find no similarity in the staining reactions of the two organelles. The temporary nature of the contractile vacuole also argues against such an origin. Contractile vacuoles can form only in regions of low viscosity. When a *Blepharisma* is transected at a level where the viscosity is high (as shown by a sluggish Brownian movement), the viscosity of the "new" posterior end is at first high. But it soon decreases, and only then do contractile vacuoles form. Just how the vacuoles form is not known. No excretion crystals have been observed in *Blepharisma* (Moore, 1934); and whether or not they have anything to do with vacuolar function even when present, as they do in other ciliates, is questionable.

No experiments have been performed on the concentration of osmotically active materials in the vacuolar fluid of *Blepharisma*. In *Amoeba proteus*, which has a vacuolar system much like that of *Blepharisma*, an osmolality of 3.2×10^{-2} was found for the vacuolar fluid, 1.01×10^{-1} for the protoplasm, and 8×10^{-3} for the medium (Schmidt-Nielsen and Schrauger, 1963). If one accepts the value for the protoplasm, these results suggest that active cellular transport is required to accumulate fluid in the vacuole. In this case, however, the method of measurement (vapor pressure of frozen or boiled amoebas) may have altered the osmolality of the protoplasm.

The vacuole of *Blepharisma* contracts rather slowly—from one-and-a-half contractions per minute to one contraction every three minutes

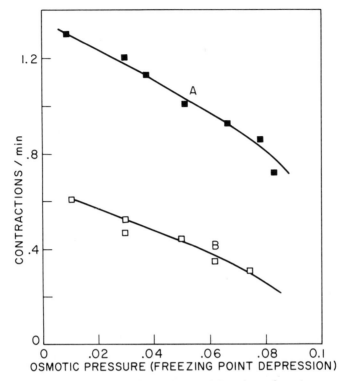

Fig. 6.13. The relation between the osmolality of a medium (measured by freezing-point depression) and the activity of *Blepharisma*'s contractile vacuole. The two curves represent trials on two different animals. Data from Zanyin Gaw, 1936.

(Fig. 6.13), depending on the temperature and osmolality of the surrounding medium (Zanyin Gaw, 1936). The primary vacuole appears to reach a constant size before each contraction. Inasmuch as Zanyin Gaw used a rather strange salt medium (potassium nitrate, potassium basic phosphate, magnesium sulfate, and ferric chloride), it would be interesting to reinvestigate the effects of osmolality on contraction rate in a medium more akin to that in which *Blepharisma* is normally found. Zanyin Gaw observed that none of his blepharismas (species not stated) survived exposure to a medium with a freezing point depression of 0.1° C or more (1.24 atmospheres osmotic pressure). In the balanced medium used in my own laboratory, *Blepharisma* will survive and grow at 3.9 atmospheres, and can withstand still higher pressures for a time.

The contractile vacuole of a *Blepharisma* acclimated to 30 or 40 × UO and then placed in distilled water is unable to cope with the influx of water, and the cell bursts within 15 minutes (see Chapter 4). But when blepharismas thus acclimated are placed in a balanced medium of unit osmolality, they swell but do not burst (Giese and Benedetti, 1971). Apparently, even the small amount of salt (1 × UO) in the culture medium is sufficient to prevent bursting, although some swelling occurs.

When the contractile vacuole is removed from a *Blepharisma* by transection, a new one must be reconstructed quickly if the cell is to remove the water continually entering through its surface membrane and food vacuoles. According to Suzuki (1957), a new contractile vacuole appears very soon after the wound closes (time not specified). This occurs in all kinds of fragments, regardless of size or constitution and of whether a macronucleus is present. Given the *de novo* origin of the vacuole in normal cells, this rapid regeneration is not surprising.

In dividing cells, a second contractile vacuole appears in the posterior end of the proter (anterior member) at an early stage, approximately 30 minutes after the first signs of the macronuclear elongation preparatory to division (Suzuki, 1957). The vacuole is therefore ready to function long before the proter and opisthe separate from one another.

LITERATURE CITED

Ackerman, E. 1952. Cellular fragilities and resonances observed by means of sonic vibrations. J. Cell. Comp. Physiol. 39: 167–90.

Asterita, H., and D. Marsland. 1961. The pellicle as a factor in the stabilization of cellular form and integrity: Effects of externally applied enzymes on resistance of *Blepharisma* and *Paramecium* to pressure-induced cytolysis. J. Cell. Comp. Physiol. 58: 49–62.

Auclair, W., and D. Marsland. 1958. Form-stability of ciliates in relation to pressure and temperature. Biol. Bull. 115: 384–96.

Dunham, P. B., and F. M. Child. 1960. Ion regulation in *Tetrahymena*. Biol. Bull. 121: 129–40.

Finean, J. B. 1966. The molecular organization of cell membranes. Progr. Biophys. 16: 143–70.

Gelfan, S. 1927. The electrical conductivity of protoplasm and a new method of its determination. Univ. Calif. Publ. Zool. 29: 453–56.

——— 1928. The electrical conductivity of protoplasm. Protoplasma 4: 193–200.

Giese, A. C. 1968a. Cell physiology. Philadelphia, 671 pp.

——— 1968b. The effect of hydrostatic pressure and heavy water upon regeneration in *Blepharisma*. Exp. Cell Res. 52: 370–78.

Giese, A. C., and T. Benedetti. 1971. Reacclimation to low salt levels of *Blepharisma* acclimated to high salt levels, as measured by rate of regeneration. Physiol. Zool. **44**: 1–8.

Giese, A. C., and B. K. McCaw. 1963. Effect of metabolic and other inhibitors on regeneration in *Blepharisma undulans*. Exp. Cell Res. **32**: 130–46.

Giese, A. C., S. G. Smith, and J. Berry Dau. 1965. Effect of osmotic pressure, ionic imbalance, and pH upon the regeneration rate in *Blepharisma*. Exp. Cell Res. **39**: 145–60.

Haye, A. 1930. Über den Exkretionsapparat bei den Protisten, nebst Bemerkungen über einige andere finere Strukturverhaltnisse der untersuchten Arten. Arch. Protistenk. **70**: 1–86.

Hilden, S. A. 1969. Sodium and potassium levels in *Blepharisma intermedium*. Ph.D. dissertation, Stanford University. 129 pp.

———— 1970. Sodium and potassium levels in *Blepharisma intermedium*. Exp. Cell Res. **61**: 241–54.

Hilden, S. A., and A. C. Giese. 1969. Effect of salt concentration on regeneration rate in *Blepharisma* acclimated to high salt levels. J. Protozool. **16**: 419–22.

Hirshfield, H. I., A. M. Zimmerman, J. V. Landau, and D. Marsland. 1957. Sensitivity of UV-irradiated *Blepharisma undulans* to high-pressure lysis. J. Cell. Comp. Physiol. **49**: 287–94.

Jennings, H. S. 1904. A method of demonstrating the external discharge of the contractile vacuole. Zool. Anz. **27**: 656–58.

Kitching, J. A. 1967. Contractile vacuoles, ionic regulation, and excretion. *In* Research in protozoology (T. T. Chen, ed.), I, 307–36. New York.

Marsland, D. A. 1958. Cells at high pressure. Sci. Am. **199** (Oct.): 36–43.

Moore, I. 1934. Morphology of the contractile vacuole and cloacal region of *Blepharisma undulans*. J. Exp. Zool. **69**: 59–104.

Nadler, J. E. 1929. Notes on the loss and regeneration of the pellicle of *Blepharisma undulans*. Biol. Bull. **56**: 327–30.

Prabhakara Rao, A. V. S. 1963. Extrusion of a protein pigment complex from *Blepharisma undulans*. J. Protozool. **10**: 204–7.

Schmidt-Nielsen, B., and C. R. Schrauger. 1963. *Amoeba proteus*: Studying the contractile vacuole by micropuncture. Science **139**: 606–7.

Smith, F. D. 1935. On the destructive mechanical effect of the gas bubbles liberated by the passage of intense sound through a liquid. Phil. Mag. Sci., Ser. 7, **19**: 1147.

Suzuki, S. 1957. Morphogenesis in the regeneration of *Blepharisma undulans japonicus* Suzuki. Bull. Yamagata Univ. Nat. Sci. **4**: 85–191.

Tschakotine, S. 1936. Quoted by T. Jahn and E. G. Bovee in Motile behavior in Protozoa. *In* Research in protozoology (T. T. Chen, ed.), I, 155.

Wrzesniowski, A. 1869. Ein Beitrage zur Anatomie der Infusorien. Arch. Mikr. Anat. **5**: 25–48.

Zanyin Gaw, H. 1936. Physiology of the contractile vacuole in ciliates. Arch. Protistenk. **87**: 185–93.

CHAPTER SEVEN

Capsule Shedding

In 1929 Nadler reported that salts of the alkaloids strychnine, morphine, codeine, cocaine, and novocaine could induce *Blepharisma* to shed a pigmented "capsule" shaped like itself. Considerable interest was immediately taken in this observation because it was thought that the cell's pellicle had been shed, leaving the cell's surface "open" and its interior more accessible to chemicals. However, electron microscopy has demonstrated that the pellicle, which gives *Blepharisma* and other ciliates their characteristic shapes, is not removed; the only thing shed is a capsule containing a fairly orderly array of pigment granules (Kennedy, 1966). The capsule consists of the granules themselves, the membranes surrounding the granules, and possibly some additional material (see Chapter 3).

Although capsule shedding is not as striking an event as the removal of the pellicle would be, it is interesting because nothing comparable has been seen in other cells, except in the related spirotrich *Stentor coeruleus*, whose pigment is akin to that of *Blepharisma* (see Chapter 11). In *S. coeruleus* various monovalent salts (for example) will induce the shedding of a capsule much like *Blepharisma*'s. Strychnine sulfate, on the other hand, only induces the shedding of fragments containing the pigment granules, and still other chemicals will bring forth only a halo of pigment. Other species of *Stentor* are not known to shed capsules or pigment at all (Tartar, 1957, 1961).

Events in Capsule Shedding

To induce capsule shedding, one immerses the *Blepharisma* in an effective solution (Table 7.1), for example, in 0.09% (0.00104 M) strychnine sulfate. Usually, the cell contracts rather violently; and a deeply pink capsule appears around it like a halo, retaining the shape of the

TABLE 7.1
Agents Tested as Causes of Capsule or Pigment Shedding

Effect	Effective agents	Ineffective agents	Source
Capsule or flakes formed	strychnine sulfate morphine sulfate codeine sulfate cocaine hydrochloride novocaine	caffeine citrate brucine apomorphine mercury succinate picrotoxin phenacetin quinine hydrochloride CCl_4, saponin, nicotine veronal veratrine	Nadler, 1929
	Janus green B	—	Weisz, 1950
	neutral red	—	Hirshfield, unpub.
	eserine salicylate puromycin	—	Giese, unpub.
Pigment and protein extruded	sodium chloride sodium sulfate potassium sulfate ammonium sulfate magnesium sulfate EDTA	potassium chloride ammonium chloride calcium chloride magnesium chloride sucrose glucose barium chloride	Prabhakara Rao, 1963
	choline chloride		Giese, unpub.
	exposure to 0° C	—	Giese and Grainger, 1970
Oxidized pigment and membranes extruded	prolonged exposure to dim light	—	Giese, 1938 Kennedy, 1966

Blepharisma but larger. After contracting for a while, the cell works its way out of the capsule, generally through the representations of the mouth opening and the cytopyge in the capsule (Figs. 7.1 and 7.2). After shedding, blepharismas are much lighter in color than controls but almost never colorless. Though more pyriform in shape than before, they swim in a normal manner, form vacuoles, and react to stimuli.

There is no further reaction to the strychnine sulfate in the solution that first induced capsule shedding. However, if the blepharismas are rinsed with a nutrient medium, kept in it for a few hours, and then immersed again in the same concentration of strychnine sulfate as before, they will once again shed capsules, although the second capsule is not as complete or as deeply pigmented as the first one. Capsule shedding has been induced in this manner three times in succession; the blepharismas become less pigmented, more fragile, and more difficult to handle after each shedding (McCaw and Giese, unpublished).

Repeated capsule shedding can also be induced by consecutive increases in the concentration of strychnine sulfate applied. If blepharismas from which capsules have been shed once are placed in a strychnine concentration sufficiently higher than the first, another capsule will be shed; and a still higher concentration sometimes induces a third shedding. The quantitative increases needed to induce the second and third sheddings have not been determined because the experimental results are rather variable (McCaw and Giese, unpublished).

Possible Physiological Reasons for the Action of Strychnine Sulfate

It is known that strychnine sulfate inhibits several enzyme systems in mammalian cells, such as choline esterase and carbonic anhydrase (Goodman and Gilman, 1970); and that both sodium barbital and chloral hydrate act as antidotes to strychnine action on these enzymes. We have therefore tried to determine whether sodium barbital and chloral hydrate are also antidotes to strychnine action in *Blepharisma*. However, sodium barbital at all concentrations tested, when used in conjunction with 0.07% or 0.09% strychnine sulfate, caused the cytolysis of the blepharismas (*B. japonicum* v. intermedium). Chloral hydrate had the same effect (Giese and Breeden, unpublished).

If strychnine sulfate affects blepharismas by inhibiting the action of choline esterase, which occurs in ciliates (Seaman, 1951), it should be possible to induce capsule shedding in *Blepharisma* with eserine, which is known to inhibit some choline esterases. Eserine salicylate does induce capsule shedding, but it must be used at concentrations of 0.15 to 0.2% to be effective—hardly the weak concentrations that would be enough to act on enzymes (Fig. 7.3). At the higher concentration of eserine, 49 out of 60 blepharismas tested shed capsules, eight cytolyzed, and three were apparently unaffected (Giese and Breeden, unpublished).

If eserine induces capsule shedding in *Blepharisma* by inhibiting choline esterase and thus blocking the hydrolysis of acetylcholine, the application of acetylcholine alone should also induce shedding. However, when blepharismas are exposed to various concentrations of acetylcho-

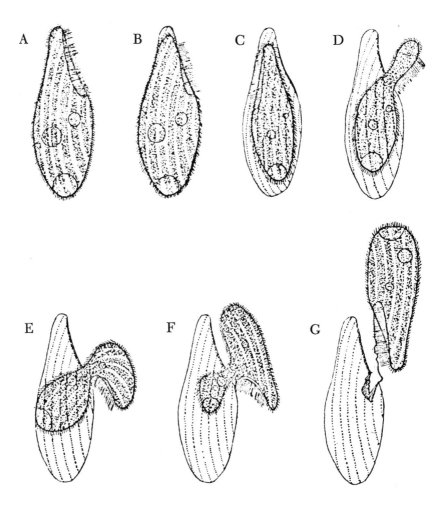

Fig. 7.1 (*above*). The process of capsule shedding in *Blepharisma*. A normal cell appears at *A*. When strychnine sulfate is added to the medium, the cytoplasm shrinks away from the outer pellicle, which forms the pigmented capsule. The animal leaves through the cytostome of the capsule and eventually returns to its usual shape; but because of protein loss and mechanical damage it is quite fragile and will cytolize easily. From Nadler, 1929.

Fig. 7.2 (*opposite, above*). Two stages in the capsule shedding of *B. japonicum* v. intermedium (corresponding to drawings *C* and *D* in Figure 7.1). Shedding was induced by a .09% solution of strychnine sulfate. Photo by Ray Velarde.

Fig. 7.3 (*opposite, below*). The comparative effects of strychnine sulfate and eserine salicylate on capsule shedding in *B. japonicum* v. intermedium. From unpublished data of McCaw and Giese.

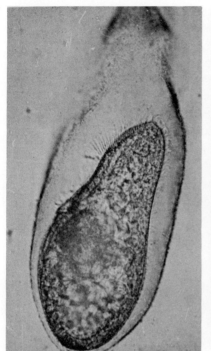
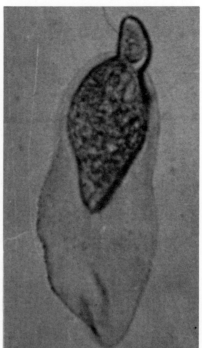
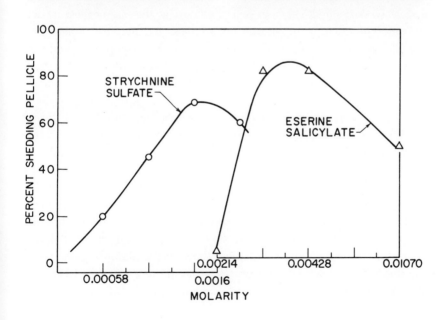

line, the capsule is shed only in concentrations so high (approaching 1%) as to have little significance theoretically, since at these concentrations almost any substance might act as an osmotic irritant. Furthermore, the shedding occurs in flakes rather than as an intact capsule. Urea, similarly, is effective only in very high concentrations (Giese and Rutherford, unpublished).

If the effect of various agents that induce shedding is a specific chemical action, the rate of shedding should decrease if the temperature is lowered. However, when blepharismas are subjected to strychnine sulfate at 13° C the capsule seems to be shed about as readily as at 25°, although my timing is not precise because the reactions are so rapid. It is not possible to make determinations at lower temperatures (e.g. 5° C) because the pigment is always shed immediately when blepharismas are immersed in a very cold medium.

Effect of Agents Other than Alkaloids

We have so far discussed only the alkaloids as agents that induce pigment shedding in *Blepharisma*, but there are others. For example, immersion in 0.9% NaCl will induce a rapid expulsion of pigment and protein. Various salts have been tested, but only the chlorides and sulfates of sodium, potassium, ammonium, and magnesium (all isotonic to 0.9% NaCl) are effective; sucrose and glucose at the same concentration are not. The effect is apparently not osmotic, but perhaps depends on specific cations and anions. With all these solutions the protein and pigment usually come out in solution; only at salt concentrations less than 0.9% NaCl equivalent will a capsule occasionally develop (Prabhakara Rao, 1963).

Most of the pigment extractable by salt treatment is released during the first five minutes of treatment. In one experiment with 0.9% NaCl, 35.6% of the pigment (determined colorimetrically) was extruded; a second treatment yielded 12% more, a third 9% more, and a fourth 6% more. However, the cells were progressively injured by each successive treatment (Prabhakara Rao, 1963). The addition of calcium to the 0.9% solutions nullifies their pigment-shedding effect. Conversely, binding the calcium with EDTA (ethylene diamine tetra-acetic acid, a chelating agent for divalent cations) will allow the solution to once again induce the discharge of pigment and protein. The binding effect of EDTA, in turn, can be overcome if additional calcium is added. Prabhakara Rao suggests that calcium in the cell membrane is removed by the cations or anions (or both), permitting a leakage of cell contents.

That the anion of a monovalent salt as well as the cation may play a role in evoking pigment discharge is suggested by my experiments with choline chloride. When blepharismas were placed in a solution of choline chloride isotonic with 0.9% NaCl, they swam backwards, emitting a spiral trail of pigment particles somewhat like an airplane's vapor trail. Even 50% of this concentration of choline chloride had the same effect. The choline cation ($C_5H_{15}NO_2$) is a large one and is not known to penetrate cell membranes, suggesting that the chloride ion is the active one in this case.

I have found that a sudden immersion of *Blepharisma* in a medium chilled to 5° C often causes pigment shedding. And immersion in a medium at 0° (ice water) invariably induces shedding of the pigment-protein complex, forming a colloidal solution of the pigment. Most of the pigment is extruded in the first 30 seconds; a little more comes out if the blepharismas are kept at 0° for up to two minutes, after which they begin to die (see Chapter 11). Blepharismas slowly chilled to 5° in the refrigerator do not discharge pigment (see Chapter 6), and stocks can be stored at this temperature. Exposing blepharismas to successively higher temperatures from 25° up to 70° will not induce shedding.*

Among the most interesting reagents that induce pigment extrusion in *Blepharisma* is puromycin. In a culture medium containing a 0.05% concentration of puromycin, violent contractions are induced in the blepharismas (*B. japonicum* Suzuki #5 and *B. japonicum* v. intermedium). Capsules soon form, but at first the blepharismas appear to be imprisoned inside them. If left in the puromycin solution the blepharismas rupture, emitting colorless globules all along the body. However, when I diluted such a solution about fourfold with nutrient medium soon after the contractions began, practically all the blepharismas emerged successfully from their red capsules, usually through the rather small mouth apertures; in some cases they struggled for 10–15 minutes before emerging. Occasional blepharismas emerged completely free of pigment, others had scattered pink areas, and a few more were still light pink in color. By the next morning all the blepharismas had developed some

---

* Treatment with electric shocks (65 volts, 0.8 milliamperes) after the manner of Dryl (1958) does not induce pigment shedding but will cause cytolysis at the anode (Giese and Breeden, unpublished).

pink pigment, even while remaining in the diluted solution of puro-mycin. Possibly, the bacteria present in the medium (*Pseudomonas ovalis*, and perhaps others) had inactivated the puromycin.

Since blepharismas are pigmented one would expect light waves to have some effect on capsule shedding. However, when I exposed deeply pigmented cells to bright light they were killed. (In extremely brilliant light from an argon plasma arc capsules were shed.) By contrast, in dim light (about 150 foot-candles for 4–8 hours), the blepharismas became distinctly grey-blue in color owing to the photooxidation of the pig-ment (see Chapter 11). If these blue blepharismas were further exposed to dim light, they gradually lost the blue pigment, although several days of exposure were required (Giese and Grainger, 1970). In no case did any of the three stocks tested (*B. americanum*, *B. japonicum* v. interme-dium, and *B. japonicum* Suzuki #5) shed pigmented capsules under any intensity of light.

The gradual loss in blue color of blepharismas exposed to dim light is the result of their shedding blue pigment granules, as has been ob-served by electron microscope in *B. americanum* (Kennedy, 1966). Light is generally too mild an irritant to cause the shedding of a complete capsule; but with prolonged exposure it gradually induces the shedding of practically all the pigment, granule by granule. Since the red pigment is always renewed in cells that carry on a normal metabolism, it is pos-sible that new red pigment forms in small amounts in the blue granules, eventually inducing the shedding of those granules.

Many other agents may cause shedding of the pigment/protein com-plex, of fragments, or even of an entire capsule. For example, after red-pigmented *Blepharisma* are centrifuged a number of pale cells can be seen under the microscope. If none were present before the treatment, they must have been induced to shed pigment by agitation or during handling.

Jytte Nilsson found that when blepharismas were exposed to alcian blue, a dye used to stain mucus, "they immediately became surrounded by a 'cloud' of material (extruded by the ciliate) in which the dye be-came adsorbed; the ciliate moved within this structure in clear fluid. If the structure was punctured, the dye solution came into direct contact with the ciliate; this most often resulted in the death of the ciliate. If, however, the ciliate within the blue 'capsule' was transferred to normal culture medium, the ciliate left the capsule and swam about, apparently unharmed. On the following morning the ciliate had divided, and food vacuoles were present. The whole process may be that of protection, resembling early cyst formation. No pigment granules were extruded with the material stained by alcian blue, so, although the process resembles the 'capsule shedding' obtained with strychnine sulfate, it appears to be less drastic" (Nilsson, unpublished).

Blue and Albino Blepharismas

Dim light will turn red blepharismas blue, and a group of blue-pigmented cells (*B. japonicum* v. intermedium and *B. japonicum* Suzuki #5) that I tested did not shed capsules when treated with drugs like puromycin or strychnine sulfate. Instead, the blue pigment granules were shed into the medium as a diffuse cloud. Only rarely were capsules, portions of capsules, or flakes shed; yet the blue blepharismas contracted as suddenly as red ones. The concentration of the drugs was substantially the same, and red blepharismas introduced into the puromycin solution immediately after the blue ones formed capsules at once. Perhaps the oxidation of red pigment to blue binds the membranes of the pigment granules to the protoplasm in a way that prevents their discharge. The occasional discharge of a capsule from one cell in a suspension of blue blepharismas may come from an organism still containing red pigment (see Chapter 11).

Albino blepharismas also fail to shed a capsule or flakes on being subjected to strychnine sulfate. One might anticipate this result, since there is almost no pigment for the albinos to shed (Brutinel and Giese, unpublished). Moreover, a concentration of puromycin that will induce immediate contraction and capsule formation in red blepharismas induces no contraction in white ones. Perhaps the capsule forms only in red blepharismas because only the red pigment (as suggested by Kennedy, 1966) interacts with the inducing drug in the right way. The question is still open.

Fine Structure of the Shed Capsule

Electron microscopy shows that the capsule shed by *Blepharisma americanum* under the action of strychnine sulfate is an amorphous structure made up largely of extruded membranes containing pigment granules still arranged as in living cells but in a less orderly manner (Fig. 7.4). The pigment of *Blepharisma* is already known to exist in the

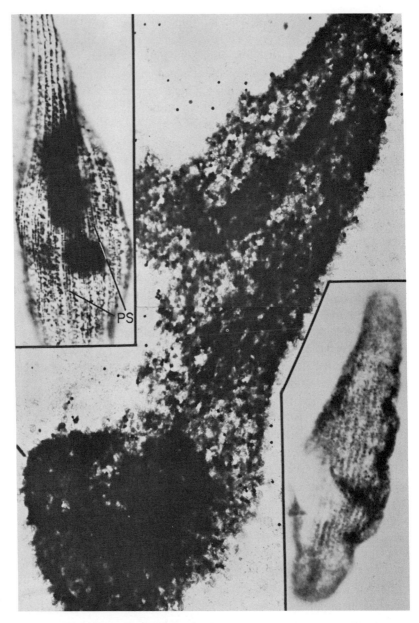

Fig. 7.4. *Upper left*: a shed capsule; the characteristic pigment stripes (PS) show up clearly under Protargol staining (× 1,500). *Center*: a capsule whose granules are deeply stained with uranyl acetate (× 3,100). *Lower right*: a capsule stained by the Chatton-Lwoff process (× 1,500). From Kennedy, 1966.

cell in membrane-bound granules (see Chapter 3), and observation suggests that the entire granule and its membrane are usually extruded when the capsule is shed. Sometimes the granular membrane attaches to the cell membrane and the pigment alone leaves the cell; when this happens rapidly or violently, as it does after exposure to an alkaloid, the pattern of granules characteristic of the cell is essentially maintained after extrusion (Kennedy, 1966).

Electron micrographs of blepharismas from which the capsule has been removed by alkaloid treatment show that the pellicle is not extruded. It remains intact and looks much like that of a normal cell, except that in spots some membranes from the extruded pigment granules are attached to the cell membrane (Kennedy, 1966).

Variations in Capsule Shedding

As the concentration of strychnine sulfate in a medium is increased, the number of blepharismas in a sample who shed their capsules increases to a maximum and then declines as an increasing proportion of the cells cytolyze and die without shedding (Fig. 7.2). The concentration of strychnine sulfate at which a maximal number of blepharismas shed their pellicles without cytolyzing can be used to compare the effectiveness of the alkaloid in inducing capsule shedding in various species and in different stocks of the same species (Table 7.2). From the comparison, several conclusions emerge. The manner of capsule shedding differs in various stocks and seems characteristic of each stock or variety of *Blepharisma*, at least under the conditions employed. Although early tests on *B. japonicum* Suzuki #5 and *B. japonicum* v. intermedium suggested that the large stocks might shed intact pellicles easily, this was not confirmed, since the large Niigata and Suzuki #3 stocks of the same species shed their capsules in many small pieces.

The tendency of *Blepharisma* to cytolyze when exposed to strychnine sulfate is partly a result of the cell's fragility after shedding a capsule. In some cases the blepharismas become pear-shaped when the capsule is shed, as if unable to maintain their characteristic elongate shape. Cytolysis proved quite common in *B. americanum* (Stanford stock): of 85 cells tested in 0.05% strychnine sulfate, 12 lost some pigment, 29 lost the capsule in small pieces, and 34 simply cytolyzed. Attempts to handle, or even touch, these cells after the capsules had been shed were frequently followed by cytolysis. *B. japonicum* v. intermedium, by contrast, quite often sheds capsules whole and seldom cytolyzes.

TABLE 7.2

Capsule Shedding Induced by Strychnine Sulfate in
Several Species of *Blepharisma*

Species and stock	Average size	Most effective strychnine sulfate concentration[a]	Manner of shedding
B. japonicum:			
Suzuki #3	318 × 96 μm	0.05%	Capsule wrinkles and is shed in many pieces; more color lost than in Niigata; keeps shape pretty well.
Suzuki #5	315 × 95	0.07	Some as in Suzuki #3, but individual cells show great diversity in reaction.
Niigata	293 × 95	0.05	Capsule wrinkles and is shed in many pieces, which cling to the cell; cells tend to assume a spherical form.
Intermedium	294 × 76	0.09	Crawls out of the intact capsule, retaining its shape fairly well.
B. stoltei, Nara	224 × 78	0.05	Capsule loosens and cell assumes spherical form; capsule shed cleanly.
B. americanum, Stanford G	149 × 43	0.03	Capsule shed in small pieces; cells lose shape, become very fragile, and cytolyze readily.
B. musculus, seshachari	147 × 56	0.04	Capsule shed in small pieces; cells fragile and cytolyze readily.
B. undulans	176 × 27	0.05–0.07	Capsule formed and cell assumes spherical form; difficulty getting out of capsule; if successful, capsule shed in one piece; many cytolyze.

[a] At approximately 25° C.

All *Blepharisma*, regardless of stock, lose some of their pigment on treatment with strychnine sulfate. (The most striking case is the Suzuki #3 stock of *B. japonicum*, whose capsules are often deep red in color.) However, in practically no case is all of the pigment removed, even if three successive exposures to strychnine sulfate are followed by shedding. Also, some blepharismas treated with strychnine sulfate lose pigment granules without shedding a capsule at all (Weisz, 1950; Inaba et al., 1958).

Acclimation to the Induction of Capsule Shedding

The induction of capsule or pigment shedding by strychnine sulfate in part depends on the suddenness (shock?) of *Blepharisma*'s encounter with the alkaloid. When blepharismas were successively exposed to solutions of 0.001%, 0.005%, and 0.01% for half-hour periods and were finally placed in 0.05%, they did not shed capsules; cells of the same stock but not acclimated in this manner did shed capsules when placed in some of the same 0.05% solution at the same time (Giese and McCaw, unpublished). This compares with *Blepharisma*'s similar acclimation to lowered temperatures, as described earlier.

Surface Damage After Capsule Shedding

The surface properties of *Blepharisma* are altered when a capsule is removed. A decapsulated *Blepharisma* bulges and becomes pyriform, as if the strength of some girdle holding it in shape had decreased. Quantitative measurements of this change are considered in Chapter 6. A needle applied to the surface of a decapsulated *Blepharisma* sticks to it, and it is much more difficult to cut the cell immediately after the capsule has been shed. This change becomes even more pronounced after a second capsule is shed (McCaw, unpublished). Since considerable protein is present in a capsule, it is likely that its removal has caused some chemical change in the cell surface. Under the electron microscope, however, no change can be seen in the physical structure of the pellicle to account for the altered properties of the cell surface after decapsulation.

To measure the damage suffered by decapsulated blepharismas, we compared the regeneration and division rates of treated cells to those of controls. In regeneration experiments it was necessary to cut the blepharismas first and then treat the pieces with strychnine to induce shedding; once a capsule has been shed the cells are difficult to handle and almost impossible to cut, not only because they are fragile but also because of their irregular shape and their stickiness. Cut halves shed a capsule more readily than whole blepharismas because of the large aperture through which the cut piece can swim out. It will be seen from Figure 7.5 that the rate of regeneration is considerably delayed by capsule shedding, the more so the longer the *Blepharisma* stays in the strychnine sulfate solution.

When *Blepharisma* is exposed to strychnine sulfate at various times after cutting, regeneration is retarded about equally in each case. Thus 50% regeneration for controls takes approximately 5.4 hours, whereas 50% regeneration of strychnine-treated (0.05% for 30 minutes) posterior halves of *Blepharisma* exposed at 0.25, 1.2, and 3 hours after cutting

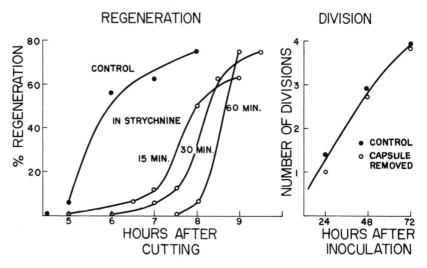

Fig. 7.5. The effect of capsule shedding on *Blepharisma*'s regeneration and growth. From unpublished data of McCaw and Giese.

took 7.9, 7.4, and 7.4 hours, respectively. It appears that strychnine damage is nonspecific and comparable at all stages in regeneration (Giese and McCaw, unpublished).

The division rate of a decapsulated *Blepharisma* is not markedly different from that of controls. The average generation time of *Blepharisma* (15–25 hours at 25° C) is quite long compared to the regeneration time, and repair of the cell surface appears to have been accomplished by the time division occurs.

It may appear surprising that regeneration should be delayed by capsule shedding, whereas division is apparently unaffected. However, during regeneration a postperistomal fragment must reconstruct all its organelles from the materials already at hand, since without a mouth it cannot obtain new supplies from the medium. Consequently, the task of regenerating the material shed after strychnine sulfate treatment is probably more formidable for the fragment than for the entire cell.

In conclusion, it appears that any agent affecting the pigment granules in *Blepharisma* can cause the shedding of a capsule. *Stentor coeruleus*, which has a photosensitizing pigment akin to that of *Blepharisma*, reacts to some salts much like *Blepharisma* (Tartar, 1957). Other protozoan cells subjected to the same agents do not so react, presumably because they lack the structures that give rise to the capsule.

LITERATURE CITED

Dryl, S. 1958. Photographic registration of movement of Protozoa. Bull. Acad. Polon. Sciences **6**: 429–30.

Giese, A. C. 1938. Reversible bleaching of *Blepharisma*. Trans. Amer. Microsc. Soc. **57**: 77–81.

Giese, A. C., and R. M. Grainger. 1970. Studies on the red and blue forms of the pigment of *Blepharisma*. Photochem. Photobiol. **12**: 489–503.

Goodman, L. S., and A. Gilman. 1970. The pharmacological basis of therapeutics. New York, 1294 pp.

Inaba, F., R. Nakamura, and S. Yamaguchi. 1958. An electron-microscopic study of the pigment granules of *Blepharisma*. Cytologia **23**: 72–79.

Kennedy, J. R., Jr. 1966. The effect of strychnine and light on pigmentation in *Blepharisma undulans* Stein. J. Cell Biol. **28**: 145–53.

Nadler, J. E. 1929. Notes on loss and regeneration of the pellicle in *Blepharisma*. Biol. Bull. **56**: 327–30.

Prabhakara Rao, A. V. S. 1963. Extrusion of a protein pigment complex from *Blepharisma undulans*. J. Protozool. **10**: 204–7.

Seaman, G. R. 1951. Localization of acetylcholinesterase activity in the protozoan *Tetrahymena geleii* S. Soc. Exp. Biol. Med. **76**: 169–70.

Tartar, V. 1957. Reaction of *Stentor coeruleus* to certain substances added to the medium. Exp. Cell Res. **13**: 317–32.

——— 1961. The biology of *Stentor*. New York, 413 pp.

Weisz, P. 1950. On the mitochondrial nature of the pigmented granules in *Stentor* and *Blepharisma*. J. Morphol. **86**: 177–84.

CHAPTER EIGHT

Morphogenesis

Problems of morphogenesis have been extensively studied with protozoans because these organisms lend themselves admirably to the purpose, requiring only the simplest of instruments and laboratory facili-
ties (though they demand great skill from the experimenter). Furthermore, at room temperature the regeneration and recovery of protozoans
are rapid, generally taking a day or less; thus numerous experiments are
possible. The literature on morphogenesis has been periodically reviewed (Balamuth, 1940; Weisz, 1954; Tartar, 1967). The extensive review by Tartar considers the major problems of morphogenesis in various classes of Protozoa and includes a critical analysis of the studies.
Ciliates in particular have been favorite objects for morphogenetic
studies, and of the ciliates *Stentor* has been used most extensively. The
literature on *Stentor* has also been reviewed in detail in a comprehensive
study (Tartar, 1961), with additions in a recent review article (Tartar,
1967).

Many of the earlier investigators who studied regeneration and morphogenesis in ciliates were concerned with the formation of a whole
organism from a part by the cooperation of macronucleus and cytoplasm. They considered the macronucleus to be indispensable for morphogenesis, but did not direct their attention to the kinety system, which
exercises an important role in ectoplasmic differentiation. More recent
studies (Lwoff, 1950; Weisz, 1951, 1954) have presented evidence that
the kinetosomes are self-producing and are able to develop into cortical
organelles other than cilia, such as trichocysts; some evidence to the
contrary has also been offered (Yusa, 1963; Ehret and Haller, 1963).

Early experimental studies on the mechanism of ciliate morphogenesis (Tartar, 1941; Yagiu, 1951a–b, 1952, 1956) did not touch on the in-

By Shōichirō Suzuki, Yamagata University, Japan.

duction and control of morphogenesis. In some of the lower invertebrates a causal analysis of morphogenesis has been made possible
through a knowledge of physiological gradients and induction phenomena. Subsequent studies in this vein have also been made with ciliates,
mainly with spirotrichs such as *Stentor* (Tartar, 1958, 1959a, 1966b;
Uhlig, 1962), *Condylostoma* (Suhama, 1961), *Blepharisma* (Suzuki,
1957; Eberhardt, 1962), and *Spirostomum* (Eberhardt, 1962). This
chapter, for the most part, presents an experimental analysis of this
kind, concentrating on the induction and control mechanisms of morphogenesis in *Blepharisma japonicum*.

Morphogenesis in Binary Fission

Binary fission in *B. japonicum* takes place every 15–20 hours at 25° C,
and the time required for the completion of each cell division averages
two hours and a half at 20° C. A cell in the prefission stage may be recognized by its comparatively large and expanded posterior half, and
also by an increased branching of the kineties in the boundary of its
V-area.* The subsequent process of binary fission and stomatogenesis
may be divided into the following four stages.

Stage I. This is the interval from the first appearance of the adoral
anlage to the beginning of macronuclear contraction, although the macronucleus retains an essentially vegetative configuration throughout the
stage. In the initial phase of stomatogenesis for the future posterior
daughter cell, kinetosomes multiply rapidly in the V-area posterior to
the peristome (Fig. 8.1, *A, B*). The new kinetosomes, bearing minute
cilia, form many transverse rows, each consisting of approximately ten
granules connected by a slender fibril. The kinetosomes located at the
right are somewhat larger than the others and are connected anterio-
posteriorly by a longitudinal fiber. The kinetosomes in this longitudinal
row will later become the basal granules of the cilia that form the undulating membrane along the right margin of the peristome. The ones
arranged transversely will form the cilia of the membranelles.

---

* The V-area is the ventral, V-shaped part of a *Blepharisma* or similar ciliate, posterior to the peristome. The V-area is important in morphogenetic events because at
critical times (for example, before cell division) the kinetosomes of its kineties multiply rapidly. Similarly, the kinetosomes in the V-area of a postperistomal piece of a
Blepharisma multiply to form the anlage (forerunner) of the missing mouth organelles in a regenerating cell. If the V-area is removed from such a fragment, an
anlage will still form from the kinetosomes dividing in other kineties, but it will
appear much more slowly.

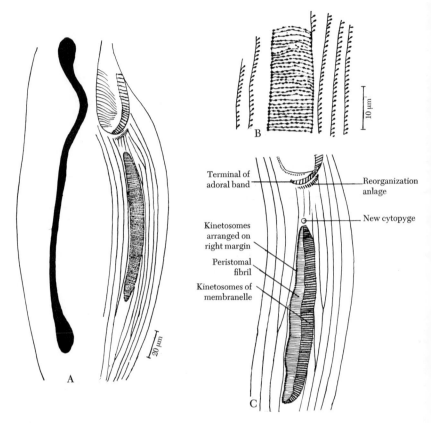

Fig. 8.1. The development of a new posterior peristome during binary fission in
B. japonicum. A, early stage of differentiation in the V-area. *B*, enlarged view of
the kinetosomes in *A. C*, oral differentiation in the V-area of a Stage II divider. After
Suzuki, 1957.

Paralleling the formation of new feeding organelles in the future posterior daughter cell is a reorganization of the original oral area of the
cell, which will become part of the anterior daughter cell. A short band,
or adoral anlage, called the "regeneration anlage" (Eberhardt, 1962)
arises in close proximity to the posterior terminal of the left peristomal
margin.

Stage II. From the beginning of macronuclear contraction to the
period immediately before the macronucleus is fully condensed. During this stage the ventral side of the cell in a side view appears flattened.
A new contractile vacuole makes its appearance on the ventral side near

the anterior end of the developing adoral anlage. The cilia arising from the kinetosomes in the V-area grow longer and become more visible at this stage, and the floor of the developing oral area grows to a width twice that of the preceding stage. As the enlargement of the peristomal area progresses, the kinetosomes in the left-hand transverse rows move further to the left, leaving naked fibers between themselves and the longitudinal rows of granules on the right margin (Fig. 8.1, *C*). The kinetosomes in the right-hand row appear on first inspection to be single large granules, but they are actually clusters of two or more granules. The reorganization anlage in this stage becomes more distinct than in the previous stage, appearing as a short band of membranelles that is almost contiguous to the distal end of the original adoral band.

Stage III. Middle stage, from the beginning of macronuclear coalescence into a single spherical mass to the period just before the macronucleus begins to reelongate. The developing posterior oral area forms a distinct longitudinal oral groove, and the cilia arising from the kinetosomes aggregated along the left peristomal margin begin to form the presumptive membranelles.

The old anterior oral organelles are partially dedifferentiated by this time. First the undulating membrane disappears, separating into its component cilia; then the membranelles grow much shorter, probably because of partial dissolution. The terminal spiral of the membranellar band begins to untwist, and the depression of the gullet gradually rises to become a shallow groove extending from the posterior end of the original oral groove. The reorganization anlage now connects directly with the old membranellar band. At the same time, according to Eberhardt (1962), a new ciliary row arises near the left side of the site of the old undulating membrane, which has already disappeared; this is the anlage of a new undulating membrane. At this stage the reorganizing anterior oral area closely resembles the posterior one, both having a new membranellar band composed of short cilia and both having no visible undulating membrane. A visible fission line begins to form near the end of this stage.

Stage IV. From the reelongation of the macronucleus to the complete separation of the daughter cells. At the beginning of this stage the macronucleus reelongates. At the same time, a "growing zone" (a narrow area encircling the midbody between the proximal ends of the two developing oral areas) begins to elongate to form the posterior half of the anterior daughter cell (see Fig. 2.1). The fission line developing along the posterior end of the growing zone becomes clearer, and cytoplasmic constriction may be seen along it. At first the line appears as a clear band without pigment granules, but it assumes the appearance of a slender line as constriction proceeds.

The completion of the anterior (reorganizing) and posterior (developing) peristomes is synchronous. At first both are straight grooves, each bordered by a membranellar band but lacking other feeding organelles. By the end of this stage, however, the new gullets are invaginated, and their membranellar bands form new terminal spirals; new undulating membranes become visible shortly before the completion of cell division. As the cytoplasmic constriction progresses, the new contractile vacuole migrates toward the division line, eventually lying at the posterior end of the presumptive anterior daughter cell.

Oral Replacement

In *B. japonicum* oral replacement takes place in small cells that have just finished regeneration and have disproportionately small peristomes, in recently excysted cells, in exconjugants before the first division, and often in ordinary vegetative cells, perhaps after some unfavorable circumstance.

Oral replacement is characterized by a regression of the original feeding organelles and the simultaneous redifferentiation of new oral organelles in conjunction with macronuclear reorganization (Fig. 8.2). The replacement process is identical with the reorganization of the anterior feeding organelles in binary fission, but it differs from binary fission in that the new oral area, which develops in the V-area, unites directly with the old one after the original mouthparts are resorbed. Oral replacement may be divided into four arbitrary stages analogous to those of division.

Stage I. Cells in this stage may be recognized by the appearance of adoral anlagen in the V-area contiguous to the original oral area. The macronucleus presents no externally discernible changes.

Stage II. The macronucleus begins to condense into a short, sausage-like body with somewhat enlarged ends. The micronuclei leave their original location near the macronucleus to scatter in the cytoplasm surrounding the macronucleus. Some of them swell, and chromatic granules (chromosomes) become visible within them. The component cilia of the adoral anlagen grow longer, and the pellicle of the new oral area forms

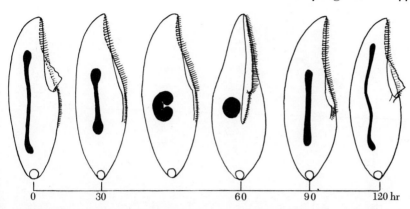

Fig. 8.2. Macronuclear behavior during oral replacement in *B. japonicum*. This is very similar to behavior during division. From Suzuki, 1957.

a longitudinal groove. Paralleling this differentiation, the original oral organelles begin to dedifferentiate.

Stage III. Cells in this stage may be recognized by their spindle-shaped bodies (fourth drawing in Fig. 8.2). The macronucleus eventually condenses into a single roundish mass. At the same time, some of the micronuclei form metaphase spindles similar to those present in vegetative division. In the meantime the gullet, the terminal spiral of the membranellar band, and the undulating membrane of the original peristome are fully resorbed, and the old oral areas complete their union.

Stage IV. The stage of macronuclear reelongation. A new cytopharynx begins to invaginate at the posterior end of the new oral groove, forming the terminal spiral of the membranellar band. Near the end of this stage a new undulating membrane appears along the right margin of the oral groove.

Regeneration

The course of regeneration differs in the anterior and posterior halves of a bisected organism.*

Anterior. Regeneration in an anterior fragment produced by excising the posterior half of the body, which contains the posterior quarter of the peristome (Fig. 8.3, A). After the wound closes, the cut end of

* Some information on laboratory techniques for transection, excision of parts, and regeneration in *Blepharisma* is given in Chapter 9.

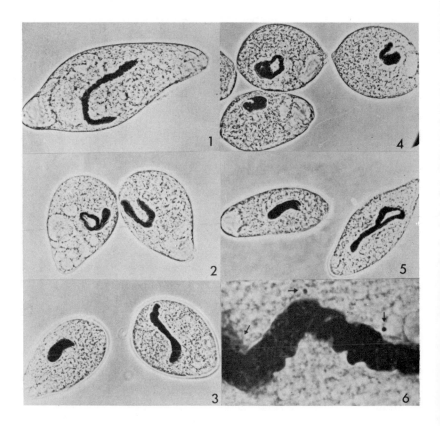

Fig. 8.3. Various aspects of regeneration in *Blepharisma*. In microphotos 1–12 (from Parker and Giese, 1966) Feulgen stain has been used to darken the macronucleus. (Whole-cell photos are × 220; nuclear photos are × 1,000.) *1*. A normal cell of *B. japonicum* v. intermedium. *2*. Postperistomal fragments one hour after cutting, showing Stage I macronucleus (× 220). *3*. Regenerating fragments after two hours, macronuclei in Stages I and III. *4*. Fragments after three hours, Stage II macronuclei. *5*. After six hours the cells have almost completed regeneration; the macronuclei are in Stages III and IV. *6*. Enlarged view of a Stage I macronucleus that has begun to coil; the arrows indicate micronuclei. *7*. Macronucleus in late Stage I, beginning secondary coiling. *8*. Stage II macronucleus. *9*. Stage III macronucleus; the arrows indicate four micronuclear metaphase spindles. *10*. In some cases a Feulgen-positive material (arrow) is extruded from the condensing Stage II macronucleus. *11–12*. As is obvious in this series of micrographs, the macronuclear cycle is not always completely coordinated with the other processes of a regenerating cell; in this unusual case the Stage IV macronucleus had not completely reorganized by the time the regenerated cell began its first division. Drawing *A* shows regeneration in an anterior fragment retaining most of its mouthparts; a new adoral anlage has begun to form, and the cell will undergo oral replacement as soon as it has regenerated. *B*, regeneration in a postperistomal fragment like those in 1–12. Drawings from Suzuki, 1957.

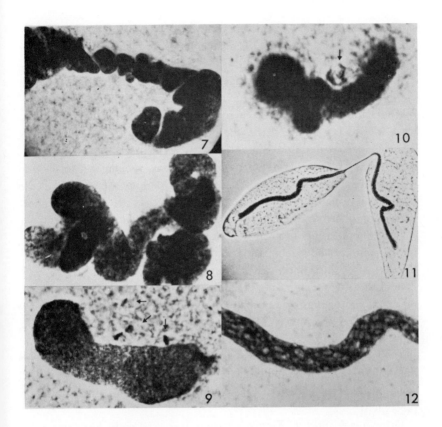

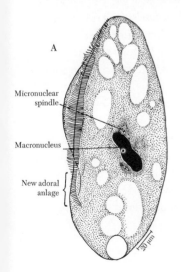

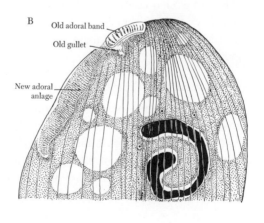

A

Micronuclear
spindle

Macronucleus

New adoral
anlage

30 μm

B

Old adoral band

Old gullet

New adoral
anlage

the fragment gradually extends to reform the posterior half of the body. A new contractile vacuole, arising near the cut end of the peristome, migrates to a terminal position. The cut peristome is compensated for by a short longitudinal groove that forms on the pellicle posterior to the cut end, and a new adoral anlage arises along the groove's left margin. In the middle stage, while macronuclear condensation and micronuclear mitosis are taking place, the original anterior feeding organelles undergo partial dedifferentiation and subsequently redifferentiate. In a later stage of regeneration, the macronucleus reelongates to assume its normal configuration, and oral organelles such as the gullet and the undulating membrane are completed much as they are during the reorganization of the anterior peristome in binary fission.

Posterior. Regeneration in a posterior fragment produced by excising the anterior body, including the larger part of the peristome (Fig. 8.3, *B*). After the wound closes, a longitudinal groove forms in the pellicle of the V-area, and a new adoral anlage arises along its left margin. Again, stomatogenesis proceeds in conjunction with macronuclear condensation and micronuclear mitosis. As adoral differentiation proceeds, the remnants of the old gullet and undulating membrane disappear and the old membranelles undergo partial dedifferentiation. The developing oral area is then united with the remnant of the old oral area. In all other respects regeneration is essentially the same as it is in oral replacement.

Drawings *A* and *B* in Figure 8.3 are to the same scale, but appear different because the anterior part of a living *Blepharisma* is rather flat and has a smaller quantity of cytoplasm than the posterior part. In a fixed specimen the rounded posterior half of the body flattens out and expands considerably, becoming many times the apparent size of the anterior body.

Encystment and Excystment

Dedifferentiation and redifferentiation also occur in the cystment cycle, which is treated in Chapter 10. However, it might be mentioned here that the crucial question of whether the kinetosomes all disappear during encystment or whether they are carried over to help form the newly redifferentiated organism has not been answered for *Blepharisma* or for any of the other ciliates studied.

The Fission Line

In *Blepharisma* the fission line becomes visible as a clear unpigmented band at the beginning of Stage IV of division. The line takes a course cutting the principal oral primordium leading into the future posterior daughter cell. At the same time, the growing zone begins to elongate to form the posterior half of the future anterior daughter cell, and cytoplasmic constriction proceeds along the fission line. These external features of division suggest that the origin and the development of the fission line may be related to the developing adoral and growing zones. One can test this impression by experimentally removing one or more portions of a dividing cell—in this case the adoral zone (both old and new), the growing zone, or the presumptive division line.

Excision of the original oral area, regardless of the stage of division, does not prevent the continued differentiation of the new adoral zone, and a fission line appears at the usual position. Division is completed in normal fashion, and new oral organelles then regenerate in the anterior daughter cell. Similarly, after excision of the developing adoral zone at any stage the organism completes division in approximately normal time, and a new adoral zone then begins to differentiate in the posterior daughter cell at the site of the original one. Thus the kineties remaining in or adjacent to the V-area can acquire morphogenetic potential after a period of surface reorganization. Evidently neither the original oral area nor the developing adoral zone is directly related to the continuance or completion of division. When the developing adoral zone of the prospective posterior daughter cell is excised at a very early stage of division, however, cytoplasmic division is often retarded; perhaps the growing zone is disturbed by this operation.

An oblique or longitudinal cut across the presumptive path of the fission line and bisecting the growing zone into dorsal and ventral halves was used to test the relation of the ventral region of the growing zone to the formation of the fission line. In this case, each fragment is macronucleate and has either the dorsal half (d) or ventral half (v) of the bisected growing zone. When the cut is made in Stage I of division, the ventral fragments are able to complete division within the time expected for division of intact animals regardless of the size of v. By contrast, the dorsal fragments never divide when d is smaller than v, but will do so

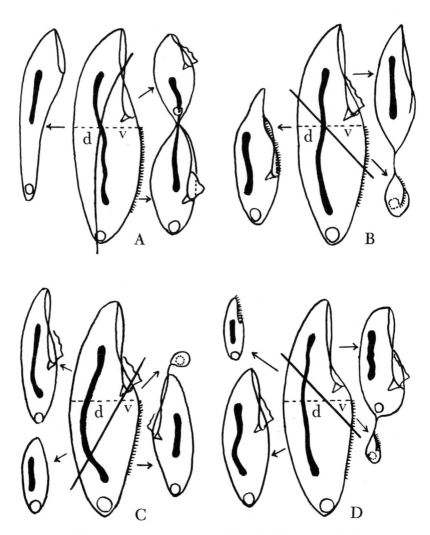

Fig. 8.4. Oblique transections made during Stage I of division to split the presumptive path of the fission line (dotted line) into dorsal (*d*) and ventral (*v*) segments. A and B are cuts in which *d* < *v*; in C and D, the reverse is true. Although the macronucleus is not always divided into equal parts, regeneration occurs whenever any sizeable fragment of it is present. When division occurs, the macronucleus condenses and reelongates as it does during the division of an intact cell (only the final macronuclear form is shown in these drawings). When the cell material remaining between the cut plane and the fission line is very small (ventral pieces in C and D), the subsequent division produces one nonviable amacronucleate cell. Notice also that when a cell segment on one side of the fission line does not contain any part of the old peristome or the new adoral anlage, the cell that develops from it after division does not produce a new set of oral structures. From Suzuki, 1957.

if d is larger (Fig. 8.4). This experiment suggests that by Stage I of division the growing region associated with the ventral half of the presumptive fission line has already initiated a change leading to the formation of a functional fission line, or that some presumptive potential produces a fission line in this region. The dorsal half, however, does not form a fission line, nor is it able to initiate such a change.

It has also been shown that in Stage I of division the excision of the ventral third to two-thirds of the growing zone interferes with division, even if the presumptive fission line is left intact. Not only do the developing adoral anlagen disappear, but macronuclear condensation and the formation of a new contractile vacuole for the anterior daughter cell fail to occur. These blepharismas remain in what is essentially a vegetative condition, as though division had never begun. But even the removal of the entire presumptive fission line region at Stage I does not prevent division. The existence of an invisible but functional fission line at such a very early stage of division is ruled out by these results, and it is evident that the growing zone plays a very important role in morphogenesis.

All fragments in Stages II and III of division are able to complete division regardless of the type of transection. Presumably, the cytoplasmic change related to the formation of a fission line has by this time extended to the dorsal half of the cell and gradually pervaded the entire region associated with the presumptive path of the fission line. In Stage II, also, neither the removal of the presumptive path of the fission line nor the excision of the growing zone interferes with the completion of division. In Stage III, however, when the entire growing zone is removed and the fission path is left intact, or vice versa, the differentiation of oral organelles proceeds normally but cytoplasmic division is retarded. At this stage, apparently, the growing zone has acquired more influence on the continuation of cytoplasmic constriction than has the presumptive fission line path.

In Stage IV of division, the growing zone elongates to its full length and forms a posterior half for the presumptive anterior daughter cell. Simultaneously, a clear fission line becomes visible and completes its differentiation functionally as well as morphologically. When the fission line is excised at this stage and the two cells are held together until fused, the cytoplasmic constriction is arrested completely, resulting in a perfect telobiotic homopolar union of the daughter cells (Fig. 8.5).

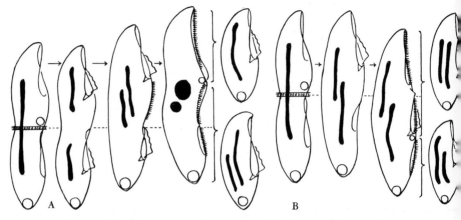

Fig. 8.5. Removal of the fission line during Stage IV of division. The two daughter cells form a complete fusion complex. The actual site of the primary fission line is indicated by a broken line, and excised area by crosshatching. Division may occur in either the anterior region (*A*) or the posterior region (*B*). From Suzuki, 1957.

At the time of division in such fusion complexes, the fission line is never formed at the site of the original path, but instead to the rear of the anterior or posterior peristome. When the line arises in the anterior half, a newly developing peristome fuses with the original posterior peristome to form a single oral area for the posterior daughter cell. When the division line occurs in the posterior half, the original anterior and posterior peristomes fuse into a single peristome for the anterior individual. Rarely, two fission lines form, and if the divisions in each half of the fusion complex are close to synchronous, a chain of three or four future daughter cells may be formed. In this case, the original anterior daughter cell usually seems to be physiologically dominant over the posterior one, since the latter undergoes only one division during two divisions of the former. In fact, the posterior component sometimes dedifferentiates and is resorbed into the anterior component.

These results show that the path of the fission line is determined uniquely both in time and in space: a missing portion cannot be reconstituted, nor is there any potential for forming an altogether new line at the old location. Fission lines always arise just posterior to the oral area, forming a boundary that divides the *Blepharisma* into anterior and posterior halves. This characteristic property ensures the independent development of a new oral area for the presumptive posterior daughter cell, even though the posterior adoral anlage appears long before the fission line cuts the posterior kineties. Similar results have been obtained by Tartar (1964) in homopolar tandem grafts on *Stentor coeruleus*.

The Morphogenetic Roles of Nuclei

Three independent morphogenetic processes—regeneration, oral replacement, and binary fission—always proceed in conjunction with a macronuclear cycle of condensation and reelongation to the vegetative state, and are also associated with the mitosis of the micronuclei. This coincidence suggests that the nuclear apparatus in *Blepharisma* has a fundamental initiating and controlling function during any sort of ectoplasmic reorganization. During conjugation, the condensed macronucleus degenerates, to be replaced by a new macronucleus derived from the synkaryon. The macronucleus is apparently an essential factor in morphogenesis, whereas the micronuclei are considered to be dispensable for regeneration in most if not all ciliates. Our analysis of morphogenesis certainly requires that we clarify the functions of the nuclei at various stages of *Blepharisma*'s life cycle.

Indispensability of the macronucleus and the role of the micronuclei. The question of whether a micronucleus is necessary for regeneration and other morphogenetic events has long attracted the attention of investigators. Dawson (1920) and Reynolds (1932) in *Oxytricha* and Chen (1940) in *Paramecium* reported normal division in all amicronucleate races. By contrast, Taylor (1923) and Reynolds (1932) in *Euplotes* and Tittler (1938) in *Uroleptus* observed that the presence of both macronuclear and micronuclear materials is necessary for division or regeneration. Moore (1924) in *Blepharisma undulans*, Reynolds (1932) in *Oxytricha*, Schwartz (1934, 1935) in *Stentor coeruleus*, and Suzuki (1957) in *Blepharisma japonicum* found that micronuclei alone cannot support regeneration.

In this study, the morphogenetic capability of micronuclei was investigated by using fragments that contained micronuclei only. This is readily accomplished in *B. japonicum*, since the micronuclei divide into two groups scattered near the ends of the filiform macronucleus in Stage IV of division; the two distal extremities at this stage inevitably contain some micronuclei but no macronuclear materials, and they are easily cut off (Fig. 8.6). An anterior fragment so obtained cannot replace the old oral organelles unless it contains part of the macronucleus; but the posterior fragment will complete stomatogenesis even in the ab-

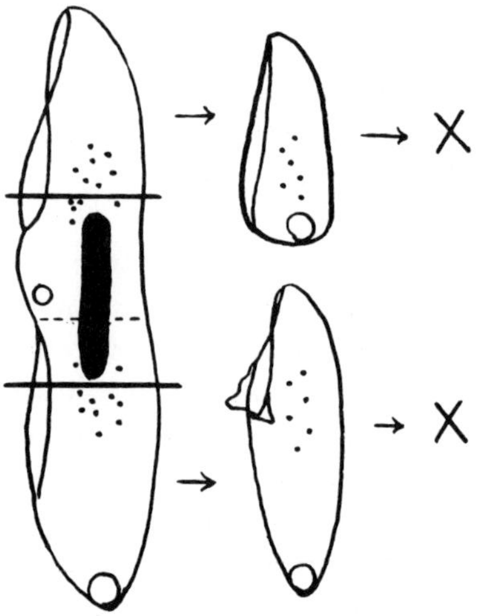

Fig. 8.6. Transection in Stage IV of division to produce amacronucleate fragments containing micronuclei. Broken line indicates the fission line. X symbols indicate degeneration.

sence of the macronucleus, provided it contains oral anlagen that have already started differentiation. Since the micronucleate anterior fragments show no signs of form regulation or regeneration, the restoration of normal form that occurs in the posterior fragment cannot have been mediated by its micronuclei. However, neither anterior nor posterior micronucleate fragments will survive for long without a macronucleus. The macronucleus may therefore be considered essential for regeneration and other morphogenetic events in *Blepharisma*.

The equivalence of macronuclear fragments. Weisz (1949b) claimed that the macronuclear nodes of *Stentor* are equivalent during the early stage of its vegetative cycle, but that the posterior nodes gradually lose their morphogenetic potential in later stages. He also proposed that in *Blepharisma* (Woods Hole strain) the middle nodes of the macronuclear chain lose their morphogenetic potential after the middle stages of division (Weisz, 1949a). He considered that in both organisms this functional difference of the macronuclear nodes does not preexist but is correlated with the position of the nodes within the cell: that is, the nodes acquire high or low morphogenetic potential according to whether they are close to or distant from the highly differentiated oral organelles. However, in *Blepharisma* the oral organelles are level with the midsection of the macronucleus, which should therefore acquire high morphogenetic potential rather than losing it. Furthermore, in *B. japonicum* and many other species of *Blepharisma* the dividing macronucleus forms a compact mass, and no part of it disappears or degenerates (Suzuki, 1957).

To test for functional differentiation in parts of the macronucleus, blepharismas both in vegetative and in different divisional stages were transected into three macronucleate fragments so as to contain anterior, middle, and posterior pieces of the macronucleus (the anterior one-sixth to two-fifths, the central one-fifth to two-thirds, or the posterior one-sixth to two-fifths of the macronucleus, respectively). All the fragments, from both dividing and vegetative cells, always completed regeneration, irrespective of the size of the fragment, the length of the macronuclear piece contained, and the portion of the macronucleus involved. In dividing cells the fragments containing a presumptive division line completed division, and oral organelles regenerated in each of the daughter cells.

Experiments have shown that in *Stentor* (Lillie, 1896; Morgan, 1901; Burnside, 1929; Schwartz, 1935; Weisz, 1948; Tartar, 1959b), *Condylostoma* (Yagiu, 1951a), *Spirostomum*, and *Dileptus* (Sokoloff, 1924), a relatively small portion (as little as one-fortieth) of the macronucleus suffices for regeneration. Below the critical size, however, regeneration fails (Morgan, 1901). We may thus regard the ciliate macronucleus as composed of many "subnuclei," each including at least one complete genome. The subnuclei are derived from the diploid synkaryon formed during conjugation, and presumably develop into a macronucleus by a rapid replication of chromatin in the macronuclear anlagen (Weisz, 1950a; Seshachar and Dass, 1953). Any one of the macronuclear anlagen is able to complete a macronucleus; yet in *B. japonicum* and *B. americanum*, the macronucleus is formed by the fusion of several macronuclear anlagen. It appears that a fragment of reasonable size cut from a fully developed macronucleus is genetically and functionally equivalent to the whole polyploid macronucleus.

Another question requiring attention is why conjugants or early exconjugants fail to regenerate when transected, since each of them must surely contain a full genome in its macronuclear anlagen. Yet until the anlagen show Feulgen-positive reactions they will not support regeneration, and even if the cells are transected when the first positive reactions appear regeneration is very slow. A possible explanation for these facts in molecular terms is given in Chapter 9.

The macronucleus during binary fission and oral replacement. Just how the macronucleus mediates the formation of the cytostome in *Blepharisma* may perhaps be elucidated by experiments in which the macronucleus is removed at various times during division or oral replacement. If the removal occurs at late Stage II division, the cell completes cytoplasmic division, but the daughter cells fail to develop their main feeding organelles completely. Cells emacronucleated at Stage III complete cytoplasmic division and finish both the reorganization of the old oral organelles and the formation of new ones in the normal way. However, the amacronucleate products of the division can neither ingest food materials nor survive longer than four to six days after the operation, during which time the oral organelles dedifferentiate. That formation of the oral area fails in late Stage II and succeeds in Stage III suggests that the macronucleus exerts its effect at an early stage of division.

Similar results are obtained from enucleation experiments carried out during the middle stages of oral replacement. The enucleated individuals complete reorganization and reassume an apparently normal morphology with complete oral organelles; but they cannot ingest food, and die after a few days.

The relation between the macronucleus and the morphogenetic potential of the cytoplasm can be seen more clearly by observing cases in which the blepharismas are bisected into longitudinal halves at different stages of division, the dorsal fragments containing macronuclei and the amacronucleate ventral ones having both original and developing oral areas (Fig. 8.7). The results of this experiment may be summarized as follows.

1. The amacronucleate ventral fragments of Stage I and Stage II dividers are unable to continue division. The developing adoral anlage for the future posterior daughter cell stops growing at the moment of the longitudinal cut. Reorganization of the original oral area never begins in the fragments of Stage I dividers, and it proves abortive in Stage II fragments.

2. The amacronucleate ventral fragments of Stage III dividers complete division and finish reorganization of the old oral area and formation of the new oral area. The daughter cells, though amacronucleate,

Fig. 8.7. Longitudinal cutting to produce amacronucleate ventral and macronucleate dorsal fragments. *A*, Stage I of division. Neither half can divide; the ventral fragment retains its old feeding organelles and resorbs the developing oral anlage. *B*, Stage II. The macronucleate dorsal fragment completes division and oral formation, whereas the ventral fragment cannot. *C*, If the cut is made at Stage III, both halves are able to complete division and oral formation. From Suzuki, 1957.

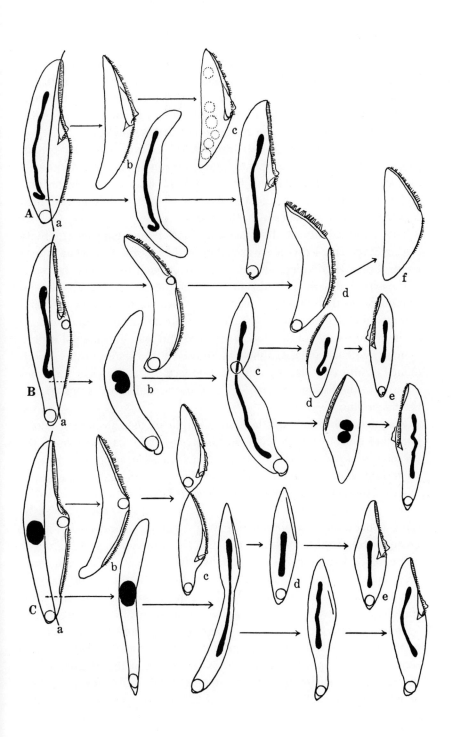

appear normal in morphology; but they do not live longer than three or four days, indicating that the macronucleus is essential not only for the initiation but also for the maintenance of stomatogenesis and fission-line formation, even though it is dispensable for the completion of cyto-plasmic division and the later formation of oral organelles.

3. An amacronucleate dorsal fragment of a Stage I divider cannot continue division, but it is able to regenerate a new oral area and revert to a single normal individual. In contrast, dorsal macronucleate fragments of Stage II and Stage III dividers complete division and then regenerate oral organelles in both daughter cells.

The dispensability of the macronucleus for morphogenetic activity during Stage III of division was tested further by the following experiments. Stage III dividers were transected through the region posterior to the expected path of the fission line, with the developing adoral band as a guide, so that either the whole or an anterior fraction of the band was included in the anterior piece. The position of the macronuclear mass in the middle stage of division is not fixed and may be changed experimentally with a needle. As shown in Figure 8.8, the results of this experiment fall into two classes: those in which the macronuclear mass lies anterior to the fission line (*a–d*), and those in which it lies posterior to the fission line (*e–h*).

Fragments that include the entire length of the developing adoral band are able to restore complete oral structures irrespective of the presence of a macronucleus (*a* and *e*); and those lacking more than the posterior half of the adoral band are unable to do so, again regardless of whether they are macronucleate (*b* and *c*) or amacronucleate (*d, f, g,* and *h*). In macronucleate fragments, however, division is followed by the regeneration of a normal cell with a complete oral area. Finally, posterior fragments retaining more than the posterior half of the developing adoral band regenerate normally whether they are macronucleate (*f, g,* and *h*) or not (*b, c,* and *d*). In two cases (*a* and *e*), the posterior terminal region was also removed from the transected cell, and these fragments, too, were able to complete formation of the oral organelles.

In the middle stage of division (beginning of Stage III), the kineties of the V-area differentiate into primitive oral organelles that will subsequently develop into the definitive form even in the absence of the macronucleus. Amacronucleate fragments remain viable for a few days, as in some other ciliates (Tartar and Chen, 1941; Yagiu, 1951a), and

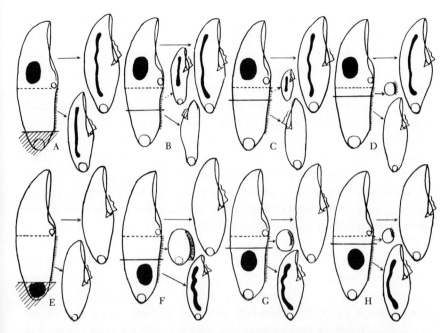

Fig. 8.8. Division and stomatogenesis in the macronucleate and amacronucleate fragments of Stage III dividers. Fission lines, cut planes, and excised regions are indicated, respectively, by broken lines, solid lines, and shading. Length between the fission line and the cut plane in each fragment is as follows (P equals the length of the adoral anlage): a and e, P; b and f, one-half P; c and g, one-fourth P; d and h, one-sixth P. After Suzuki, 1957.

stomatogenesis goes on during this time, apparently as a continuation of the development of preexisting oral anlagen. Amacronucleate fragments cannot complete the formation or regeneration of oral organelles when the posterior half of the developing adoral anlage is removed at this stage, and the regeneration of macronucleate fragments is always confined to fragments bearing anlagen that have already been organized into primitive organelles. Once set in motion, morphogenesis continues but ultimately fails of completion without the macronuclear influence. The possible nature of this influence will be considered in Chapter 9.

The macronucleus during conjugation. During conjugation the old macronucleus condenses into an encapsulated mass and degenerates, and a new one then develops from anlagen originally derived either from a synkaryon or from parthenogametes (see Chapter 2). The anlagen exhibit different responses to the Feulgen reaction before and after the extinction of the old macronucleus. To elucidate whether the morphogenetic function of the prospective macronucleus is in fact correlated with the biochemical change underlying response to the Feulgen reaction, the following experiments were carried out. Conjugating pairs at different stages of either normal or "parthenogenetic" conjugation were separated with a steel needle, and one of each pair was fixed and stained, the other being used for the experiment. Other pairs were allowed to separate and completed their nuclear reorganization normally, after which one exconjugant was fixed and stained and the other used for the experiment. In both cases, the stained cells were used as controls to ascertain the stage in conjugation and the nuclear condition of each pair at the time of the operation. The living cells were either transected into two fragments or had their oral areas excised (Suzuki, 1957).

The fragments produced during the first pregamic division of normal conjugation regenerated completely, whereas those produced during stages in which the conjugants contained haploid micronuclei were nonviable. In all cases, the fragments proved viable only after the macronuclear anlagen in the exconjugant had become strongly positive to the Feulgen reaction, and usually after the disappearance of the old macronucleus. Apparently, the old macronucleus was no longer able to mediate regeneration, whereas the macronuclear anlagen, even a single one, could do so. The time required for regeneration was inversely proportional to the length of time elapsed between conjugation and transection: the later the fragment was transected, the shorter the time. A possible explanation for this in molecular terms will be considered in Chapter 9.

The fragments produced during parthenogenetic conjugation were usually viable, and more often so than those obtained from normal exconjugants. The macronuclear anlagen appeared even when the conjugants had been separated and transected during the first or second divisions of their micronuclei, and they developed parthenogenetically from the progeny of the diploid nuclei produced by the second micronuclear division. As in the case of true conjugation, regeneration did not occur as long as the macronuclear anlagen remained negative to the Feulgen stain. And again, the time required for regeneration after the operation varied inversely with the development of the macronuclear anlagen.

Progressive Specification of the Oral Anlage

The discrepancy in morphogenetic ability between the anterior and posterior halves of the adoral anlagen suggests that the differentiation of presumptive feeding organelles begins early in division, probably before Stage III. To test this hypothesis, some cells were cut at Stage I or II of division, and others when the anlagen were fully formed but the cells were still regenerating oral organelles. In a divider, the developing anlage of the posterior cell, which eventually separates from the anterior daughter cell, was bisected into an anterior piece belonging to the anterior daughter and a posterior piece belonging to the posterior daughter. In a regenerating *Blepharisma* the anlage was simply bisected into an anterior piece and a posterior piece.

When the operation is carried out in Stage I of division or regeneration, both anterior and posterior fragments that have more than about two-thirds of the original anlage will complete a perfect set of oral organelles, without adding a new adoral anlage. Fragments with less than a quarter of the old anlage, however, cannot complete the oral organelles without elongating the small piece of anlage. Only a membranellar band is completed, and the undulating membrane and gullet will not form unless the anlage is able to extend and provide the necessary structures (Fig. 8.9). In Stage II of division, the posterior quarter of the adoral anlage is able to form a short but complete oral area without elongation, but the anterior quarter will only form a membranellar band.

These experiments demonstrate that the separate structures of the adoral anlage are not yet determined in Stage I of division and regeneration, inasmuch as the removal of the posterior portions of the anlage (which are destined to form the terminal spiral of the membranellar band, the undulating membrane, and the gullet) does not interfere with the completion of the oral organelles. But whenever the remaining posterior portion of the anlage is small in size, the oral organelles other than the membranellar band are never formed unless the remaining anlage first elongates. Therefore, the regulation of stomatogenesis is determined by the length, or polarity, of the adoral anlage. It is also reasonable to suppose that the determination of the regions of the anlage may occur during Stage II, since even a small posterior portion of the anlage can develop directly into a set of oral organelles at this stage

194   *Morphogenesis*

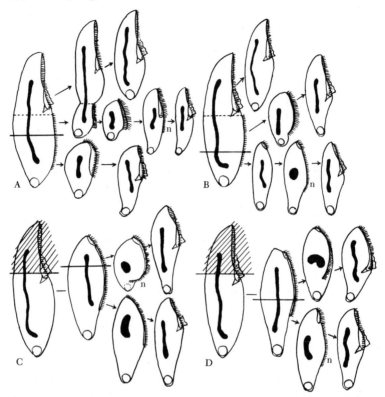

Fig. 8.9. Transections (solid lines) through the oral anlage in Stage I of division (*A* and *B*) and in an early stage of regeneration (*C* and *D*). The anlagen are cut into anterior and posterior pieces in different ratios of length (1:2 in *A* and *C*; 3:1 in *B* and *D*). In some cases oral formation occurs only after the missing anlage has been replaced by a new one (*n*). The presumptive fission line is indicated by a broken line, and excised areas are shaded. From Suzuki, 1970.

without elongation. This assumption coincides, broadly speaking, with the conclusion stated by Tartar (1957), who pursued the problem of the progressive specification of determination in the oral anlage in *Stentor coeruleus.*

Morphogenetic Function of the Oral Area and the V-Area

Oral differentiation in blepharismas always occurs in the V-area, which contains specialized kineties. An analogous type of stomatogenetic area has been observed in *Stentor* (Weisz, 1951), *Condylostoma* (Tartar, 1941; Yagiu, 1951a), and *Spirostomum* (Eberhardt, 1962). If the specialized kineties in the V-area are excised, some of the adjacent ones may acquire morphogenetic properties. But although the kineties of the V-area are "dominant" over other body kineties in that they replace missing organelles, they cannot initiate stomatogenetic activity unless the existing oral organelles are either excised or are undergoing the dedifferentiation incidental to division and oral replacement. These facts suggest that an intact oral area will always inhibit the morphogenetic potential of the V-area.

Inhibition of the stomatogenetic activity of the V-area. Excision of the gullet, either alone or together with the posterior parts of the peristome, always results in regeneration and the induction of a new adoral anlage in the V-area; this happens whatever the extent of the excision, but the length of the anlage formed is proportional to that of the excised parts (Fig. 8.10). When the anterior part of the peristome alone is excised, the results vary with the extent of the excision. The excision of the whole peristome, the anterior three-quarters of the peristome, or the corresponding anterior regions of the body induces a new adoral anlage in the V-area. These facts indicate that the morphogenetic activity of the V-area must be initiated by the removal of the oral area, but not by just the diminution of the body volume. And it should be noted that excision of the anterior part involving half or less of the peristome never induces regeneration until the cell's next division.*

When the *Blepharisma* with such a cut peristome enters the division stage, the future anterior daughter cell undergoes reorganization, producing a short anlage at a region adjacent to the posterior end of the remaining oral area in much the same way as in normal division (Fig. 8.10, *c*). Since the time required for the onset of regeneration is proportionate to the length of the remaining peristome, it appears that the inhibiting function of the oral area depends on its length. About half the peristome length seems to completely inhibit oral differentiation in the V-area.

Induction and inhibition phenomena during stomatogenesis. In the above-mentioned experiments the inhibitory influence of the peristome can be removed by excising the anterior three-quarters of the peristome. This suggests that the inhibitory influence may also be removed when the peristome is moved to the other side of the cell from the V-area. It

---

* Eberhardt (1962), in similar experiments with *Blepharisma*, noted that regeneration proceeded whether the cell divided or not. The discrepancy between his experiments and mine is probably ascribable to the difference in age of the cells used.

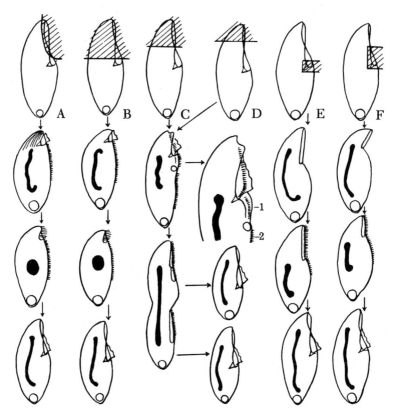

Fig. 8.10. Excision of various fractions of the oral area and the regeneration of a new peristome. The figures 1 and 2 indicate the reorganization anlage and the division anlage. From Suzuki, 1970.

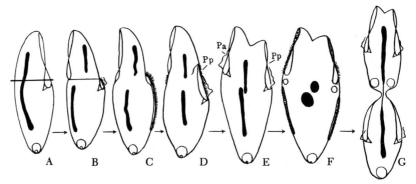

Fig. 8.11. Doublet cells may be formed by cutting the cell body somewhere along the peristome and rotating the anterior fragment 180° before allowing it to fuse. Peristome Pa is derived from the anterior segment, and peristome Pp from the posterior. From Suzuki, 1957.

is also reasonable to suppose that other body kineties might acquire a stomatogenetic potential like that of the V-area if they are moved to the rear of the peristome. To test this possibility, nondividing blepharismas were cut through the posterior part of the peristome, the anterior body was rotated 180°, and the two halves were allowed to reunite (Fig. 8.11).

When the anterior part includes three-quarters or more of the peristome, both dorsal and ventral sides will generate new oral structures. An adoral anlage forms in the V-area behind the posterior quarter of the original peristome, and this new ventral peristome gradually shifts toward the anterior pole of the cell (unless it fuses with the old anterior peristome fragment owing to detorsion of the cut halves). The larger anterior peristome section also regenerates, producing a short adoral anlage in the former dorsal kineties. Thus a doublet cell is formed, with a peristome and a V-area on either side of the cell body.

When a doublet cell divides, two adoral anlagen form simultaneously in the twin V-areas. Twin contractile vacuoles and cytopyges are also formed for the future anterior daughter doublet, but fuse to form a single opening in the final stage of division. Thus once the V-area has differentiated and formed a doublet, similar doublets are produced at every successive division. With repeated divisions, however, the doubled peristomes gradually develop individuality. The doublet first assumes a form presenting the external appearance of a parabiotic homopolar fusion of two cells, which are defined by a longitudinal groove developing on the pellicle. Then the cell becomes a foot-to-foot telobiotic form, and finally splits into two single-peristome cells.

When the anterior body, including the whole peristome, is rotated at the level of the anterior end of the V-area, the region posterior to the oral area and that anterior to the plane of fusion grow to form a new V-area (Fig. 8.12). However, a new adoral anlage develops only after cell division. At the division, two adoral anlagen are produced, one in the new V-area posterior to the peristome and the other in the original V-area. Thus the division produces a single anterior daughter and a doublet posterior daughter. If the anterior three-quarters of the peristome is excised after the whole peristome has been translocated in this way, two adoral anlagen arise before cell division; but the one in the small V-area associated with the remaining part of the original peristome is much smaller than the one in the original V-area (Fig. 8.13). Later the two reorganize to equal sizes, still without cell division.

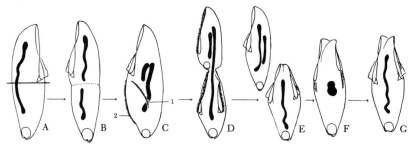

Fig. 8.12. When the anterior body is rotated just posterior to the peristome, two adoral anlagen arise during division; one from the original V-area (C, 1) and one from the new V-area (C, 2). The resulting posterior doublet later adjusts the length of its peristomes by oral replacement. From Suzuki, 1957.

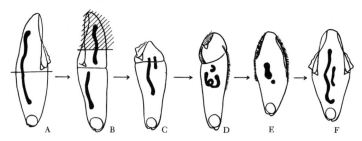

Fig. 8.13. The anterior half of the cell is rotated as in Figure 8.12, but this time most of the peristome is excised as well. In this case a doublet cell will develop even before the cell divides. From Suzuki, 1957.

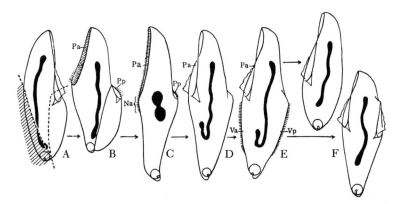

Fig. 8.14. Homopolar transplantation of the V-area to the back of the cell; the original peristome is divided into two unequal fragments (Pa and Pp). Pa regenerates and forms a short adoral anlage (Na), whereas Pp degenerates (in C and D). Before division (e–f) two adoral anlagen arise, one in the new V-area (Va) posterior to Pa and the other in the old V-area posterior to Pp. Division produces one singlet and one doublet. From Suzuki, 1957.

Another test along these lines is the translocation of an amacronucleate ventral fragment (including the whole V-area and about one-fourth of the peristome) to the dorsal region of the cell (Fig. 8.14). Regeneration of the two peristomal pieces is synchronous, and doublets are produced just as they are when the entire anterior region (including three-quarters of the peristome) is rotated. But in most cases only the anterior peristomal piece regenerates a normal structure, and the translocated V-area is unable to initiate the oral organelles until the cell begins to divide.

The results of these experiments can be interpreted in terms of the relation between the V-area and regeneration. Because translocation of the larger part of the peristome leads to the development of a new adoral zone in the V-area, it is natural to suppose that the inhibiting effect normally exerted by the peristome on the stomatogenetic potential of the V-area has been removed. But if the whole peristome is translocated, the original V-area is unable to initiate oral differentiation unless the anterior three-quarters of the peristome is excised (presumably removing its inhibitory influence on the V-area), or until the cell enters the division stage, which is accompanied by reorganization of the peristome.

Another example of this interrelation between regeneration and the V-area is seen when the V-area, implanted into the dorsal region of the cell, fails to initiate oral regeneration until the cell divides or undergoes oral replacement. If the inhibitory effect is based on the interrelationship of the oral area and the V-area when aligned anterio-posteriorly, the inhibition should be removed when the whole oral area is translocated to the other side; but this is not the case. These results suggest that an intact oral area can still inhibit the V-area, even from the opposite side of the organism, so long as it lies anterior to the V-area.*

The inhibitory influence of the peristome decreases during division; consequently, adoral differentiation in the V-area becomes possible despite the development of an intact anterior oral area during the process. Essentially, stomatogenesis in a dividing cell is the same as the process of regeneration in a fragment lacking all or part of the oral area. Moreover, a translocated anterior peristome is able to regenerate any missing portions and form a new V-area; and the doublet cells produced in the subsequent division are for a time able, by induction, to produce simi-

* However, it is possible that the oral differentiation in the V-area of the posterior body may have been caused by mechanical injury to the oral area rather than by alteration of the spatial relation between the oral area and the V-area.

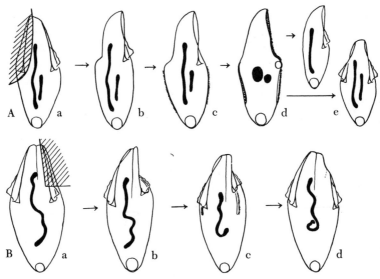

Fig. 8.15. The removal of peristomes in doublets (excised regions are shaded). Oral structures will not regenerate when all of one peristome is removed, as in A; but during division a new adoral anlage arises from the associated V-area (*c*), forming a doublet posterior daughter cell. If only three-quarters of one of the peristomes is removed, as in B, two new anlagen arise, and the peristomes are replaced without division. From Suzuki, 1957.

lar double forms, during successive divisions. This is another illustration of the oral area's function in organizing the specialized kineties of a new V-area: the kineties induced by the fully formed oral area may acquire morphogenetic potential, but the actual initiation of morphogenetic activity is still controlled by the oral area itself. In sum, the anterior oral area seems to control both the induction and the inhibition of the V-area.

These interrelations between the oral area and the V-area were confirmed by a separate regeneration experiment using doublet cells (Fig. 8.15). Complete removal of the oral area on one side of the doublet did not initiate regeneration; and only after the doublet began to divide were adoral anlagen formed posterior to both the intact and the cut peristomes. It is clear that the stomatogenetic activity of the V-area below the excised oral area was inhibited by the intact oral area on the other side, and only began when that oral area dedifferentiated before division. However, if the anterior three-quarters of either peristome is excised, the remaining fragment of the peristome shifts forward, bringing the anterior half of its concomitant V-area level with the intact peristome on the other side. Immediately after this, the repair of the missing oral area and the reorganization of the intact oral area begin simultaneously, producing an adoral anlage in each of the associated V-areas. This suggests that regeneration of a cut oral area, in itself, can induce the reorganization of an intact one.

Similar examples have been reported by Tartar (1958) for *Stentor*. When one set of mouthparts is removed from a *Stentor* doublet produced by grafting, or if a small *Stentor* with mouthparts excised is grafted to a larger cell, a regeneration anlage appears first on the cut (or grafted) side, and an induced anlage then appears on the intact (or host) component. *Stentor* also responds with anlage formation, division, or reorganization when dividing or regenerating cells are fused with vegetative cells (Tartar, 1966a–b).

Polarity in the V-Area

Structural polarity of the oral area. As we have seen, the orientation of oral and aboral differentiation in *Blepharisma* follows the intrinsic polarity of the body kineties, particularly the polarity of the V-area; and anlagen always develop posterior to the structures they reproduce. It would seem that for this reason the extensive, and dominant, oral areas should lie toward the extreme anterior end of the cell. Nevertheless, the main oral organelles—undulating membrane, adoral spiral, and gullet— always begin to form at the posterior end of a developing oral area. More conclusively, when two oral areas fuse end to end, the anterior oral organelles dedifferentiate (except for the membranellar band) and prepare to initiate oral replacement, while the posterior oral structures remain and serve as feeding organelles.

Influence of the anal region on the structural polarity of the oral area. To determine whether the differentiation of *Blepharisma*'s feeding organelles is influenced by the position of the anal region, we must first establish the relationship between the regeneration capacity of the anal region and the anterio-posterior polarity of the cell. A simple way to do this is to compare the time required for the regeneration of a cytopyge in two different cases: one in which the whole posterior body is removed, and one in which only a small posterior region including the cytopyge is removed. (Since it is difficult to distinguish a newly completed cytopyge from an unfinished one, the time required for the first discharge of the contractile vacuole following regeneration should be the figure recorded.) The result is straightforward: the greater the extent of the excision, the greater the time required for completion of a functional cytopyge. Thus the potential for cytopyge formation is clearly highest at the anal pole and diminishes anteriorly.

This characteristic seems to be general in other ciliates that have been studied in detail. Uhlig (1959) demonstrated in *Stentor coeruleus* an axial gradient in foot formation that was highest at the posterior end and also proved strongest on the ventral side, where the oral anlage is formed. The same results have been reported for *S. coeruleus* by Tartar (1956, 1961), and have since been reconfirmed by Uhlig (1962). Eberhardt (1962), working with *Spirostomum ambiguum*, notes that oral differentiation in this species is also closely related to the anal pole. According to him, when the developing adoral anlage is bisected into large anterior and small posterior parts at an early stage of division, the anterior part is resorbed and the posterior part continues oral differentiation.

Weisz (1948) noted that the presence of the holdfast (a posterior terminal structure) also hastens oral differentiation in *Stentor*, since middle fragments regenerate more slowly than posterior ones. And Child (1949) attributed this difference to the fact that middle fragments must carry out regeneration at both head and tail. However, Tartar (1961) has pointed out: "If the presence of a holdfast hastens oral differentiation, then stentors from which the head only is excised should regenerate sooner than animals from which head and tail are removed, but they do not."

In *Blepharisma*, the first exploratory experiment to show the relation between oral differentiation and the position of the cytopyge involved an attempt at the heteropolar fusion of macronucleate ventral and macronucleate dorsal halves cut from a single cell (Suzuki, 1957). The ventral halves were cut so as to include the posterior quarter of the peristome and the whole V-area, with or without the anal region. In the event, the fragments did fuse for a short time. But in all cases they eventually seemed to behave as though they had retained their old polarity: that is, they repelled each other and separated.

The attempt is more successful if the dorsal half of such a heteropolar fusion lacks a nucleus, in which case the fragments are able to fuse successfully in the first place. Although the heteropolar kinety systems reject each other as though they had a magnetic polarity, they are able

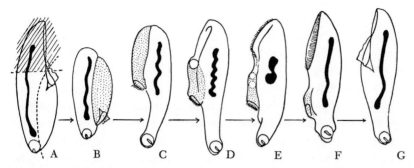

Fig. 8.16. Heteropolar fusion of macronucleate dorsal and amacronucleate ventral fragments. The shaded segment is removed (to prevent the inhibition of regeneration), the cell is cut as shown by the dotted line, and the two halves are reversed in polarity. The dorsal component, seeming to ignore the amacronucleate half, elongates to form a tail-like projection (about three hours after the operation). Eventually, the ventral component degenerates, and regeneration then occurs on the dorsal surface (*e–g*). From Suzuki, 1957.

to initiate regeneration independently when associated with a macronucleus. Apparently, the macronuclear ventral fragment is able to induce a new adoral anlage in the original V-area without being influenced by the amacronucleate dorsal fragment.

By contrast, when the ventral fragment is amacronucleate and the dorsal part is macronucleate, the ventral fragment will not begin oral differentiation within the region of heteropolarity; but the dorsal part produces a normal oral area along the line of union even though its original V-area has been translocated (Fig. 8.16). Oral formation apparently occurs preferentially in the macronucleate fragment, and the resulting oral area inhibits stomatogenetic activity in the heteropolar amacronucleate fragment just as a previously existing peristome would.

This series of experiments shows clearly that in heteropolar combinations a macronucleate segment will dominate one without a macronucleus in controlling regeneration. However, a macronucleate ventral segment will complete the formation of a normal oral structure, provided the intact anal region of the dorsal segment is not near the small fragment of remaining peristome.

When the original anal region of the dorsal segment does lie too near the anterior end of the peristome fragment, stomatogenetic activity in a macronucleate ventral segment may be curiously affected by not one but two antagonistic anal poles: the new cytopyge regenerates at the posterior end of the ventral segment, and the old one in the amacronu-

leate part of the dorsal segment (Fig. 8.17). In the end, this translocation leads to a "bipolar" peristome with two sets of oral organelles, one
at each end. The peristomal groove is bordered by two separate undulating membranes on one side and a continuous series of membranelles on
the other, so that the two ends are mirror images of one another (Fig.
8.18). At the same time the *Blepharisma* as a whole assumes the external
appearance of two cells forming an anterior fusion, even to the extent
of developing a cytoplasmic constriction at the union of the two peristomes. However, the gullet of the reversed peristome is incomplete; and
the anterior body half containing the reversed organelles gradually
shrinks and is eventually either resorbed by the posterior half or cast
away as an amacronucleate fragment.

The reversed oral area just described cannot maintain itself, but it
is able to coexist for a time with a normal oral area in a single *Blepharisma* when the two heteropolar oral areas are structurally independent. As
shown in Figure 8.19, the anterior and posterior halves of the original
peristome, juxtaposed by fold fusion, will reorganize into two independent peristomes through successive oral replacements. It is note-
worthy that only the original posterior portion regenerates a normal
oral area, whereas the anterior half forms a reversed structure with organelles directed toward the anal region (Fig. 8.20).

Thus a bistomal doublet cell with one normal and one reversed oral
structure is obtained. The reversed peristome cannot gather or engulf
food, since its membranelles retain their intrinsic polarity and beat outward, and since its gullet is incomplete. When the doublet divides, two
sets of adoral anlagen arise, one in the original V-area behind the normal peristome and the other in the new V-area formed behind the reversed peristome. These develop into a similar pair of normal and reversed peristomes in the posterior daughter cell. Since the doublets will
yield analogous doublets for as long as two or three generations, it is
evident that even the useless reversed oral area can induce a differentiation of oral organelles in the kineties that lie behind it and stand in
homopolar relation to it.

*Antagonistic function of the V-area and the anal region in polarity
determination.* It is possible that the induction of a bipolar peristome
by the antagonistic effects of a ventral V-area and the anal region of an
amacronucleate dorsal part depends on the anterio-posterior length of
the V-area. To test this, a ventral macronucleate part (including a

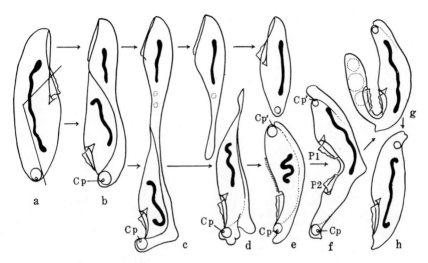

Fig. 8.17 (*above*). Heteropolar fusion of dorsal and ventral fragments, with the original cytopyge (Cp) in the dorsal fragment. When the ventral half, with a small, amacronucleate part of the dorsal half attached, is pulled away from the larger, macronucleate part of the dorsal component (*c–d*), a new cytopyge forms (Cp'), and oral regeneration occurs on the ventral fragment (*e*). The new peristome is bipolar (P1 and P2), but the "mirror" half (P2), nearest the original cytopyge, eventually degenerates. From Suzuki, 1957.

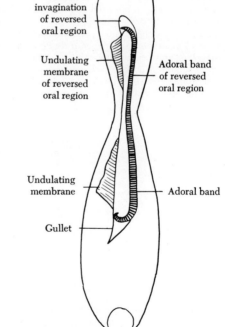

Original cytopyge

Gulletlike invagination of reversed oral region

Undulating membrane of reversed oral region

Adoral band of reversed oral region

Undulating membrane

Adoral band

Gullet

Cytopyge

Fig. 8.18. Schematic drawing of a bipolar cell with normal and inverted structures. From Suzuki, 1957.

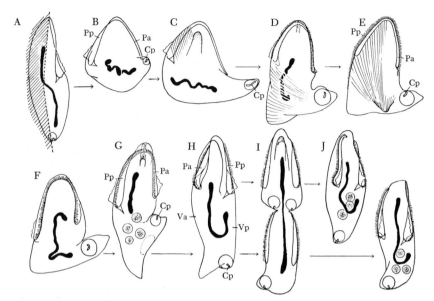

Fig. 8.19. Fold fusion of a cell. The dorsal region is cut away (shaded area in *A*), and the cell is folded back so that the anterior end fuses with the posterior near the cytopyge. After fusion the cell assumes a roughly triangular shape (*B*), with corners falling in the middle of the peristome and in the anterior part of the V-area. The anterior (Pa) and posterior (Pp) sections of the peristome are now heteropolar. Ectoplasmic shifting straightens the V-area, forming a new posterior body, and the midsection of the original peristome becomes a new anterior pole (*C–D*). Eventually a new peristome is developed from Pp by oral replacement; at the same time Pa develops new oral organelles at its posterior end, reversing its polarity. The cytopyge moves to the rear of the cell, and the new V-areas Va and Vp form behind the peristomes (*E–H*). The eventual doublet cell has only one functioning peristome, and its later divisions (*I–J*) will produce similar cells for two or three generations. From Suzuki, 1957.

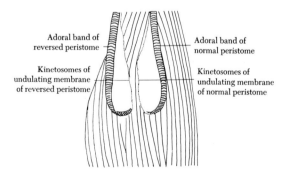

Fig. 8.20. Posterior end of the normal and reversed peristomes in a doublet produced by fold fusion. From Suzuki, 1957.

V-area) was fused in heteropolar orientation with a dorsal amacronucleate part containing the anal region. When the ventral part of the cell includes the entire V-area, the reversal of the anterio-posterior axis is partial and results in the formation of a bipolar peristome. But if the ventral part of the cell is shortened so as to include only the anterior half of the V-area, the effect of the anal region dominates the polarity of the developing or reorganizing peristome, and a completely reversed peristomal structure results (Fig. 8.21). The size of the dorsal fragment has no influence on the results.

This antagonistic interaction between the V-area and the anal region is also revealed clearly by experiments with heteropolar combinations of sister cells. The backs of animals in the middle stage of division were excised longitudinally and the specimens were folded back to make a heteropolar fusion of the anterior and posterior daughter regions. After the complexes had fused, the greater part of the peristome and the posterior body, including the anal region, was excised from one of the components. In every case, regeneration took place in the injured component, accompanying oral replacement in the intact mate. It is worthy of note that the regeneration induced oral replacement in spite of the heteropolar relation of the kinety systems in the two members.

When the deletion of the V-area is less than half the area of the whole posterior body, both the intact and the injured peristomes transform into bipolar structures in most cases (Fig. 8.22, A), presumably because the regeneration of the cytopyge and the contractile vacuole precedes that of the peristome; therefore, each of the peristomes is influenced by the anal regions lying next to it. When deletion of the V-area is greater than half the area of the posterior body, however, the injured component is unable to produce either a cytopyge or a contractile vacuole (Fig. 8.22, B). In this case, the intact peristome maintains its freedom from the influence of its fusion mate; but the regenerated peristome of the injured component becomes a completely reversed structure, since the inherent polarity of the V-area is unable to prevail over the reorganizing influence of the reversed anal region. Thus normal and reversed peristomes are produced in parallel in one cell.

As all these examples indicate, the polarity of oral organelles such as the undulating membrane and the adoral terminal spiral is determined in the peristomal field in relation to the direction of the cytopyge. At the same time, the differentiation of the undulating membrane and the

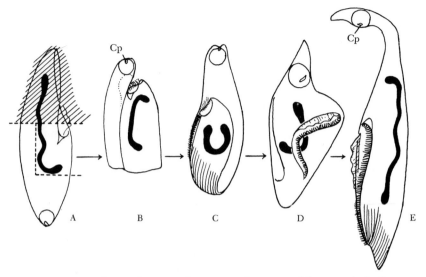

Fig. 8.21. Heteropolar combination of a macronucleate ventral fragment including the anterior half of the V-area and an amacronucleate dorsal fragment including the anal region. The shaded region in *A* is removed, the remaining fragment is cut approximately as shown by the dotted lines, and the ventral fragment is inverted before the fragments are allowed to fuse, placing the remaining peristome next to the cytopyge (Cp). Regeneration occurs in the ventral component, and a completely reversed peristome appears (*D*). At the same time a tail-like projection is formed toward the anal pole of the cell. From Suzuki, 1957.

membranellar band is fixed, respectively, on the intrinsic right and left margins of the peristome. Accordingly, in a reversed peristome the transverse relation of the undulating membrane and the membranellar band is also reversed when observed from a new posterior pole. Clearly, the anterior-posterior axis of the peristome is changeable, depending on the position of the anal region, whereas the transverse axis is fixed in relation to the intrinsic polarity of the kineties, which are arranged according to the "rule of desmodexy" (Chatton and Lwoff, 1935).

Summary

In conclusion, the experiments described here allow certain generalizations about the four essential morphogenetic processes: cell division, conjugation, regeneration, and encystment.

1. The kinetosomes in the ectoplasm are self-duplicating units that

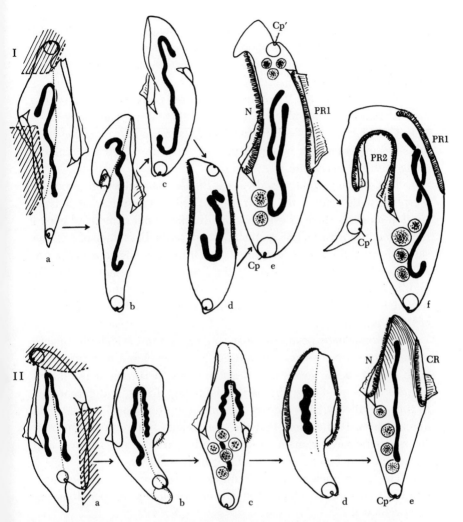

Fig. 8.22. The removal of anal and oral regions (shaded) from one half of a para-biotic heteropolar fusion complex (dotted line indicates the fusion area). In Se-quence I the greater part of the peristome and less than half the posterior body are removed. The injured component regenerates its missing structures (PR1 and Cp'), and the intact component undergoes oral replacement at the same time (*b–d*). The regenerated peristome is bipolar, and the normal peristome (N) of the intact com-ponent soon becomes bipolar as well (PR2). In Sequence II the greater part of the peristome and more than half the posterior body are removed. The injured half regenerates its mouthparts, but not its cytopyge. Here, too, regeneration of the injured component is accompanied by reorganization of the intact organelles; but the regenerated peristome is completely reversed rather than bipolar, whereas the reorganized peristome (N) is normal in structure and orientation. In both sets of drawings food vacuoles are shown at stages in which the cell has at least one intact peristome and can feed normally. From Suzuki, 1957.

produce the cilia. However the pattern and polarity of the cortex play a decisive role in all the morphogenetic processes.

2. The peristome is either reorganized or developed anew in each morphogenetic process.

3. The kineties of the V-area subtending the peristome take an active part in organizing the anlage of a new peristome during morphogenesis.

4. The kineties adjacent to the V-area acquire the morphogenetic potential of inducing a new peristome if the entire V-area is removed along with the peristome.

5. The growing zone in a dividing *Blepharisma* plays an important morphogenetic role; if the ventral one-third to two-thirds of it is excised at an early stage of cell division, division is not completed even if the presumptive fission line is intact. At an intermediate stage of cell division, however, division is completed even if the growing zone or the presumptive fission line is excised. If the fission line is removed after the middle stage, division again fails, presumably because the line has been fully determined by this time and cannot be reinduced in the remainder of the cytoplasm.

6. Micronucleate postperistomal fragments from which the macronucleus is removed soon after cutting fail to develop a new peristome. Such fragments, however, may develop a new peristome if the macronucleus is removed after the peristomal anlage has fully differentiated. In this case the peristome never becomes fully functional and later dedifferentiates. It is evident that the micronuclei alone can neither initiate regeneration nor maintain an already partially regenerated peristome initiated before removal of the macronucleus.

7. The macronucleus is thus required both to initiate and to maintain the peristome in blepharismas from which the old peristome has been removed.

8. All portions of the macronucleus in a *Blepharisma* are equivalent in inducing a new peristome during the various morphogenetic processes.

9. During conjugation, the induction of a new peristome in a postperistomal fragment of a conjugant fails if the old macronucleus has started to degenerate and the anlagen of the new macronuclei have not yet become Feulgen-positive; but a new peristome is induced once the anlagen become Feulgen-positive. The greater the Feulgen stainability of the anlagen, the quicker the regeneration of the peristome.

10. During division, macronuclear influence on peristomal reorganization depends on the stage of division. Removal of the macronucleus early in division prevents induction by the V-area; removal later does not, although the induced peristome never becomes fully functional except in the continued presence of the macronucleus. The macronucleus thus supports the influence of the V-area. Thus in division as in conjugation the specification of the oral anlagen is progressive.

11. The presence of a fully developed oral apparatus inhibits the induction of a peristome by the V-area. Excision of the entire peristome, its anterior three-quarters, or the corresponding anterior region of the body will remove this inhibition, and a new peristome is then produced by the V-area. A diminution of the body volume alone, without V-area removal, does not do this. By the appropriate manipulation of these potentials and inhibiting influences it is possible to make doublet and bipolar cells.

12. The oral area has a distinct polarity, as does the V-area. The oral area of a *Blepharisma* is always located as far anteriorly in the cell as possible, and the main oral organelles (undulating membrane, adoral spiral or membranellar bands, and gullet) are always formed at the posterior end of the peristome. This polarity can be reversed under certain circumstances. However, the relative positions of the undulating membrane and the membranelles are governed by the rule of desmodexy and are not subject to modification by experimental manipulation.

13. The anal area also influences the structural polarity of the oral area. A gradient exists such that a new cytopyge is formed sooner the further posteriorly a cell is transected to remove the old cytopyge. The polarity of the anal area affects regeneration of the oral area, and in certain combinations of dissected pieces of a *Blepharisma* it leads to the development of a bipolar peristome in the regenerant.

14. As a result of these morphogenetic potentials and gradients, the course of division, conjugation, encystment, or regeneration proceeds in an orderly manner, ensuring that a normal *Blepharisma* will be produced and maintained in accordance with the information in the genome of the organism. Deviations from this course are quickly corrected.

15. If the micronuclei seem to have been neglected in this discussion, it need only be remembered that they contain the genome of the cell, which is copied for each daughter cell during the micronuclear mitoses preceding cell division. The micronuclei are also the major

actors during conjugation, at which time the genomes of the two part-
ners are exchanged, and a new synkaryon is formed by the fusion of a
haploid migratory and a haploid stationary nucleus in each partner. The
synkaryon then divides, and among its products are the anlagen of the
new macronuclei, in which the genome replicates manyfold. Thus the
micronucleus is also the source of information for copies of the genome
in the macronucleus. In short, the micronucleus plays the important role
of genome preservation, but apparently delegates morphogenetic functions, trophic functions, and the direction of macronuclear (and possibly other) syntheses to the macronucleus.

LITERATURE CITED

Balamuth, W. 1940. Regeneration in Protozoa: A problem in morphogenesis.
Quart. Rev. Biol. **15**: 290–337.

Burnside, L. H. 1929. Relation of body size to nuclear size in *Stentor coeruleus*. J. Exp. Zool. **54**: 473–83.

Calkins, G. N. 1911a. Effects produced by cutting a *Paramecium* cell. Biol.
Bull. **21**: 36–72.

———— 1911b. Regeneration and cell division in *Uronychia*. J. Exp. Zool. **10**:
95–116.

Chatton, E., and A. Lwoff. 1935. La constitution primitive de la strie ciliaire
des infusoires: La desmodexie. C. R. Soc. Biol. Paris **118**: 1068–72.

Chen, T. T. 1940. Conjugation of three animals in *Paramecium bursaria*.
Proc. Nat. Acad. Sci. U.S. **26**: 231–38.

Child, C. M. 1949. A further study of indicator patterns in ciliate Protozoa.
J. Exp. Zool. **111**: 315–47.

Dawson, J. A. 1920. An experimental study of an amicronucleate *Oxytricha*,
II: The formation of double animals, or "twins." J. Exp. Zool. **30**: 129–57.

Dembrowska, W. S. 1938. Körperreorganisation von *Stylonychia mytilus* beim
Hungern. Arch. Protistenk. **91**: 89–105.

Eberhardt, R. 1962. Untersuchungen zur Morphogenese von *Blepharisma*
und *Spirostomum*. Arch. Protistenk. **106**: 241–341.

Ehret, C. F., and G. D. Haller. 1963. Origin, development, and maturation
of organelles and organelle systems of the cell surface in *Paramecium*.
J. Ultrastructure Res., Suppl. 6, pp. 1–42.

Hirshfield, H. I., and P. Pecora. 1956. Studies of isolated *Blepharisma* and
Blepharisma fragments. J. Protozool. **3**: 14–16.

Ishikawa, H. 1912. Wundheilungs- und Regenerationsvorgänge bei Infusorien. Arch. Entw-Mech. Org. **35**: 1–29.

Isquith, I. R., and H. I. Hirshfield. 1968. Studies of doublet *Blepharisma
intermedium* (Protozoa: Ciliata). Notulae Natur. **413**: 1–6.

Janisch, R. 1969. Morphogenesis and regeneration in the infusorian *Blepharisma undulans americanum*, I: Recovery of form after merotomy. Folia Biologica (Prague) **15**: 63–70.

Lillie, F. 1896. On the smallest parts of *Stentor* capable of regeneration: A contribution on the limits of living matter. J. Morph. **12**: 239–49.

Lwoff, A. 1950. Problems of morphogenesis in ciliates. New York, 103 pp.

McLoughlin, D. K. 1957. Macronuclear morphogenesis during division of *Blepharisma undulans*. J. Protozool. **4**: 150–53.

Moore, E. L. 1924. Regeneration at various phases in the life history of *Spathidium spathula* and *Blepharisma undulans*. J. Exp. Zool. **39**: 249–316.

Morgan, T. H. 1901. Regeneration of proportionate structures in *Stentor*. Biol. Bull. **2**: 311–28.

Peeble, F. 1912. Regeneration and regulation in *Paramecium caudatum*. Biol. Bull. **23**: 154–70.

Reynolds, M. E. C. 1932. Regeneration in amicronucleate infusoria. J. Exp. Zool. **62**: 327–61.

Schwartz, V. 1934. Versuche über Regeneration und Kerndimorphismus der Ciliaten. Nachr. Ges. Wiss. Göttingen, Mathphysik. VI, N.F. **1**: 143–55.

——— 1935. Versuch über Regeneration und Kerndimorphismus bei *Stentor coeruleus*. Arch. Protistenk. **85**: 100–139.

Seshachar, B. R., and M. S. Dass. 1953. Evidence for the conversion of desoxyribonucleic acid (DNA) to ribonucleic acid (RNA) in *Epistylis articulata* From (Ciliata: Peritrichida). Exp. Cell Res. **5**: 248–50.

Sokoloff, B. 1924. Regenerationsproblem bei Protozoen. Arch. Protistenk. **47**: 143–252.

Suhama, M. 1961. Experimental studies on the morphogeneis of *Condylostoma spatiosum* Ozakiet Yagiu. J. Sci. Hiroshima Univ. Sec. B. **20**: 33–81.

Suzuki, S. 1957. Morphogenesis in the regeneration of *Blepharisma undulans japonicus* Suzuki. Bull. Yamagata Univ. Nat. Sci. **4**: 85–192.

——— 1970. Experimental morphology on *Blepharisma japonicum*. Shizen **19**: 1–35. In Japanese.

Tartar, V. 1941. Intracellular patterns: Facts and principles concerning patterns exhibited in the morphogenesis and regeneration of ciliate Protozoa. Growth **5** (Suppl.): 21–40.

——— 1956. Further experiments correlating primordium site with cytoplasmic pattern in *Stentor coeruleus*. J. Exp. Zool. **131**: 75–122.

——— 1957. Deletion experiments on the oral primordium of *Stentor coeruleus*. J. Exp. Zool. **136**: 53–74.

——— 1958. Induced resorption of oral primordia in regenerating *Stentor coeruleus*. J. Exp. Zool. **139**: 1–32.

——— 1959a. Specific inhibition of the oral primordium by formed oral structures in *Stentor coeruleus*. J. Exp. Zool. **139**: 479–505.

——— 1959b. Some effects of altered nucleo-plasmic ratio in *Stentor coeruleus*. (Abst.) Anat. Rec. Suppl. **134**: 645.

——— 1961. The biology of *Stentor*. New York, 413 pp.

———— 1964. Morphogenesis in homopolar tandem grafted *Stentor coeruleus*. J. Exp. Zool. **156**: 243–52.

———— 1966a. Synchronization of oral primordia in *Stentor coeruleus*. J. Exp. Zool. **161**: 53–62.

———— 1966b. Induced division and division regression by cell fusion in *Stentor*. J. Exp. Zool. **163**: 297–310.

———— 1967. Morphogenesis in Protozoa. *In* Research in protozoology (T. T. Chen, ed.), II, 1–116. New York.

Taylor, C. V. 1923. The effect of removal of the micronucleus. Science **58**: 308.

Tittler, I. A. 1938. Regeneration and reorganization in *Uroleptus mobilis* following injury by induced electric currents. Biol. Bull. **75**: 533–41.

Uhlig, G. 1959. Polaritätsabhängige Anlagenentwicklung bei *Stentor coeruleus*. Z. Naturforsch. **146**: 353–54.

———— 1962. Entwicklungsphysiologische Untersuchungen zur Morphogenese von *Stentor coeruleus* Ehrbg. Arch. Protistenk. **105**: 1–109.

Weisz, P. B. 1948. Time, polarity, size, and nuclear content in regeneration of *Stentor* fragments. J. Exp. Zool. **107**: 269–88.

———— 1949a. The role of the macronucleus in the differentiation of *Blepharisma undulans*. J. Morph. **85**: 503–18.

———— 1949b. The role of specific macronuclear nodes in the differentiation and maintenance of the oral area in *Stentor*. J. Exp. Zool. **111**: 141–56.

———— 1950. On the morphogenetic role of the macronucleus during conjugation in *Blepharisma undulans*. J. Exp. Zool. **114**: 293–304.

———— 1951. An experimental analysis of morphogenesis in *Stentor coeruleus*. J. Exp. Zool. **116**: 231–57.

———— 1954. Morphogenesis in Protozoa. Quart. Rev. Biol. **29**: 207–29.

Yagiu, R. 1951a. Studies on *Condylostoma spathiosum* Ozakiet Yagiu, III: The relationship of the quantity of the macronucleus and power of division. J. Sci. Hiroshima Univ., Ser. B. **12**: 122–30.

———— 1951b. Studies on *Condylostoma spathiosum* Ozakiet Yagiu, IV: The relationship between an injury and the power of division. J. Sci. Hiroshima Univ., Ser. B. **12**: 131–39.

———— 1952. Studies on *Condylostoma spathiosum* Ozakiet Yagiu, V: Abnormal phenomenon caused by being kept in fresh water. J. Sci. Hiroshima Univ., Ser. B. **13**: 92–109.

———— 1956. Studies on morphogenesis in ciliates, II: The individuality of the macronucleus in maintenance of the peristome. J. Sci. Hiroshima Univ., Ser. B. **16**: 61–72.

Yusa, A. 1963. An electron-microscope study on regeneration of trichocysts in *Paramecium caudatum*. J. Protozool. **10**: 253–62.

CHAPTER NINE

The Molecular Biology of Regeneration

It is established that both the macronucleus and the ectoplasm of a ciliate are essential to its regeneration (Balamuth, 1940a–b; Weisz, 1954; Tartar, 1967), but the manner in which each produces its effects at the molecular level is still unknown. However, a number of experiments on *Blepharisma* have suggested a possible scheme of the molecular events that occur during regeneration, and we may postulate the following: The injury caused by cutting a cell releases some substance that stimulates the cell's macronucleus to produce messenger RNA (mRNA); and the mRNA, in turn, evokes the protein syntheses required to replace the missing organelles. At the same time, the lysosomes release enzymes that hydrolyze the cellular proteins, thereby liberating the amino acids needed for protein synthesis. It is possible that lipid synthesis is also induced. Since energy transferred by ATP is required for all these synthetic processes, the cell must have reserves of glycogen and other nutrients to provide it.

It is known that soon after a *Blepharisma* is transected kinetosomes begin to multiply in the V-area of the posterior fragment, forming the anlage of the new peristome (see Chapter 8). The peristome as first regenerated is too small, but it is subsequently enlarged by oral replacement. This implies that some message from the ectoplasm, and perhaps specifically from the peristome, has caused the macronucleus to construct additional organelles in the peristome until it is proportional to the size and needs of the cell (Fig. 9.1).

If DNA replication somewhere in the *Blepharisma* (macronucleus, micronucleus, or kinetosomes) plays a role in regeneration, then specific inhibitors of DNA synthesis should delay or stop regeneration, possibly by delaying the formation of the additional kinetosomes needed in the process. The same is true of RNA synthesis and protein synthesis.

All three of these processes, and the action of inhibitors on them, can be detected autoradiographically by using precursor substances labeled with carbon 14 (e.g., ^{14}C-thymidine in the case of DNA); an inhibitor will slow down or stop the incorporation of these precursors. The same methods will show whether DNA, RNA, or proteins must be synthesized to complete the macronuclear cycle. And if the macronuclear liberates mRNA into the cytoplasm of regenerating cells it should be possible to get autoradiographic evidence of the process.

It is self-evident that energy is required for regeneration. One might therefore expect starvation to delay or stop regeneration, since a post-peristomal fragment cannot feed during regeneration and must depend entirely on the stored nutrient reserves it contains. Even in a well-nourished fragment, metabolic inhibitors might prevent the flow of energy necessary for regeneration and so retard or stop it. Since ATP is synthesized by two major pathways—anaerobic and aerobic—it should be possible to determine by specific inhibitors for each pathway which of the two is essential for regeneration, or whether both are.

Finally, it is evident that physical conditions retarding chemical reactions—cold, increased osmotic pressure, hydrostatic pressure (Giese, 1968b), ionic imbalance in the suspending medium, etc.—should reduce the rate of regeneration. Conditions that accelerate the rate of chemical reactions, of course, should also hasten regeneration.

DNA Replication During Regeneration

DNA is present in the micronuclei, in the macronucleus, and possibly in the kinetosomes. The presence of DNA in two or three separate organelles greatly complicates any attempt to interpret the significance of various experiments, and the interpretations are therefore likely to be highly speculative. The micronuclei divide during regeneration in *B. japonicum* (Suzuki, 1957) and in *B. japonicum* v. intermedium (Parker and Giese, 1966); but this is probably incidental to regeneration, inasmuch as amicronucleates regenerate normally (see Chapter 8). The macronucleus of the same species undergoes a complex cycle of change during regeneration, coiling upon itself singly, then doubly, and finally forming a compact ellipsoid of rotation (Parker and Giese, 1966). However, it does not divide or increase in bulk. Whether these events are a requirement for regeneration or a consequence of it is also unknown. In any case, the macronuclear cycle is a convenient marker of events.

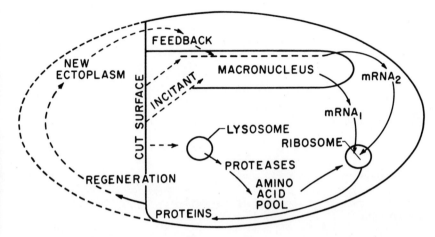

Fig. 9.1. Schematic diagram of possible molecular events in the regeneration of
Blepharisma. An incitant from the cut surface of the cell provokes RNA synthesis
in the macronucleus. The messenger RNA induces protein synthesis on the ribosomes,
which draw on an amino-acid pool resulting in large part from hydrolysis of the
old cellular proteins. The hydrolysis itself is carried out by proteases produced by
the lysosomes, which also seem to be affected by incitants from the cut surface.
A feedback reaction from the regenerated peristome, which is usually undersized,
provokes oral replacement until the new mouthparts are proportional to the rest
of the cell.

There is evidence that the kinetosomes of some ciliates contain DNA,
and some evidence that the DNA replicates during division (see references in Giese, 1970). This is in keeping with the independent replication
of kinetosomes in *Blepharisma* and with their function in regeneration
(a ciliate deprived of its ectoplasm does not regenerate; see Tartar,
1967). The size of the new peristomal anlage, in fact, depends directly
on the number of new kinetosomes formed.

When postperistomal fragments of blepharismas taken from cells that
have just divided (and so are in synchrony with one another) are tested
for the incorporation of ^{14}C-thymidine into DNA, the macronucleus is
seen to take in no more tracer than the surrounding cytoplasm takes in.
But if the blepharismas are taken at random from a population of cells,
and are thus in various stages of the division cycle, some cells show an
increased amount of tracer in the macronucleus, indicating DNA replication. Since the incorporation of ^{14}C-thymidine in this case is sporadic,
it is most likely a result of cutting some cells that are replicating or
about to replicate their DNA (Giese, 1970).

One might expect DNA replication to occur in the kinetosomes of a

TABLE 9.1

Effect of Various Conditions on the Macronuclear Cycle in *Blepharisma*

Condition	Known effect	Effect on macro-nuclear cycle	Source
Size of fragment	Smaller size inhibits cycle		Giese et al., 1963
Species differences		No marked effect	Giese and McCaw, 1963a
Starvation	Removes available energy reserves	Delays	Unpublished
Temperature	Rate of reaction	Cold delays; heat accelerates	Giese and McCaw, 1963a
Hydrostatic pressure	Delays most syntheses	Delays	Giese, 1968b
Far UV light	Affects synthesis of DNA and RNA	Delays	Giese and Lusignan, 1961a; Giese, 1971
X-rays	Affect nucleic acid synthesis	Delay	Giese and Lusignan, 1961b
Metabolic inhibitors:			
KCN	Inactivates cytochrome oxidase	None	Giese and McCaw, 1963b
Sodium azide	Inactivates cytochrome oxidase	None	
Iodoacetic acid	Inactivates glycolytic enzymes	None	
Macronuclear synthesis inhibitors:			
Puromycin	Inhibits protein synthesis	None	Giese, 1970
Actinomycin D	Inhibits RNA synthesis	Delays	
Phleomycin, naladixic acid	Inhibit DNA synthesis	Delay	
RNA-ase	Hydrolyzes RNA	Delays	

NOTE: Most experiments were performed on *B. japonicum* v. intermedium in a constant-temperature room (25° C), except where temperature was a variable.

regenerating *Blepharisma*, which always multiply to form the anlage for the new peristome. However, the resolution of ^{14}C-compounds is very low because of the long pathway the tracer radiation must follow, and one cannot detect the specific incorporation of ^{14}C-thymidine in bodies as small as kinetosomes. I have also used ^{2}H-thymidine, which gives better resolution; but its radioactive emanations have only a short path in protoplasm and cannot be detected at the surface of a large cell like *Blepharisma* (Giese, 1970, 1971). There is, therefore, no direct autoradiographic evidence that thymidine is incorporated into kinetosomal

DNA during regeneration, or that DNA synthesis occurs in kinetosomes. But it is quite possible that the scattered incorporation of tracer often detected throughout *Blepharisma*'s macronucleus and cytoplasm results from just such a process.

As noted earlier, we can gain indirect evidence of the importance of DNA synthesis to regeneration by applying specific inhibitors to a regenerating cell. For example, the regeneration of blepharismas is retarded in the presence of naladixic acid or phleomycin, both inhibitors of DNA synthesis (Giese, 1970; Fig. 9.2). The concentration of these substances required to delay regeneration is much higher than that required to stop the replication of the bacterium *Escherichia coli*, but this may simply mean that *Blepharisma*'s surface is less permeable to the inhibitors. Both naladixic acid and phleomycin also retard the macronuclear cycle (Figs. 9.3, 9.4; Table 9.1).

Regeneration is strongly retarded by mercaptoethanol; and in marine eggs this substance is known to prevent the division of centrioles, which are homologous to the kinetosomes of ciliates. Accordingly, mercaptoethanol may affect *Blepharisma* by preventing kinetosome replication, which would delay the formation of the anlage of the new peristome. If this inhibitor is allowed to act for some time after a *Blepharisma* is cut, its effect is much more striking than if it is applied only briefly (Giese, 1970; Fig. 9.5). Mercaptoethanol also delays the macronuclear cycle (Fig. 9.4).

RNA Synthesis During Regeneration

Postperistomal fragments of *Blepharisma* that are placed in a solution of ^{14}C-uridine soon incorporate this tracer into the RNA they are synthesizing, mainly in the macronucleus (Giese, 1970). Pulse-labeling shows that the RNA formed in the macronucleus gradually leaks into the cytoplasm, and after about ten hours the cytoplasm is almost as heavily labeled as the macronucleus. There is no evidence to indicate whether messenger, transfer, or ribosomal RNA is being synthesized, but the fact that the RNA moves rapidly from the macronucleus into the cytoplasm suggests mRNA. This is the more likely because ^{14}C-uridine is most readily incorporated into the macronucleus when the cut fragment is placed into the tracer solution soon after cutting rather than several hours later.

Actinomycin D, an inhibitor of DNA-dependent RNA synthesis, also retards regeneration (Fig. 9.6). The effect is most striking if the inhibitor

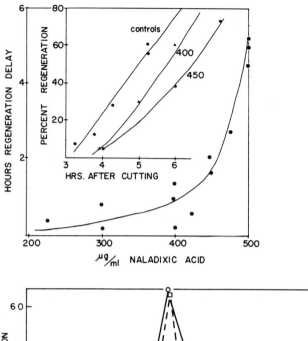

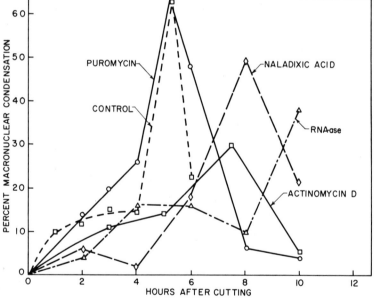

Fig. 9.2 (*above*). Regeneration delay in *B. japonicum* v. intermedium resulting from exposure to naladixic acid, an inhibitor of DNA replication. From Giese, 1970; by permission of the Academic Press.

Fig. 9.3 (*below*). Delay of the macronuclear cycle during regeneration by the application of various inhibitors: naladixic acid (450 μg/ml) throughout regeneration; RNA-ase (20 μg/ml) for the first half-hour after cutting; and actinomycin D (250 μg/ml) for 2.5 hr after cutting. Puromycin at a concentration that normally delays regeneration does not affect the macronuclear cycle. From Giese, 1970; by permission of the Academic Press.

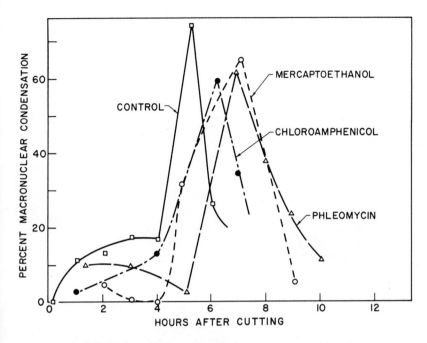

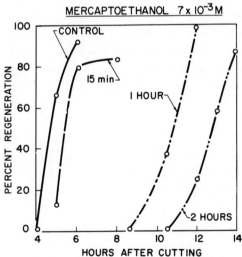

Fig. 9.4 (*above*). Delay of the macronuclear cycle resulting from the application of mercaptoethanol (0.25%), chloramphenicol (.002 *M*), and phleomycin (60 μg/ml); each concentration is one that normally delays regeneration. The mercaptoethanol was applied only during the first hour of regeneration, and the other solutions throughout regeneration. From Giese, 1970; by permission of the Academic Press.

Fig. 9.5 (*below*). The retardation of regeneration by mercaptoethanol applied after cutting and left for varying lengths of time. From Giese and McCaw, 1963b.

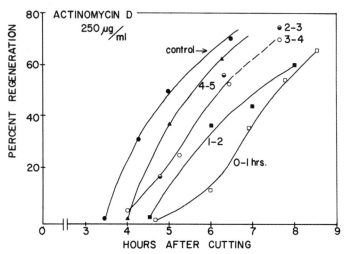

Fig. 9.6. The retardation of regeneration by actinomycin D applied for one hour at various times after cutting. From Giese, 1970; by permission of the Academic Press.

is applied immediately after cutting, or if the blepharismas are cut while immersed in the inhibitor solution; and it is progressively diminished after longer intervals. After even one or two hours the cell has accumulated enough mRNA to start the protein synthesis needed for regeneration. An inhibitor applied at this point may slow down the formation of more RNA; but the effect on regeneration will be small, since much of the protein synthesis is already completed. Actinomycin D also reduces the incorporation of ^{14}C-uridine into RNA (Table 9.2).

The enzyme RNA-ase, which most readily hydrolyzes RNA not attached to other compounds (that is, idle mRNA, transfer RNA, or ribosomal RNA), is known to penetrate amoebas and other cells, probably by pinocytosis. Although ciliates are supposedly unable to take in material by pinocytosis, the regeneration of *Blepharisma* fragments is greatly retarded by RNA-ase, especially if the cells are cut in a solution of the enzyme. Under these circumstances, or if exposure comes immediately after cutting, the enzyme enters and reduces the pyronin (RNA-specific) stainability of the cells; but applied even two hours later it has no effect (Fig. 9.7). If the mRNA is in fact selectively removed by RNA-ase, presumably because of its greater lability, the effect of RNA-ase is apparently much like that of actinomycin D (Giese, 1970).

My experiments show that the exposure of postperistomal fragments to UV radiation retards regeneration in *Blepharisma*, the more so as the UV dose is increased (Fig. 9.8). For a given dose, the retardation of regeneration is greatest if the fragments are irradiated immediately after cutting and decreases as the interval between cutting and irradiation is lengthened (Giese, 1971; Fig. 9.9). The action spectrum for UV retardation resembles the absorption spectra of nucleic acids (Fig. 9.10) but does not distinguish between RNA and DNA (Giese et al., 1965b).

We know that both DNA synthesis and RNA synthesis are sensitive to UV radiation, DNA synthesis generally being the more vulnerable. In the foregoing experiments DNA synthesis in the kinetosomes is possibly retarded by UV radiation, which would thus slow down regeneration. However, the retardation of DNA synthesis in cells is usually subject to photoreactivation (Rupert, 1964), whereas the retardation of regeneration in *Blepharisma* is not. It therefore seems more likely that the inhibiting effect of UV radiation results from its reduction of RNA synthesis, particularly since my tests indicate that the incorporation of ^{14}C-uridine in RNA is decreased by UV irradiation (Table 9.3; Giese, 1971).

The greater effectiveness of UV radiation on postperistomal fragments when applied soon after cutting the cell is also best interpreted as an inhibition of mRNA synthesis. If the *Blepharisma* fragments are irradiated soon after cutting, mRNA synthesis is immediately retarded or stopped, and regeneration cannot begin. As the cell recovers, mRNA

TABLE 9.2

Effect of Actinomycin D on the Incorporation of ^{14}C-uridine
During Regeneration in *B. japonicum* v. intermedium

Time after cutting	Counts over macronucleus	Counts near macronucleus	Counts far from macronucleus	Cells strongly labeled
0.5–3.0 hr:				
Controls	24.0 ± 5.8	11.4 ± 2.7	8.2 ± 2.4	59.8 ± 19.4%
Treated cells	7.0 ± 5.5	4.2 ± 2.9	3.6 ± 2.4	14.2 ± 20.9
3.0–5.5 hr:				
Controls	29.6 ± 10.2	10.6 ± 6.7	4.0 ± 2.8	48.0 ± 143.3
Treated cells	7.4 ± 6.2	4.0 ± 1.2	2.8 ± 1.1	13.0 ± 23.9

SOURCE: Giese, 1970. Cells were treated with tracer and actinomycin (at 250 μg/ml) for three hours in each of five series of experiments. The counts given are averages of six strongly labeled cells in an area of 88 μm^2. In other series I exposed the cells to inhibitor and tracer for only one hour, but in this case the tracer incorporated in the inhibited cells was too little to give a count. The background count was 0–3 per 88 μm^2, the higher figures usually occurring when the total count was higher.

TABLE 9.3

Incorporation of Carbon Tracers into RNA, DNA, and Protein
During Regeneration in *B. japonicum* v. intermedium

Treatment	Count in macronucleus	Count near macronucleus	Count in cytoplasm	Strongly labeled cells[a]
	^{14}C-uridine[b] (0–2.5 hr)			
Control	24 ± 4	13 ± 3	8 ± 3	83%
UV$^c_{3,200}$ at once	21 ± 2	11 ± 4	5 ± 2	55
	^{14}C-uridine[d] (0–3 hr) irradiated at various times			
Control	96 ± 16	65 ± 10	54 ± 11	100
UV$_{4,400}$	59 ± 13	42 ± 10	34 ± 7	100
UV$_{4,400}$ 4 hr later	58 ± 10	50 ± 11	35 ± 8	100
	^{14}C-uridine[d] (0–3 hr) irrad. whole; cut at various times			
Control	95 ± 18	72 ± 19	47 ± 13	100
UV$_{4,400}$ cut at once	72 ± 11	51 ± 9	41 ± 4	100
UV$_{4,400}$ cut 4 hr later	79 ± 15	52 ± 13	41 ± 11	100
	^{14}C-thymidine[d] (0–5 hr)			
Control	84 ± 15	27 ± 11	6 ± 4	60
UV$_{4,000}$	8 ± 7	2 ± 3	0.3 ± 2	12
	^{14}C-leucine[e] (0–3 hr)			
Control	83 ± 19	82 ± 23	83 ± 22	90
UV$_{5,000}$	48 ± 26	47 ± 13	42 ± 11	77

SOURCE: Giese, 1971. All counts give the number of labels in an area of 88 μm².
  [a] Approximately 25 ± 5 cells/expt.   [d] Concentration 20 μCi/ml.
  [b] Concentration 5 μCi/ml.   [e] Concentration 10 μCi/ml.
  [c] UV at 265 nm, dose in ergs/mm².

synthesis begins, and regeneration proceeds belatedly. By contrast, when the fragments are not irradiated until after mRNA synthesis has proceeded for a while, the fact that some of the mRNA is destroyed and its synthesis reduced or stopped does not prevent regeneration from beginning and proceeding as far as possible with the mRNA already synthesized.

Actinomycin D, RNA-ase, and UV radiation all delay the macro-nuclear cycle at doses that also delay regeneration (Figs. 9.3, 9.11). Whether the retardation of the macronuclear cycle is the cause of the delay in regeneration or the result of it is not evident from the data.

It is interesting that although the regeneration rate is almost the same for all the *Blepharisma* species tested (Giese and McCaw, 1963a), the division rates of these species are quite different (see Chapter 4). The reason for this is not evident, but it may rest on the relative importance

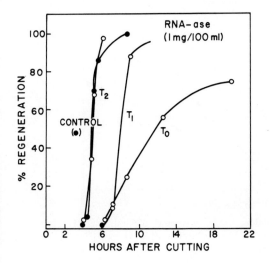

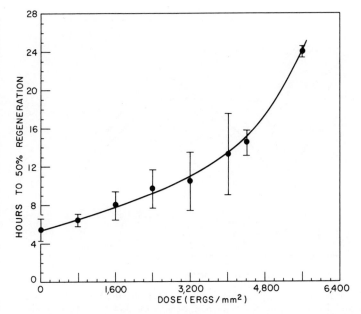

Fig. 9.7 (*above*). Retardation of regeneration by RNA-ase. T_0, cells cut in RNA-ase solution. T_1, cells exposed one hour after cutting. T_2, cells exposed two hours after cutting. From Giese and McCaw, 1963b; by permission of the Academic Press.

Fig. 9.8 (*below*). Effect of increasing doses of UV (wavelength 265 nm) on regeneration in *B. japonicum* v. intermedium (zero dose is the control). Vertical lines represent standard deviations. From Giese, 1971; by permission of the Academic Press.

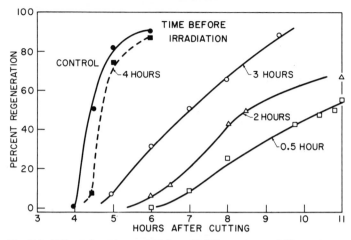

Fig. 9.9. Effect of a constant UV dose (3,200 ergs/mm², 265 nm; intensity about 15 ergs/mm²) delivered at various times after cutting. From Giese, 1971; by permission of the Academic Press.

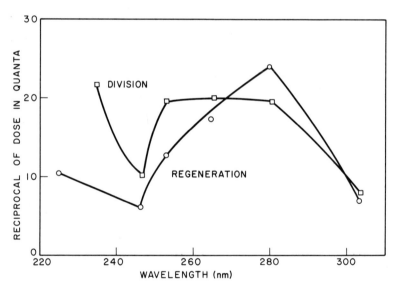

Fig. 9.10. The relative efficiency (action spectrum) of different UV wavelengths on regeneration and division, expressed as the reciprocal of the dose required to produce a ten-hour delay of time to 50% regeneration or time to complete division. The dose in ergs has been converted to quanta. From Giese et al., 1965b.

Fig. 9.11 (*opposite, above*). Effect of two doses of UV (265 nm) on macronuclear condensation during regeneration. From Giese, 1971; by permission of the Academic Press.

Fig. 9.12 (*opposite, below*). The retardation of regeneration by puromycin. The cut cells were immersed for one hour at the indicated time after cutting. From Giese, 1970; by permission of the Academic Press.

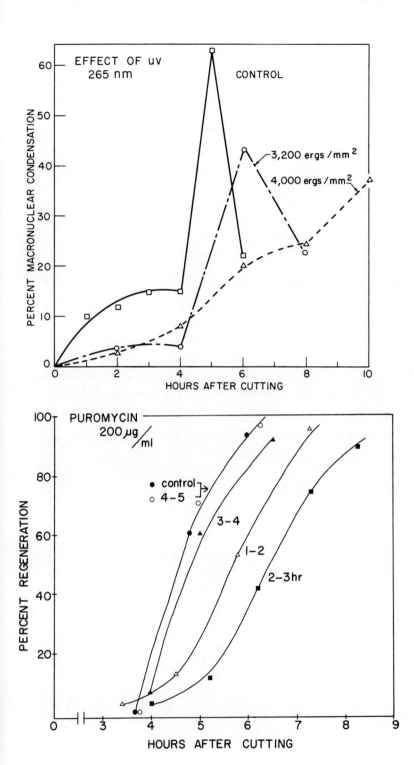

of RNA and DNA synthesis in the two events. During regeneration, RNA synthesis in the macronucleus is quite prominent and continues through the entire period of regeneration, whereas DNA synthesis seems to be minor and secondary (Giese, 1971). During division, on the other hand, DNA synthesis in the macronucleus is prominent (at least in *B. japonicum* v. intermedium), continuing for at least seven hours (Minutoli and Hirshfield, 1968). The dividing macronucleus undergoes the same cycle of changes as in regeneration, but in addition it must increase in size and split about equally between the two daughter cells. It is possible that DNA synthesis takes more time in some species than in others, but no data are available for any other species.

Protein Synthesis During Regeneration

Postperistomal pieces of *Blepharisma* that are placed in ^{14}C-amino acids incorporate the tracers equally well throughout their structure, and the protein synthesis indicated by this incorporation continues for all five hours of regeneration. When the fragments are treated with puromycin, which inhibits protein synthesis, the incorporation of tracers is reduced (Table 9.4). Puromycin retards regeneration (Fig. 9.12), but

TABLE 9.4

Effect of Puromycin on Incorporation of Tracers into *Blepharisma* During Regeneration

Time after cutting	Counts over macronucleus	Counts near macronucleus	Counts in cytoplasm	Strongly labeled cells
Controls:				
0–3.5 hr	40	42	42	70%
0–3.5	49	41	34	58
0–3.5	37	46	36	73
0–3	86.3	86.6	91.0	100
3–6	93.3	93.0	93.0	100
Treated cells:				
0–3.5 hr	17	24	15	32
0–3.5	24	21	21	32
0–3.5	31.5	30	25	39
0–3	39.3	42.3	40.0	100
3–6	39.0	38.0	37.6	100

SOURCE: Giese, 1970. Sum of counts for 88 μm^2 in each of five cells. Protein hydrolysate at 10 $\mu Ci/ml$ (Schwarz Bioresearch) in first three series of experiments; ^{14}C-leucine at 20 $\mu Ci/ml$ (Cal. Biochem.) in last two. The data cited are from illustrative experiments rather than summaries of all of them.

does not affect the macronuclear cycle, which seems to continue at much the same rate as in controls (see Fig. 9.2). Chloramphenicol, an inhibitor that is also supposed to interfere with protein synthesis, delays the macronuclear cycle (see Fig. 9.4); however, this substance is thought to interfere with RNA synthesis as well (see references in Giese, 1971).

Metabolic Energy Sources for Regeneration

Postperistomal fragments of *Blepharisma* do not appear to require oxygen for regeneration, since they complete the process about as rapidly as controls even when placed in a nitrogen atmosphere containing less than 10^{-3} mm Hg of oxygen. Apparently, anaerobic pathways can supply all the energy needed for regeneration. Most protozoans, including *Blepharisma*, will tolerate relative anaerobiosis (low oxygen) for prolonged periods (Beadle and Nilsson, 1959), provided there is enough food available to permit survival.

If oxygen is not required for regeneration in *Blepharisma*, then inhibiting the enzyme cytochrome oxidase, which passes electrons to oxygen, should not retard regeneration. HCN and azide, at concentrations known to stop respiration by this means in most cells, were tried and had no effect on the rate of regeneration (Giese and McCaw, 1963b). High concentrations of both these poisons do retard regeneration, but when they do the blepharismas are usually in a precytolytic state. Indeed, almost any chemical in a high enough concentration will have much the same effect (McCaw, 1962).

However, if anaerobic pathways furnish the energy for regeneration in *Blepharisma*, inhibiting them should retard or stop regeneration. Tests have indicated that this is indeed the case. For example, iodoacetate, which inhibits anaerobic respiration even at a concentration as low as $2.5 \times 10^{-4} M$, markedly retards regeneration (Fig. 9.13). The same effect is produced by dinitrophenol, which uncouples the enzymes that transfer the energy liberated during metabolism and permit the formation of high-energy phosphate bonds (Giese and McCaw, 1963b). High-energy phosphate compounds are necessary for regeneration, and those produced by *Blepharisma*'s anaerobic pathways appear sufficient. This does not mean that the energy liberated by aerobic reactions is not also used when available, but only that anaerobic liberation suffices whenever aerobic liberation is suppressed. By contrast, cell division will not take place unless oxygen is present. Apparently, some of the synthetic reactions occurring in cell division are different, even though morphogenesis is similar in both processes (see Chapter 8).

Since most agents that affect the rate of regeneration also retard the macronuclear cycle of condensation and reelongation, the effect of iodoacetate on that cycle was tested and was found to be relatively slight (Giese, 1970; Fig. 9.14). The greatest macronuclear condensation occurred a bit later than in the control, but the difference was well within the error of the measurements; elongation was delayed about an hour. It would seem that iodoacetate also affects regeneration at some point other than the macronuclear cycle.

Some investigators have preferred to starve ciliates before regeneration experiments because it is much easier to see the organelles in starved specimens. However, *Blepharisma* fragments recover and regenerate most rapidly if they come from well-fed cells. Fragments from cells in various stages of starvation show a progressive retardation of the process, and those cut after four days of starvation fail to regenerate. Even starved blepharismas that are fed bacteria just before cutting will usually recover their capacity to regenerate at a normal rate

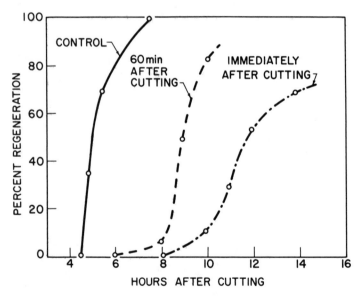

Fig. 9.13. The retardation of regeneration by iodoacetate ($2.5 \times 10^{-4}\ M$) applied at different times. After treatment for 15 minutes the cell fragments were washed in balanced salt solution. From Giese and McCaw, 1963b; by permission of the Academic Press.

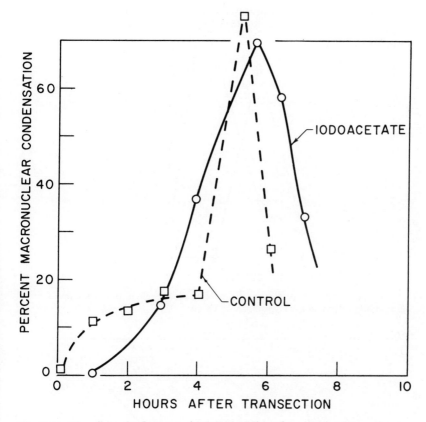

Fig. 9.14. The effect of iodoacetate ($2.5 \times 10^{-4}\,M$) on the macronuclear cycle during regeneration. From Giese, 1970; by permission of the Academic Press.

only after the food has been digested and incorporated in the cell (Giese and McCaw, 1963a). The macronuclear cycle is also delayed by starvation (Moreton and Giese, unpublished; Fig. 9.15).

Postperistomal fragments of *Blepharisma*, unless starved for a few days, regenerate fully even in a medium completely without food organisms. Furthermore, the rate of regeneration is the same whether the fragments are placed in a balanced salt solution or in an axenic nutrient medium. Thus regeneration can occur using only stored reserves.[*]

[*] Since protozoan cells vary in their content of food reserves, some are able to regenerate even when starved. Weisz (1954) points out that glycogen reserves are required for regeneration in *Stentor*, which fails to regenerate without glycogen even when oil droplets remain; but Tartar (1961) did not find this to be general for *Stentor*.

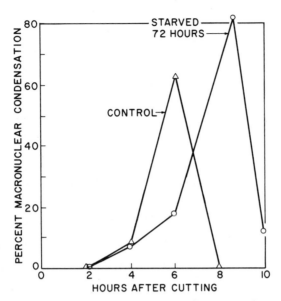

Fig. 9.15. The effect of starvation on the macronuclear cycle in *B. japonicum* v. intermedium. From data of Moreton and Giese.

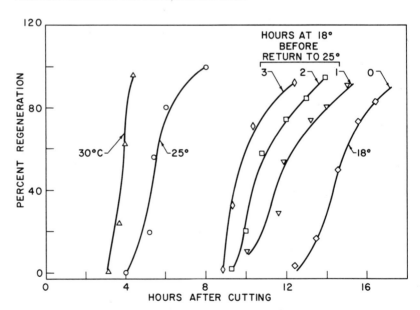

Fig. 9.16. The regeneration of postperistomal fragments at 30°, 25°, and 18° C, and at 25° after various periods of exposure to 18° immediately after cutting. Data from Giese and McCaw, 1963a; by permission of the Academic Press.

Effect of Temperature on Rate of Regeneration

Blepharisma grows well between 15 and 30° C. Above 30° it grows more slowly, and below 15° it does not grow at all unless the cells are acclimated for long periods (see Chapter 4). Regeneration takes place over much the same range: slowly at 13° and most rapidly at 30°. At 35° blepharismas regenerate more slowly than at 30°. If the cut cells are kept at 25° and placed at 30° later, regeneration is even faster (Giese and McCaw, 1963a).

Blepharismas kept at 25° C, cut and placed at 40° for five minutes, and then returned to 25°, regenerate at a much reduced rate. The retardation is the same regardless of whether the fragments are exposed to the higher temperature immediately after cutting (15 minutes) or as much as four hours later. It does increase progressively with longer exposure to 40°, but the data are too variable to reveal a systematic pattern. If the transected blepharismas are placed at a lower temperature after cutting, their regeneration is slowed in proportion to the time spent at the lower temperature (Fig. 9.16). Apparently, some reaction needed for regeneration is being slowed down by temperatures markedly higher or lower than that to which the cells are acclimated (Giese and McCaw, 1963a).

When *Blepharisma* fragments are placed at 5° C they shed a cloud of pigment and contract to a rounder shape, just as whole cells do. Also, a good many fragments cytolyze almost immediately: when I exposed two groups of 30 fragments to 5°, seven recovered in one case and 16 in the other. The fragments that recover regenerate at about the same rate as controls when returned to 25°. If cultures of *Blepharisma* are slowly acclimated to 5°, the cells do not shed pigment; and if they are cut and placed at 25°, they regenerate at about the same rate as those acclimated to 25° (Giese and McCaw, 1963b).

When blepharismas are cut and kept at lower or higher temperatures, the macronuclear cycle that accompanies regeneration is retarded or speeded up. Macronuclear contraction and elongation proceed continuously and in the same manner as at 25° C, and no one stage is selectively inhibited. The cycle takes about five hours at 25°, and about 25 hours at 13°; at 30° it is accelerated by three hours (Giese and McCaw, 1963a).

The temperature coefficients for complete regeneration in the ranges

13–18°, 18–25°, and 25–30° are, respectively, 6.9, 3.9, and 1.6 (Giese and McCaw, 1963a). These values resemble those obtained for many other biological processes and in many other organisms, although significantly lower coefficients have been reported for regeneration in *Stentor* (Weisz, 1948). At present, one cannot say whether regeneration is delayed by temperature change because some macromolecular reaction is selectively stopped by high or low temperature, or whether an altered temperature increases or decreases the rate of other necessary reactions in the cell and thus throws them out of step with the regenerative process.

Role of the Macronucleus in Regeneration

If the macronucleus of *Blepharisma* is removed from a fragment immediately after cutting, regeneration will not occur. If it is removed shortly after regeneration has begun, the process is completed but the cell subsequently dedifferentiates and dies. The macronucleus is therefore necessary not only for inducing regeneration but also for maintaining the differentiated organelles of the peristome (Suzuki, 1957; see Chapter 8). This fact is also apparent in experiments that involve removing the macronuclei from exconjugants. An exconjugant contains both an old macronucleus and the developing anlage of a new one. If the old macronucleus is removed soon after union and before the new one has become at least somewhat Feulgen-positive (i.e., has synthesized some DNA), the exconjugant will not regenerate if cut. The rate of regeneration increases as Feulgen stainability increases (Fig. 9.17), and fragments with fully differentiated macronuclei will regenerate as rapidly as nonconjugants with untouched nuclei (Suzuki, 1957). Thereafter, as the old macronucleus fragments and loses its Feulgen stainability, it no longer synthesizes DNA; but the new macronuclei do, becoming increasingly Feulgen-positive.

Presumably, regeneration fails when the macronucleus is removed right after transection because no mRNA can be synthesized to initiate the process. If regeneration has proceeded for several hours, by the same reasoning, it can be completed without a macronucleus because enough mRNA has been accumulated; the dedifferentiation that often occurs after this implies that the newly completed peristome is too small and must be enlarged by oral replacement. Normally, the incitement for enlargement of the peristome is probably sent to the macronucleus

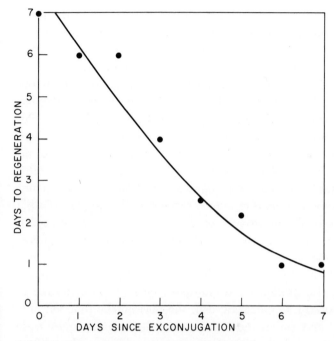

Fig. 9.17. The relation between regeneration and the state of the postconjugation nucleus in *B. japonicum*. Data from Suzuki, 1957.

by the cortex, inducing the production of mRNA to control the process of dedifferentiation and replacement. Perhaps there is always such a continuing communication between macronucleus and cortex even in a vegetative cell (see Fig. 9.1); this would mean that the macronucleus of *Blepharisma* is continuously synthesizing mRNA.

The failure of regeneration at certain stages of conjugation may also be interpreted on this basis. Conjugants transected soon after pairing, when the old macronucleus still has intact DNA, will regenerate. When the old macronucleus loses its reaction to the Feulgen stain and the new macronuclear anlagen have not yet developed one, regeneration does not occur. Presumably, the amount of DNA present at this stage is too slight to give a positive reaction to the Feulgen reagents in either macronucleus; therefore, even if the macronuclear anlagen produce mRNA, they produce so little that the regeneration of the peristome would take almost infinite time. Only as the anlagen enlarge and become Feulgen-positive are they capable of synthesizing much more mRNA. The larger and more Feulgen-positive they become, the more mRNA they can produce, and the sooner regeneration will be completed.

It has been demonstrated by Suzuki (1957) that *Blepharisma japonicum* fragments containing micronuclei but no macronucleus whatever cannot regenerate. This has been found to be true generally among the ciliates (Tartar, 1967). Micronuclei occur in large numbers in *Blepharisma*; and they contain the complete genome of the cell's DNA, which provides the genome for macronuclear DNA after conjugation. Theoretically, they should also be able to produce various types of RNA, including mRNA. But even if the micronuclei did produce mRNA after the injury or transection of an amacronucleate *Blepharisma*, the amount produced might be too small to induce regeneration in any observable time (as is true of the macronuclear anlagen in early exconjugants). It is also possible that the micronuclei are incapable of producing RNA. This has been shown to be the case in *Paramecium aurelia*: in this species the synthesis of RNA is a trophic function assigned to the macronucleus, which also produces the multiple copies of DNA needed to carry on the work of an enlarging cell; the micronuclei function only in cell division and conjugation, preserving the original DNA code (Gorovsky and Woodward, 1969). No comparable data for *Blepharisma* are available on this point.

It has been found that in metazoan nuclei DNA exists in two forms, genetic and metabolic. The genetic DNA replicates during cell division but otherwise remains inactive. The metabolic DNA, formed by multiple replication from the genetic DNA, transcribes RNA required for the metabolic functions of the cell—for example, it produces ribosomal RNA. Should the metabolic DNA need replenishing, the genetic DNA could presumably reactivate and replicate at any point in the cell's normal cycle. The probable reason for the whole arrangement is that DNA is sometimes altered during transcription; therefore, the master code is kept apart from its metabolic counterparts. Codon multiplicity in chromosomes may vary in different tissues, depending on their metabolic functions (Flamm, 1972). In ciliates the genetic DNA seems to be confined to the micronucleus; the metabolic DNA is solely in the macronucleus, where it exists in high polyploidy and presumably in high multiplicity. A ciliate probably exemplifies the extreme separation of genetic and metabolic DNA, which could be a useful trait in a cell so large and so complex morphogenetically. The presence of many pores in the macronuclear envelope of *Blepharisma*, and their absence from the micronuclear envelope (see Chapter 3), would seem to substantiate this view.

The Effect of X-rays on Regeneration

Although the investigation of this point is still incomplete, irradiation with X-rays seems to delay the regeneration of *Blepharisma*, the effect increasing with dose (Fig. 9.18). A given dose delays regeneration in air more than in nitrogen, presumably owing to the indirect effect of the injurious oxidizing radicals that are produced in the aqueous medium of the cell when oxygen is present. The effect of X-rays is greater if they are applied three hours after transection rather than within the first two hours; it declines thereafter, and by 4.5 hours after transection it has little effect (Fig. 9.19). Clearly, some critical event occurs three to four hours after transection; and since X-rays are known to affect nuclear activity and chromosomes, the nuclear events during *Blepharisma*'s regeneration are probably the critical ones. Between three and four hours, the micronuclear premetaphase reaches its peak, and macronuclear condensation is proceeding rapidly (Fig. 9.20). The micronuclear activity is thought to be incidental (see Chapter 8); but the macronuclear condensation is also delayed by X-rays in proportion to the dose administered (Giese and Lusignan, 1961b).

Since UV radiation also delays macronuclear condensation in *Blepharisma*, it seems inconsistent that UV retards regeneration most strikingly if it is applied immediately after cutting, whereas X-rays are most effective several hours after cutting. Possibly, UV affects both macronuclear condensation and RNA synthesis, the second being more important to the overall process of regeneration.

If UV radiation does reduce RNA functioning during regeneration, then it should act additively rather than synergistically with some other factor that affects RNA functioning, since both affect the same substrate. We have seen that RNA-ase delays regeneration, presumably by decomposing labile and unattached RNA. Therefore, we treated *Blepharisma* fragments with both RNA-ase and UV radiation, as well as with UV radiation alone and RNA-ase alone (Fig. 9.21). The effects of the two were indeed additive, not synergistic. A dose of UV radiation too small to retard regeneration by itself did not accentuate the effect of cutting the cells in RNA-ase solution; and a dose that could retard regeneration for several hours lengthened the effect of RNA-ase by that time.

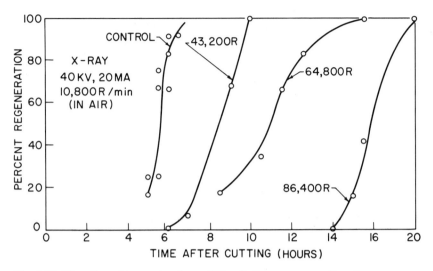

Fig. 9.18. The effect of increasing doses of X-radiation on regeneration of post-peristomal fragments in *B. americanum*. X-rays of 40 kilovolts and 20 milliamperes were applied at 10,800 roentgens/min for 4, 6, and 8 minutes; exposure occurred one hour after cutting. The fragments were kept in a normal atmosphere throughout regeneration. Data from Giese and Lusignan, 1961b.

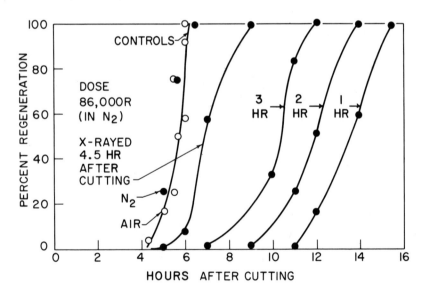

Fig. 9.19. The effect of a constant dose of X-radiation (86,000 R) applied at different times. For this test the cells were kept in a nitrogen atmosphere in order to minimize the formation of oxidizing radicals (some controls were kept in normal air). Voltage and amperage same as Figure 9.18. Data from Giese and Lusignan, 1961b.

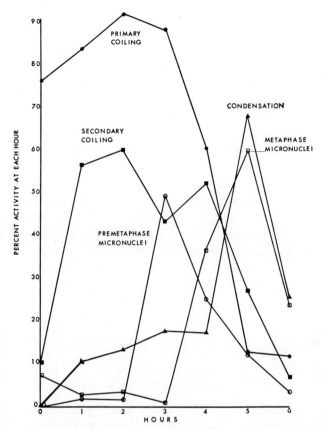

Fig. 9.20. Percentage of cells showing various nuclear activities during each hour of regeneration in *B. japonicum* v. intermedium. From Parker and Giese, 1966.

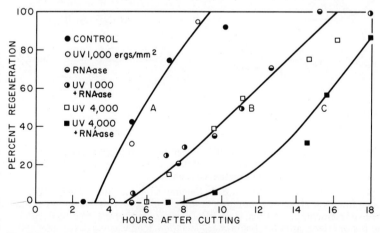

Fig. 9.21. The additive retarding effect of RNA-ase and UV (265 nm) on regeneration in *B. japonicum* v. intermedium. Unpublished data of McCaw and Giese.

Note on Laboratory Methods

Aside from the theoretical material so far discussed, readers may be interested in some of the practical aspects of regeneration experiments as described in this and other chapters (Fig. 9.22).

A flexible glass needle for cutting cells can be made by pulling a fine filament between two soft glass rods (5 mm diameter) heated in a Bunsen flame; one, heated just a little longer than the other, is the source of the needle, and the other receives the residual glass. Some students have pulled successful needles from plastics, which will not break in use as easily as glass. A long, rigid eyelash (preferably from a hog) mounted with Scotch tape on a wooden handle 3 mm in diameter also serves very well. Dr. Suzuki uses two fine, flexible steel needles for the intricate operations described in Chapter 8—one needle to hold the cell in place, and the other to cut fragments and guide them to new locations.

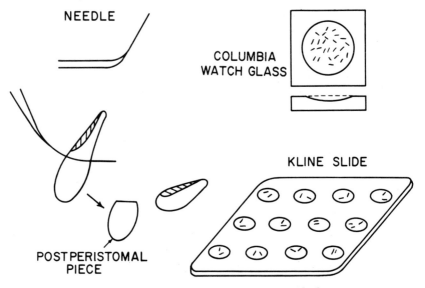

Fig. 9.22. Basic equipment for regeneration experiments on *Blepharisma*. *Left*: a cutting needle and the process of transection (the cell shown is greatly enlarged in relation to the needle). *Right*: observation containers.

Fig. 9.23 (*opposite*). Regeneration in *B. japonicum* v. intermedium. *Top left*: post-peristomal fragment about one hour after cutting. *Top right*: two hours after cutting. *Center*: two fragments about three hours after cutting. *Bottom left*: four hours after cutting. *Bottom right*: after five hours of regeneration, food vacuoles have appeared, but the peristome is still small and will later be reorganized. All photos × 350.

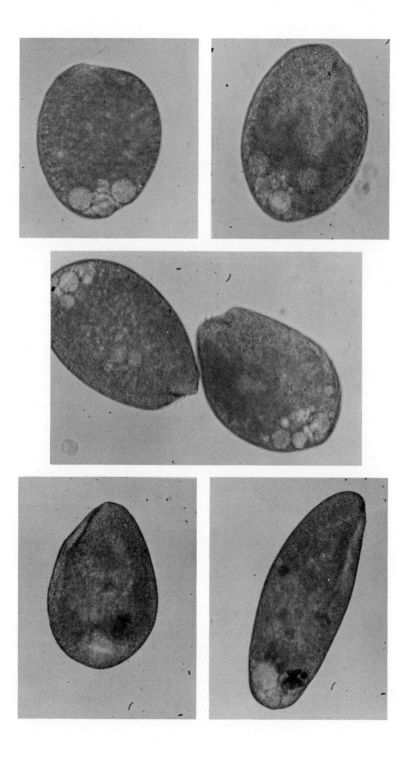

The *Blepharisma*, held in a Columbia watch glass under a dissecting microscope, is allowed to swim under the needle, which is then rocked gently from one side to the other to transect the cell. With practice, one can section almost anywhere on the organism, and the removal of the peristome is relatively easy. The resulting postperistomal fragments are placed in pairs in the twelve concavities of a Kline agglutination slide containing culture medium or balanced salt solution (see Chapter 4); each slide is moist-chambered in a Petri dish, which is itself moist-chambered in a large dish and kept at room temperature or at 25° C in an incubator.

The fragments are observed under the low power of a dissecting microscope about every half hour, and the number of fragments that have regenerated functional mouthparts (as indicated by the formation of food vacuoles) is recorded. The percentage of cells forming food vacuoles is plotted against time (e.g., as in Fig. 9.6), and the difference in hours between the times of 50% regeneration in experimental and control sets gives a measure of regeneration delay (or acceleration). *Blepharisma*'s mouthparts appear to regenerate fairly rapidly at 25° (Fig. 9.23), but the objective test is the appearance of food vacuoles. (If balanced salt solutions are used, one must add a suspension of bacteria about four hours after transection to provide for the formation of food vacuoles.)

If Kline slides are not available, a substitute can be made from a cover slip and a slide. Vaseline is liquified by heat, sucked up in a warmed fine-mouth pipette (see Chapter 4), and blown out to form a ring on the slide. The blepharismas are placed in a drop of medium on the cover slip, and the ring on the slide is inverted over this to make an all-around seal. When this technique is used the fragments may be observed under a compound microscope, and more detail is visible. Alternatively, the cover slip may be mounted with vaseline on a well slide containing a little water. Either mount is satisfactory for classroom work.

The size of a *Blepharisma* fragment affects its rate of regeneration to some extent: the larger the fragment, the more rapidly the cell regenerates; and in very small pieces the rate may be slowed still further because much of the V-area has been excised (Fig. 9.24; see also Chapter 8). Obviously, one should use pieces of about the same size for repeatable experiments; but it is difficult to cut pieces to an exact size,

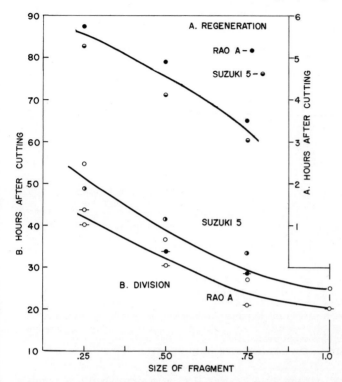

Fig. 9.24. At *A* is shown the regeneration rate of two *Blepharisma* strains cut to different volumes. At *B*, the division rates of cells regenerated from disparate fragments of this kind. From Giese, Recher, and Berry, 1963.

and a certain variability in results is unavoidable. Variations in the environment also influence regeneration. In general, one must run several series of experiments to test a point at issue.

Anterior fragments may also be used to study regeneration in *Blepharisma,* but it is more difficult to follow the course of regeneration in this case because it must be determined by the observation of oral replacement and dedifferentiation of mouthparts, which requires a high magnification. Moreover, the rate of regeneration in anterior fragments is in general slower than regeneration in postperistomal fragments. Division in a regenerated anterior fragment is also slower (Fig. 9.25), indicating that the complete replacement of missing organelles and subsequent growth to division size have taken longer. (Part of the delay certainly results from the smaller volume of anterior fragments, which

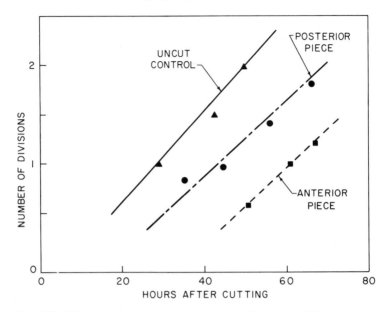

Fig. 9.25. Division rates in anterior and posterior fragments of *B. japonicum* v. intermedium. Division was used as a measure of the time required for regeneration because even the closest observations of a regenerating anterior fragment proved too subjective. In all cases the anterior fragments were smaller.

I have usually cut much as in Fig. 9.22.) In other respects, such as nuclear behavior or the incorporation of labeled nucleic acids, anterior and posterior pieces behave much the same. However, for most purposes, a postperistomal fragment is preferable to an anterior fragment (Giese, Broker, and Cheung Ho, unpublished).

Unless otherwise stated, 24 fragments were isolated in Kline slides for each experimental test. The percent regenerating was determined for each hour after cutting. Each point on a graph therefore represents the average for 24 cells. Three tests were performed to test each experimental variable unless the data were inconsistent and required more tests. Graphs usually represent one set of tests because the timing was not always the same on a series of three.

Another variable that affects the rate of regeneration in postperistomal fragments is the time since the cell's last division. If blepharismas are cut soon after division, regeneration is markedly delayed; from 8 to 16 hours after division the regeneration rate is almost constant; and from that time until a second division (about three hours more at room temperature) the rate is accelerated. It is difficult to get accurate data on this point, but the general trend is quite evident. The time required for the first postregeneration division of the cut cells is also an index of the relative rate of recovery. Those cut 2 to 4 hours after division regenerate and divide 36 hours later; those cut 8 to 16 hours after division regenerate and divide 26 hours later; and those cut very late in the division interval will regenerate more rapidly and divide 18 to 20 hours later (Kost, Gibson, and Giese, unpublished). One reason for the differences in regeneration rate during the division interval may be the amount of body substance available at the time the blepharismas are cut, there being more later in the division interval than earlier.

LITERATURE CITED

Balamuth, W. 1940a. Contributions to the problem of regeneration in protozoa. Amer. Naturalist **74**: 528–41.
———— 1940b. Regeneration in Protozoa, a problem in morphogenesis. Quart. Rev. Biol. **15**: 290–337.
Beadle, L. C., and J. R. Nilsson. 1959. The effect of anaerobic conditions in two heterotrich ciliate Protozoa from papyrus swamps. J. Exp. Biol. **36**: 583–87.
Dollinger, M., and A. C. Giese. 1957. Effect of some carcinogens upon the rate of regeneration in *Blepharisma*. Anat. Rec. **125**: 639–40.
Flamm, W. G. 1972. Highly repetitive sequences of DNA in chromosomes. Int. Rev. Cytol. **32**: 1–51.
Giese, A. C. 1968a. Cell physiology. Philadelphia, 671 pp.
———— 1968b. The effect of hydrostatic pressure and heavy water upon regeneration in *Blepharisma*. Exp. Cell Res. **52**: 370–78.
———— 1970. Macromolecular syntheses during regeneration in *Blepharisma* determined by specific inhibitor and incorporation of ^{14}C tracers. Exp. Cell Res. **61**: 91–102.
———— 1971. Nucleic acid and protein synthesis, as measured by incorporation of tracers during regeneration in UV-treated *Blepharisma*. Exp. Cell Res. **64**: 218–26.
Giese, A. C., and M. W. Lusignan. 1961a. Retardation of regeneration and division of *Blepharisma* by ultraviolet radiation and its photoreversal. J. Gen. Physiol. **44**: 543–54.
———— 1961b. Regeneration and division of *Blepharisma* following X-irradiation. Exp. Cell Res. **23**: 238–50.
Giese, A. C., and B. K. McCaw. 1963a. Regeneration rate of *Blepharisma* with special reference to temperature. J. Protozool. **10**: 173–82.
———— 1963b. Effect of metabolic and other inhibitors on regeneration in *Blepharisma undulans*. Exp. Cell Res. **32**: 130–46.

Giese, A. C., J. Recher, and B. Berry. 1963. Regeneration and division rates of different-sized fragments of *Blepharisma*. J. Exp. Zool. **154**: 239–46.

Giese, A. C., S. G. Smith, and B. J. Berry Dau. 1965. Effect of osmotic pressure, ionic imbalance, and pH upon the regeneration rate in *Blepharisma*. Exp. Cell Res. **39**: 145–60.

Giese, A. C., B. K. McCaw, J. W. Parker, and J. T. Recher. 1965. Ultraviolet sensitivity of regeneration in the genus *Blepharisma*. J. Protozool. **12**: 171–77.

Hirshfield, H. I., and A. C. Giese. 1953. Ultraviolet radiation effects on growth processes of *Blepharisma undulans*. Exp. Cell Res. **4**: 283–94.

Hirshfield, H. I., and P. Pecora. 1955. Reconstitutive events in *Blepharisma undulans* as affected by colchicine. Exp. Cell Res. **9**: 414–27.

———— 1956. Studies of isolated *Blepharisma* and *Blepharisma* fragments. J. Protozool. **3**: 14–16.

Janisch, R. 1969. Morphogenesis and regeneration in the infusorian *Blepharisma undulans americanum*, I: Recovery of form after merotomy. Folia Biologica (Prague) **15**: 63–70.

McCaw, B. K. 1962. Selected chemicals and regeneration in *Blepharisma undulans*. Master's thesis, Stanford University, 77 pp.

Minutoli, F., and H. I. Hirshfield. 1968. DNA synthesis cycle in *Blepharisma*. J. Protozool. **15**: 532–35.

Moore, E. L. 1924. Regeneration at various phases in the life history of the infusorians *Spathidium spatula* and *Blepharisma undulans*. J. Exp. Zool. **39**: 249–315.

Parker, J. W. 1967. A cytochemical investigation of the nuclear and enzymatic activities in regenerating cells of the ciliate *Blepharisma intermedium*. Doctoral dissertation, Stanford University, 160 pp.

Parker, J. W., and A. C. Giese. 1966. Nuclear activity during regeneration in *Blepharisma intermedium* Bhandary. J. Protozool. **13**: 617–22.

Rupert, C. 1964. Photoreactivation of ultraviolet damage. *In* Photophysiology (A. C. Giese, ed.), II, 283–327. New York.

Saxena, D. M. 1966. Isolation of macronuclei from the ciliates *Blepharisma intermedium* and *Spirostomum ambiguum*: The role of digitonin. Ind. J. Exp. Biol. **4**: 182–84.

Seshachar, B. R., and D. M. Saxena. 1968. DNA-dependent RNA synthesis in isolated macronuclei of *Blepharisma intermedium* (Ciliata). J. Protozool. **15**: 697–700.

Suzuki, S. 1957. Morphogenesis in the regeneration of *Blepharisma undulans japonicus* Suzuki. Bull. Yamagata Univ. Nat. Sci. No. 4. 4, No. 1: 84–192.

Tartar, V. 1961. The biology of *Stentor*. New York, 413 pp.

———— 1967. Morphogenesis in Protozoa. *In* Research in protozoology (T. T. Chen, ed.), II, 1–116. New York.

Weisz, P. B. 1954. Morphogenesis in Protozoa. Quart. Rev. Biol. **29**: 207–29.

CHAPTER TEN

Encystment and Excystment

Most species of *Blepharisma* live in fresh water and must face the hazards of streams and ponds that may dry out in summer and freeze in winter. *Blepharisma*, like other freshwater protozoans, meets such conditions by forming a cyst—that is, by adopting an undifferentiated, dehydrated, and inactive state in which its resistance to environmental variations is far greater. When favorable conditions return, the cell emerges from its cyst and continues to grow and divide.

The first protozoan cysts observed were those of the ciliate *Amphileptus* (Guanzati, 1796), and cysts of *Blepharisma* (*B. lateritium*) were first observed by Cienkowsky in 1855. Penard (1922) and Stolte (1922, 1924) were the first to illustrate stages in the encystment of *Blepharisma*. McLoughlin (1955a, b) has reviewed this early literature on encystment in detail. Cysts have been recorded in *B. seculum, B. undulans, B. musculus* v. giesei, *B. stoltei, B. americanum,* and *B. japonicum* (Stolte, 1924; Suzuki, 1954; Hirshfield et al., 1962, 1965; Isquith et al., 1965). *Blepharisma*'s cyst is ovoid or nearly spherical, and varies in size depending on the species involved (Table 10.1).

Kinds of Cysts

Some ciliates normally produce several kinds of cysts: protective resting (thick-walled), temporary resting (thin-walled), and division cysts (thin-walled). *Blepharisma* is known to form only protective resting cysts, but these vary considerably in size, reflecting the varying nutritional state of the cells in a population. Cannibal giants, for example, invariably form much larger cysts than blepharismas fed on bacteria (Ibara, 1939). *B. stoltei* has been seen to divide while still inside its cyst; however, this occurs only after excystment is virtually complete (Repak, 1968).

TABLE 10.1

Size of Cysts in *Blepharisma*

Species	Major axis	Minor axis
B. undulans	44–80 μm, usu. 55–70 μm	38–70 μm, usu. 45–63 μm
B. musculus v. giesei	60–140 μm, usu. 90–110 μm	60–125 μm, usu. 80–105 μm
B. japonicum:		
normal cell	93–170 μm, usu. 130–150 μm	78–135 μm, usu. 95–110 μm
cannibal giant	195–225 μm	132–195 μm

SOURCE: Unpublished data of Shōichirō Suzuki.

The cyst wall comprises a thick, rigid outer shell, or ectocyst, and a thin inner membrane, or endocyst. The ectocyst is rugose, containing numerous minute vacuoles, and its outer surface is brownish in color with many pitlike depressions. The endocyst is pyriform and contains a large vacuole at the bluntly pointed end near the emergence pore, where the ectocyst becomes a thin membrane (Fig. 10.1). The macronucleus of an encysted *Blepharisma* may assume various forms. In younger cysts it is elongate and irregular in shape, but in mature ones it shortens and thickens, becoming spiral, horseshoe-shaped, rod-shaped, or globular. The micronuclei remain scattered through the cytoplasm of the cyst without changing shape.

Conditions Favoring Encystment

A wide variety of conditions have been regarded by different investigators as favoring encystment in protozoans (the extensive literature has been reviewed by van Wagtendonk, 1955). For example: lack of food (some authors claim exactly the reverse); the accumulation of excretory products; changes in hydrogen-ion concentration; evaporation of the medium, resulting in a concentration of electrolytes; lack of oxygen; crowding; and low temperatures. The diversity of these factors probably arises from experiments performed with varying degrees of control. Perhaps more than anyone else, C. V. Taylor and his coworkers achieved an accurate control of the environment when working with *Colpoda duodenaria* (van Wagtendonk, 1955). In this species (now called *C. steini*, see Burt, 1940), lack of food and crowding were especially conducive to encystment and were thought to be causative (Strickland, 1940). The temperature was kept constant at 20° C; and changes in pH, accumulation of excretory products, electrolyte balance, and oxygen supply affected neither the rate nor the degree of encystment. For *Colpoda* grown axenically on a defined medium, lack of any necessary vitamin (thiamin, pyridoxin, pantothenic acid, or riboflavin) or lack of the bacterial plasmoptyzate used in the medium would induce encystment (Garnjobst, 1947).

Little comparable work has been done with *Blepharisma*; and most observations of the genus have examined various aspects of encystment as it occurs naturally in old cultures affected by a whole complex of variables. Possibly, one or more of the factors listed above may induce encystment in *Blepharisma*, but there is as yet no adequate experimental evidence to clarify matters. In any case, no controlled nutritional experiments are possible with *Blepharisma* at present because the proper medium for axenic culture of the genus is still too complex and poorly defined (see Chapter 4). However, blepharismas always seem to encyst when food is depleted after a period of plenty. In *B. americanum*, encystment is always completed once it has begun, even when fresh medium containing bacteria is added; the only exceptions I have observed are cells in the very first stages of encystment (Giese, unpublished). Encystment has not been reported in cases where food is continuously abundant.

Density of population in a culture seems to be an important factor in encystment, perhaps because metabolites and wastes accumulate more rapidly. However, I have found that washing *B. americanum* from such a culture in balanced salt solution will not prevent their encysting at

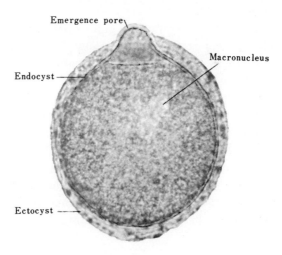

Emergence pore

Macronucleus

Endocyst

Ectocyst

Fig. 10.1. A living cyst of *B. japonicum*, × 300. From Suzuki, 1957.

about the same rate as cells in the old culture medium. These observations are not conclusive, since any crowded culture will accumulate metabolites very rapidly. Barker and Taylor (1931) thought that the accumulation of metabolites was an important cause of encystment in *Colpoda steini*; but later experiments indicated that even when the effect of metabolites is minimized by suspending the cells in a fresh balanced salt medium, *Colpoda* in an appropriate physiological state will encyst within a few hours (Taylor and Strickland, 1938, 1939).

Changes in hydrogen-ion concentration from 5.5 to 8.0 have no observable effect on the rate or percentage of encystment in *B. americanum*. To test this, I washed the cells in portions of balanced salt medium contained at the various pH values in this range. The same is true of *Colpoda steini* (Taylor and Strickland, 1938, 1939).

It has been suggested, though without adequate experimental support, that the concentration of osmotically active materials produced by evaporating a culture medium might induce encystment in *Blepharisma* (McLoughlin, 1955). However, when I tried this with *B. americanum*, encystment occurred at about the same rate and to the same degree over a range from distilled water (containing some electrolytes leached from the cells) to a medium twelve times the concentration of salts in the balanced medium usually used for washing cells. It is possible that species of *Blepharisma* from brackish or marine waters might react differently, for some other ciliates certainly do. For example, the marine hypotrich *Euplotes taylori* encysts when the medium is concentrated by evaporation and excysts when the medium is again diluted (Garnjobst, 1928).

A lowered temperature does affect the encystment of *B. americanum*. Cultures kept at 30° C never show signs of encystment. At 25° the blepharismas encyst about ten days after achieving their peak population. When cultures that have reached a maximum population at 23° are placed at 13°, by contrast, the cells encyst within 24 to 48 hours, provided most of the food bacteria in the culture have been consumed. Cultures transferred from 30° encyst within 36 hours if they have not been at the high temperature too long. Too low a temperature seems to delay encystment: at 5° no cysts appear; but abnormal, rounded cells develop, and these will encyst when warmed to 13° if they have not been kept too long at the lower temperature (Giese, unpublished). Ibara (1939) has found that lowering the temperature also provoked encystment in *B. undulans*. Stolte (1924), however, claimed that his strain of the same species (this was probably *B. stoltei*) would encyst at either low or high (30°) temperatures.

A temperature of 25° C or higher is also considered unfavorable for the encystment of *Stylonychia curvata* (Giese, 1951) and *Urostyla*. *Urostyla* cells starved at 26° get smaller and smaller without encysting; but when starved at 20° under otherwise identical conditions they encyst readily, and at 15° practically every cell in a culture encysts (Pigoń, 1961). When *Urostyla* is starved at 26° for an extended time the cells appear normal, but Pigoń and Edstrom (1959, 1961) have shown that both DNA and RNA decrease in this case. Since the DNA of normal cells remains constant even during starvation (Mirsky, 1951), the DNA in *Urostyla* must be damaged to an unusual degree by starvation. DNA repair mechanisms exist in various types of cells (Hanawalt, 1968), but the damage apparently passes a critical point in these starved *Urostyla*, precluding repair and recovery. Similar experiments have not been tried with *Blepharisma*.

Not all protozoans are as sensitive to temperature during encystment as *B. americanum*. For example, the temperature of *Didinium nasutum* cultures can be varied over a range from 16° to 39° C with virtually no effect on either the percentage or the rate of encystment (Mast and Ibara, 1923).

Stages in Encystment

Stolte (1924) described six stages in the encystment of *B. undulans* (Fig. 10.2); this was repeated by McLoughlin (1955). Repak (1968) recently described the encystment of *B. stoltei*, which corresponds closely with that described for *B. undulans* but has only four stages. The two species have different kinds of macronuclei, and consequently their encystment behavior differs in detail (macronuclear events in encystment are shown in Figure 10.3). The following account is based on Repak (1965) and Suzuki (unpublished).

Stage I (hours 1–3). The *Blepharisma* is rounded and the peristome organelles overlap the posterior end. The cell rotates around the spherical axis of the incipient cyst, and the macronucleus bends along the contours of the organism. The ciliary rows and pigment granules are still evident. Cells in this stage may be recognized by their slightly increased girth and deep color. Toward the end of this stage the macro-

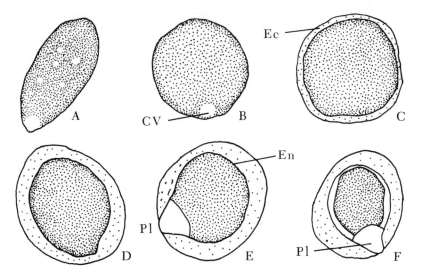

Fig. 10.2. Development of cyst walls in *Blepharisma* (× 200). CV, contractile vacuole; Ec, ectocyst wall; En, endocyst wall; Pl, fibrous plug. From Stolte, 1924; by permission Springer Verlag.

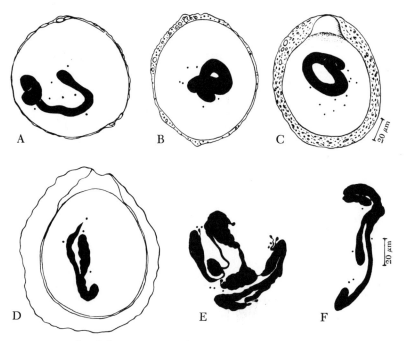

Fig. 10.3. Nuclear behavior in cysts of *B. japonicum*. A–C, late stages in encystment; D, an excysting cell just before emergence; E–F, nuclei in excysting cells. From Suzuki, 1954.

nucleus begins to contract, the peristome ceases to ingest food, and the oral organelles begin to dedifferentiate. At the same time, the blepharismas, still with visible contractile vacuoles, assume an ellipsoidal form and become inactive.

Stage II (hours 4–9). The oral structures are gradually resorbed but the body may continue to rotate. The pigment granules aggregate, making the cell appear a deeper red in color, and the contractile vacuole, active in the first stage, finally disappears, presumably with a loss of water and a corresponding increase in the density of the cytoplasm. The macronucleus becomes horseshoe-shaped, and the ectocyst wall appears. By the ninth hour most of the cells are stationary.

Stage III (hours 10–14). The cell contracts to a regular ellipsoidal shape and the cilia disappear completely. The cytoplasm shrinks away from the ectocyst wall, leaving a narrow gap, and an endocyst wall is secreted. When this process is complete, a cylindrical plug forms near the contractile vacuole. The macronucleus does not change markedly in this stage. According to Repak (1968), the pigment in *B. stoltei* appears to concentrate in the interwall space and then gradually fades until none is evident. He also states that the contractile vacuole may continue to operate even in Stage III.

Stage IV (hours 15–40). The thin outer membrane produced in the previous stage gradually develops into a thick, solid ectocyst with a rugose surface. At the same time fibrils develop between the ectocyst and the endocyst (which covers the cytoplasm and the vacuolar plug). When observed in optical section, the cyst wall appears spongelike in structure, containing numerous vacuoles; and according to Suzuki (personal communication), in some species the pigment is retained in the cell, which becomes dark red as the cyst becomes spherical and the cytoplasm homogeneous. As the ectocyst grows in thickness a large vacuole appears at one pole of the cyst.

An electron-microscope study of extracellular structures in a cyst of *B. stoltei* has been made (Repak, 1967), but the intracellular makeup of cysts has not received similar treatment. However, electron-microscope studies on *Colpoda steini* demonstrate that such internal cell organelles as the mitochondria and the endoplasmic reticulum remain differentiated in the cyst (Tibbs, 1968). The micronuclei remain scattered in the cytoplasm throughout encystment.

I have observed much the same four stages of encystment in a strain of *B. americanum*. In this species the cysts are also red when first formed; but they change to blue within 24 hours whether the cell is in light or in darkness, although this happens sooner in light. Light induces a similar photooxidation in the vegetative cells of a red *Blepharisma* (see Chapter 11). That the color change during encystment is incidental can be shown by exposing vegetative cells to light (Lite-Mite, 8 cm distant passed through a water filter; about 200 foot-candles) for several hours to photooxidize the pigment, which turns the cells blue-grey. These blue blepharismas, when placed at 13° C, encyst as readily and at the same rate as the red controls. We might consider the final change to blue pigment to be Stage V of encystment, since no further changes occur until the cell begins to excyst. Since pigment is continuously being replenished in a vegetative cell, the final change to blue in the cyst perhaps signals the inactivity of the enzyme system that normally produces the pigment.

Rate of Encystment

When the number of blepharismas encysting in a culture is plotted against time, a sigmoid curve is produced. The point of inflection of this curve marks 50% encystment and provides the most convenient means of comparing rates of encystment under different environmental conditions. At 13° C it takes about 24 hours for the cells to reach Stage I and another 12 hours to reach Stage II. Within another 12 hours, all the cells have passed through Stage III and arrived at Stage IV; some may have developed oxidized pigment, but this usually takes another 12 hours. There is some variation, and one can usually see a mixture of red and blue cysts in a 48-hour culture. At 7.5° blepharismas take eight days to reach Stage II, and only a small percentage of them encyst at all. Generally, the formation of the exocyst (Stage IV) is regarded as marking the end of encystment.

As we have seen, temperature has a marked effect on the rate of encystment, which is exceedingly slow at both 30° and 5°. These limits are poorly defined: no cysts appear at either extreme, but only abnormal rounded cells that may sometimes encyst when cooled from 30° to 13° or warmed from 5° to 13°. The favorable zone for encystment seems to lie between 13° and 18°, at least for *B. americanum* acclimated to room temperature (22°–24°).

A dim light (10–50 foot-candles) has no readily measurable effect on encystment, but stronger fluorescent light (ca. 200 foot-candles) completely prevents it, even when the blepharismas are shielded from the infrared wavelengths by a water cell and are kept at a constant temperature of 13° (Giese, unpublished).

When I exposed a concentrated suspension of *B. americanum* to a nitrogen atmosphere (obtained by evacuating to 2 mm Hg and substituting nearly pure nitrogen), widespread encystment occurred in the expected manner 24 to 48 hours after the cells were exposed to 13° in the dark. Presumably, oxygen is not necessary for encystment except in the tiny amounts remaining after the above treatment. Encystment did not occur in cultures subjected to three cycles of vacuum and gas replacement with nitrogen.

Obviously, many other factors injurious to cells might change the rate of encystment. Few of these have been tested, however, since they are seldom present in the normal environment of *Blepharisma*.

Metabolism of Cysts

A protozoan's encystment is essentially a way of going to sleep (i.e., becoming cryptobiotic) when conditions are unfavorable. This hibernation may last for days, weeks, months, or even several years; and in nature it normally carries the cells through unfavorable seasons of several months. In most protozoan cysts that have been tested, oxygen consumption falls to a low level (Pigoń, 1959; Scholander et al., 1952), but no measurements have been made on *Blepharisma*. Contractile-vacuole function ceases when a permanent cyst forms in *Blepharisma*, and no other activity is evident.

The activity of the respiratory enzyme systems probably decreases with encystment. In *B. americanum*, which readily encysts when a concentrated suspension of cells is exposed to a lowered temperature, I have found that iodoacetate ($1 \times 10^{-5} M$), fluoride ($1 \times 10^{-3} M$), and malonic acid ($1 \times 10^{-3} M$), all inhibitors of metabolic pathways, do not affect either the rate of encystment or the percentage of cells encysting; this indicates that the anaerobic systems of the cells are inactive. However, the aerobic inhibitors sodium azide and potassium cyanide (both at $1 \times 10^{-3} M$) introduce a considerable delay; so some respiration is clearly essential to the encystment process.

Tests for the activity of hydrolases and other mainly nonrespiratory enzymes during encystment have not been made in *Blepharisma*. But in the ciliate *Urostyla* many enzymes have been found to decrease as encystment proceeds (Pigoń, 1960, 1961, 1962), and this is also true of *Colpoda* (Tibbs and Marshall, 1970). It is to be expected that some enzyme systems will remain active even during encystment—for example, those involved in protein synthesis, since the cyst walls of ciliates are proteinaceous. Inhibitors of protein synthesis do affect the encystment of *B. americanum*: puromycin almost completely blocks encystment, and chloramphenicol prolongs its initiation (Giese, unpublished). Similar results have been found in amoebas (Tibbs and Marshall, 1969, 1970). The blocking of encystment by low temperature that I have described could also result from the inhibition of protein synthesis.

Histochemical Studies of Cysts

Tests on *B. stoltei* have shown that material reacting positively to per-iodic acid Schiff reagent (PAS) is present in the cytoplasm in the vegetative cell and in Stages I–III of encystment. At Stage IV the PAS-positive material disappears from the cytoplasm but appears between the endocyst and ectocyst, remaining there until the first stage of excystment, at which time it again appears in the cytoplasm (Repak, 1968; Chunosoff and Hirshfield, 1964). A PAS-positive test denotes the presence of polysaccharides: that is, per-iodic acid is an oxidizing agent that breaks 1:2 glycol carbon bonds in various carbohydrate structures, converting them to dialdehyde groups; these groups react with the leucofuchsin of the Schiff reagent (Gurr, 1961). The specific role played by polysaccharides during encystment and excystment is not known.

The macronucleus remains positive to basic fuchsin (Feulgen reaction), methyl green, and azure blue A during both encystment and excystment, suggesting that no biochemical DNA reorganization detectable in this manner is taking place. Pyronin and naphthol yellow, which test for RNA, indicate RNA presence in the cytoplasm throughout encystment and excystment. Osmic acid reagent affects cortical structures as well as some material in the cytoplasm; during encystment osmic-acid staining of the cortical structures decreases, and during excystment it increases as the cells once again differentiate (Repak, 1968).

This information is in all cases preliminary, and more tests investigating the biochemical changes occurring in an encysted cell are needed before any conclusions can be drawn.

The Survival of Cysts

The protective or permanent cysts of protozoans are known to withstand extremely unfavorable conditions. No data concerning the resistance of *Blepharisma* cysts have been published. However, since the cysts of *Blepharisma* resemble those of other ciliates that have been closely examined, some knowledge of the experimental findings for other genera may be useful.

The dried cysts of *Colpoda steini*, resting on filter paper, can withstand an hour at 106° C and a momentary exposure to 120°; if wet, they are killed at 44°. They can even be placed in liquid air for 13.5 hours with only a slight loss in viability (Taylor and Strickland, 1935, 1936). Wet resting cysts are not injured by freezing and thawing that would kill vegetative cells (Bychenkova et al., 1969). Dry cysts of *Colpoda* can also tolerate a vacuum for prolonged periods (Taylor and Strickland, 1936).

The cysts of ciliates can remain inactive for many years (Dawson and Mitchell, 1929). Survival is statistical—the more prolonged the encystment, the fewer the protozoans emerging from cysts. *Didinium* cysts have been kept for as long as ten years in the debris of a culture medium, but very few survive (Beers, 1937). *Tillina* cysts in soil are quite viable after ten years (Bridgman, 1957). Many cysts of *Colpoda steini* have been seen to excyst after a lapse of five years (Taylor and Strickland, 1936), and cysts of two other species of *Colpoda* excysted after 38 years (Goodey, 1915).

The surface available for encystment seems to determine the mortality, and possibly the survival time, of protozoan cysts. In natural ponds, for instance, cysts are almost invariably formed on debris. The cysts formed on the glass surfaces of laboratory vessels almost always suffer injury, especially after drying. Some artificial environments seem to favor encystment, however: for example, *Colpoda* that have encysted in grooves cut with a razor in a piece of cellophane will survive for many months (Taylor and Strickland, 1938).

Protozoan cysts are also highly resistant to damage by visible and UV radiation. For example, intense visible light will kill normally pigmented *Blepharisma* within a few minutes; but several times the same dose of light will do no more to newly formed cysts than change their color. The dose of far UV radiation required to kill the division cysts of *Colpoda maupasi* is greater than the dose that will kill a vegetative cell; and resting cysts are much more resistant than division cysts, especially when dry (Lozina-Lozinskii and Uspenskaja, 1968). The resistance of *Blepharisma* cysts to UV radiation of any kind has not been tested as yet.

Conditions Favoring Excystment

If encystment results from the failure of a particular metabolic enzyme owing to a lack of certain nutrients in the culture medium, then one might expect excystment to be induced by the addition of these nutrients to the medium. And in fact, experiments with *Blepharisma* indicate that the addition of a nutrient medium with a rich bacterial flora will usually induce excystment. McLoughlin (1955a, b) found that diluted whole milk and horse-dung infusion were the best materials for inducing excystment in his cultures of *Blepharisma*. The effectiveness of such complex mixtures, however, tells one little about which constituent of the nutrient supplied has activated the enzyme system involved in excystment.

More definitive experiments have been performed with *Colpoda steini*, in which sterile and highly diluted plant and animal extracts were found to induce excystment (Barker and Taylor, 1933). The simplest effective solution proved to be a mixture of $3 \times 10^{-1}\,M$ ethanol and $1 \times 10^{-4}\,M$ potassium phosphate (Strickland and Haagen-Smit, 1947). Such solutions also induce excystment in *Blepharisma*, but not with great success.

It need hardly be emphasized that all environmental conditions—temperature, oxygen, and the absence of any inhibiting factors—must favor excystment if any one factor is to touch it off. However, it has been proved that the presence of oxygen is not critical. In *Colpoda steini*, for example, the oxygen partial pressure can be reduced to 15 mm Hg without affecting the rate or degree of excystment; below this value excystment is blocked. Excystment in the same species occurs readily throughout the temperature range 11°–32° C (Brown, 1939). Further studies of *C. steini* support the view that substances favoring excystment do so by activating some enzyme in the cell (Brown and Taylor, 1938).

Metabolism During Excystment

Oxygen consumption, which falls to an unmeasurable level during encystment in most ciliates, gradually rises to the normal level during excystment (Fig. 10.4; Scholander et al., 1952; Pigoń, 1959). It would be interesting to know whether specific inhibitors of various aerobic processes could stop excystment under otherwise favorable conditions.

Little is known about the metabolism of *Blepharisma* excystment.

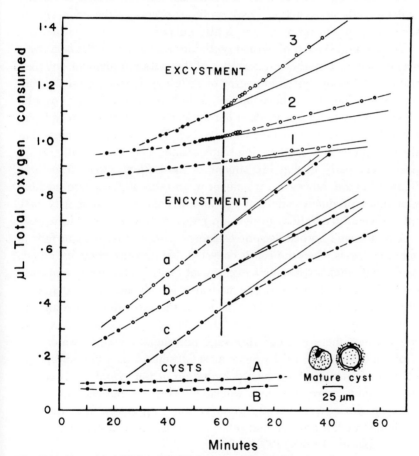

Fig. 10.4. Respiration of the ciliate *Bresslaua insidiatrix* during encystment, as measured in a microrespirometer. The vertical lines indicate the point at which the curves begin to deflect from their previous slope. A microliter (μl) is equal to .001 ml. From Scholander et al., 1952; by permission of the *Biological Bulletin*.

However, since the entire process of morphogenesis must occur before an encysted cell can regain its vegetative form, one would expect that protein and RNA synthesis take place, energized by metabolic reactions that furnish the necessary ATP molecules. RNA synthesis has not been measured during excystment, but cytochemical tests indicate that the RNA in *B. stoltei* remains unaltered throughout encystment and continues to be prominent in the cytoplasm during excystment (Repak, 1968). Messenger RNA, at least, would have to be formed to initiate protein synthesis. Whether DNA synthesis occurs as the cell's kinetosomes multiply to form anlagen is also unknown.

The reestablishment of normal synthetic reactions in a *Blepharisma* is usually signaled by the reappearance of the cell's red pigment (blepharismin). A resting cyst is blue-grey or colorless, depending on the conditions to which it has been subjected; but the blue pigment (oxyblepharismin), when present, does not appear to be reduced to red pigment during excystment (see Chapter 11). Thus we must assume that the cell is somehow synthesizing blepharismin. The red coloration reappears very early during excystment in most *Blepharisma* strains. In *B. americanum*, however, excystment in an ethanol-phosphate medium sometimes produces cells that are almost colorless, and it may take them several generations to develop pigment (Giese, unpublished).

A protozoan's normal osmotic exchange with its environment falls to very low levels when the cell is encysted. No measurements have been made with *Blepharisma*, but experiments with *Actinosphaerium* indicate that a cyst's permeability to water is only one-tenth that of a vegetative cell (Pigoń, 1955). This is not too surprising, since all protozoans lose a great deal of water when they encyst. (In *Colpoda* cysts, for instance, there is a 60% shrinkage in volume owing to water loss; Tibbs and Marshall, 1970.) Since most substances pass into and out of cells in a water solution, such dehydration of the cytoplasm is certain to slow down normal osmotic exchange. This is confirmed by a cell's behavior during excystment: water is taken up avidly from the very beginning of the process, and other materials are also known to enter the cytoplasm (Brown, 1939).

Stages in Excystment

In many respects excystment is the reverse of encystment. The process has been fully described in *B. stoltei* (Repak, 1968), and seems to have five stages. In Stage I, movement of the cytoplasm begins. Before this occurs, however, the kinetosomes multiply and form partial kineties at the surface of the encysted cell, and cilia are regenerated. In Stage II the peristome reappears, and the cell becomes pear-shaped. In Stage III the cell elongates and resumes its vegetative form, still within the cyst wall; the macronucleus resumes its elongate form, the contractile vacuole begins to function, and the cyst plug disappears, leaving a cavity in its place. Division may occur while the *Blepharisma* is still in its cyst. In Stage IV, the regenerated ciliate ruptures the endocyst membrane and squeezes out of the cyst through the open pore. In Stage V, the cell resembles a vegetative *Blepharisma* except that it is still essentially devoid of pigment and is shorter.

Morphogenesis During Encystment and Excystment

During encystment, protozoan cells dedifferentiate; and in *Blepharisma* this is most evident when the complicated feeding organelles are resorbed. The membranelles, the undulating membrane, and the somatic cilia all disappear, and the contents of the cyst appear homogeneous except for a condensed macronucleus and unaltered micronuclei scattered through the cytoplasm. The contractile vacuole may continue to function up to Stage III of encystment, but it then disappears as well. Some synthetic activity continues, however, as the cyst walls are formed (Suzuki, unpublished).

The macronucleus in *Blepharisma*, which controls most of the cell's trophic processes, changes greatly during encystment, and eventually contracts to a compact spiral, horseshoe, or sphere (see Fig. 10.2). Whether this event involves a reorganization of the macronuclear chromatin has not been determined, but there is no reason to suppose so. As excystment begins—that is, when the cell starts to rotate before emergence—the macronucleus elongates greatly and may assume various shapes (Fig. 10.3, *E–F*). Throughout the entire process the micronuclei remain inactive, lying close to the macronucleus; they may swell and change positions slightly, but no more (Suzuki, unpublished).

In some ciliates (e.g., *Colpoda steini*), the macronucleus undergoes a more radical reorganization during cystment, behaving much like the macronucleus of a dividing cell; the only differences are that half the macronucleus of a resting cyst degenerates instead of going to a daughter cell, and that the micronuclei do not undergo mitosis. For this reason, Taylor and Garnjobst (1938, 1941) suggest that the resting cyst of *Colpoda* is simply a modified form of division cyst. No such behavior has been reported in *Blepharisma*.

A recently excysted *Blepharisma* often contains a massive macronucleus with a configuration characteristic of oral replacement. And many blepharismas do undergo oral replacement after emerging from a cyst, remodeling the newly reorganized oral area into a larger one. Oral replacement after excystment is not inevitable; but it may occur from one to three times before the first binary fission of the excysted cell (Suzuki, unpublished).

The Significance of Encystment

Blepharisma cysts, like any protective cysts, allow the cells to weather unfavorable periods of drought or cold. Moreover, cysts that are blown by the wind, carried by migrating waterfowl, or the like are an effective means of dispersing a species to new bodies of water. Why then do some species of *Blepharisma* encyst readily whereas others do not? *Blepharisma*'s behavior in a natural ecology is so little known that one cannot answer this question with any certainty. Conceivably, species that do not encyst readily have adapted to large bodies of water in which a vegetative cell may never have to cope with a dry spell, whereas species that encyst normally inhabit temporary or seasonal ponds. It is also possible that non-encysting races could survive even in small bodies of water by replenishing their population with vegetative cells carried by snails or other animals migrating from pool to pool, since not all pools are likely to meet with unfavorable conditions simultaneously. If the fundamental nature of the factors that actually cause encystment could be determined, it is likely that one could induce encystment in any *Blepharisma*, regardless of species.

LITERATURE CITED

Barker, H. A., and C. V. Taylor. 1931. A study of the conditions of encystment of *Colpoda cucullus*. Physiol. Zool. 4: 620–34.
———— 1933. Studies on the excystment of *Colpoda cucullus*. Physiol. Zool. 6: 127–36.
Beadle, L. C., and J. Nilsson. 1959. The effect of anaerobic conditions on two heterotrich ciliate Protozoa from papyrus swamps. J. Exp. Biol. 36: 583–89.

Beers, C. D. 1937. The viability of ten-year-old cysts of *Didinium nasutum.* Amer. Nat. **71**: 521–25.

Bridgman, A. J. 1957. Studies on dried cysts of *Tillina magna.* J. Protozool. **4**: 17–19.

Brown, M. G. 1939. The blocking of excystment reactions of *Colpoda duodenaria* by absence of oxygen. Biol. Bull. **77**: 382–90.

Brown, M. G., and C. F. Taylor. 1938. The kinetics of excystment in *Colpoda duodenaria.* J. Gen. Physiol. **21**: 475–500.

Burt, R. L. 1940. Specific analysis of the genus *Colpoda* with special reference to the standardization of the experimental material. Trans. Amer. Microsc. Soc. **59**: 414–32.

Bychenkova, V. N., L. K. Lozina-Lozinskii, and T. Namalov. 1969. Microscopic observations of the processes of freezing and thawing in *Colpoda maupasi.* Zool. Zh. **48**: 1772–79.

Chunosoff, L., and H. I. Hirshfield. 1964. A cytochemical investigation of cysts of a species of *Blepharisma.* J. Protozool. **11** (suppl.): 90.

Cienkowsky, L. 1855. Über Cystenbildung bei Infusorien. Zeit. Wiss. Zool. **6**: 301–6.

Dawson, J. A., and W. H. Mitchell, Jr. 1929. The viability of certain infusorian cysts. Amer. Nat. **63**: 476–78.

Dreyer, G. 1903. Die Einwirkung des Lichtes auf Amöben. Mitt. Finsens. Med. Lichtinst. **4**: 81–107.

Garnjobst, L. 1928. Induced encystment and excystment in *Euplotes taylori,* sp. nov. Physiol. Zool. **1**: 561–75.

——— 1947. The effects of certain deficient media on resting cyst formation in *Colpoda duodenaria.* Physiol. Zool. **20**: 5–14.

Giese, A. C. 1938. Sublethal effects of long-wavelength ultraviolet. Science **87**: 326–27.

——— 1951. Encystment in *Stylonychia curvata.* Anat. Rec. **111**: 150 (abstr.).

——— 1967. Effects of radiation upon Protozoa. *In* Research in protozoology (T. T. Chen, ed.), II, 267–356. New York.

Goodey, T. 1915. Note on the remarkable retention of vitality by protozoa from old stored soils. Ann. Applied Biol. **1**: 395–99.

Granzati, L. 1796. Quoted from McLoughlin, 1955a.

Griffiths, A. J., and D. E. Hughes. 1968. Starvation and encystment in a soil amoeba, *Hartmanella castellanii.* J. Protozool. **15**: 673–77.

——— 1969. The physiology of encystment of *Hartmanella castellanii.* J. Protozool. **16**: 93-99.

Gurr, E. 1961. Encyclopaedia of microscopic stains. Baltimore, 489 pp.

Hanawalt, P. 1968. Cellular recovery from photochemical damage. *In* Photophysiology (A. C. Giese, ed.), IV, 203–51. New York.

Hirshfield, H. I., L. Chunosoff, and A. V. Bhandary. 1962. Macronuclear variability of *Blepharisma* associated with growth. Intern. Soc. Cell Biol. **2**: 27–56.

Hirshfield, H. I., I. R. Isquith, and A. V. Bhandary. 1965. A proposed reorganization of the genus *Blepharisma* Perty and description of four new species. J. Protozool. **12**: 136–44.

Ibara, Y. 1939. An observation on *Blepharisma undulans* with special reference to cannibalism and gigantism. Annot. Zool. Jap. **18**: 21–28.

Isquith, I. R., A. J. Repak, and H. I. Hirshfield. 1965. *Blepharisma seculum*, sp. nov., a member of the subgenus (Compactum). J. Protozool. **12**: 615–18.

Lozina-Lozinskii, L. K., and Z. I. Uspenskaja. 1968. The influence of ultraviolet irradiation (2537 Å) on infusoria *Colpoda maupasi*. Acta Protozool. **6**: 297–307.

McLoughlin, D. C. 1955a. Cystic phenomena in the ciliate *Blepharisma undulans*. J. Protozool. **2** (suppl.): 11 (abstr.).

———— 1955b. A study of cystic phenomena and of macronuclear morphogenesis in strains of the heterotrichous ciliate *Blepharisma undulans* Stein. Doctoral dissertation, Univ. Ill., 66 pp. Dissert. Abstr. **15**: 902.

Mast, S. O., and V. Ibara. 1923. The effect of temperature, food, and the age of culture on the encystment of *Didinium nasutum*. Biol. Bull. **45**: 105–12.

Mirsky, A. E. 1951. The chemical composition of chromosomes. Harvey Lect. **46**: 98–115.

Penard, E. 1922. Etudes sur les Infusoires d'eau douce. Geneva.

Pigoń, A. 1955. Permeability to water of active forms and cysts of *Actinosphaerium*. Bull. Acad. Polon. **3**: 235–39.

———— 1959. Respiration of *Colpoda cucullus* during active life and encystment. J. Protozool. **6**: 303–8.

———— 1960. Changes of enzyme activity during starvation and encystment of a ciliate (*Urostyla*): Amylase, catalase. Acta Biol. Cracov. Ser. Zool. **3**: 59–70.

———— 1961. Changes in the respiratory activity during starvation and encystment of a ciliate (*Urostyla*). Acta Biol. Cracov. Ser. Zool. **4**: 33–45.

———— 1962. Changes of enzyme activity during starvation and encystment of a ciliate (*Urostyla*): Cathepsin, acid phosphatase. Acta Biol. Cracov. Ser. Zool. **5**: 179–97.

Pigoń, A., and J. E. Edström. 1959. Nucleic acid changes during starvation and encystment in a ciliate (*Urostyla*). Exp. Cell Res. **16**: 648–56.

———— 1961. Excystment ability, respiratory metabolism, and RNA content in two types of resting cysts of *Colpoda cucullus* O. F. Müller. J. Protozool. **8**: 257–60.

Repak, A. J. 1967. Electron microscopic observations on the extracellular structures of the resting cyst of *Blepharisma stoltei*. Trans. Amer. Microsc. Soc. **86**: 417–21.

———— 1968. The encystment and excystment of the heterotrichous ciliate *Blepharisma stoltei* Isquith. J. Protozool. **15**: 407–12.

Scholander, P. F., C. L. Clapp, and S. L. Sveinsson. 1952. Respiration studies on single cells, II: Observations on the oxygen consumption in single protozoans. Biol. Bull. **102**: 178–84.

Stolte, H. A. 1922. Verlauf, Ursachen, und Bedeutung der Encystierung bei *Blepharisma undulans*. Verh. Deutsch. Zool. Ges. **27**: 79–81.

———— 1924. Morphologische und physiologische Üntersuchungen an *Blepharisma undulans* Stein. Arch. Protistenk. **48**: 245–301.

Strickland, A. G. R. 1940. The effect of concentration of *Colpoda duodenaria* on the time required for encystment in food-free medium. Physiol. Zool. **13**: 356–65.

Strickland, A. G. R., and A. J. Haagen-Smit. 1947. Chemical substratum inducing excystment of the resting cysts of *Colpoda duodenaria*. J. Cell. Comp. Physiol. **30**: 381–90.

Suzuki, S. 1954. Taxonomic studies on *Blepharisma undulans* with special reference to macronuclear variation. J. Sci. Hiroshima University, Ser. B, Div. 1, **15**: 205–20.

Taylor, C. V., and L. Garnjobst. 1939. Reorganization of the silverline system in the reproductive cysts of *Colpoda duodenaria*. Arch. Protistenk. **92**: 73–90.

———— 1941. Nuclear reorganization in resting cysts of *Colpoda duodenaria*. J. Morph. **68**: 197–213.

Taylor, C. V., and A. G. R. Strickland. 1935. Some factors in the excystment of dried cysts of *Colpoda cucullus*. Arch. Protistenk. **86**: 181–90.

———— 1936. Effects of high vacua and extreme temperatures on cysts of *Colpoda cucullus*. Physiol. Zool. **9**: 15–26.

———— 1938. Reactions of *Colpoda duodenaria* to environmental factors, I: Some factors influencing growth and encystment. Arch. Protistenk. **90**: 396–409.

———— 1939. Reactions of *Colpoda duodenaria* to environmental factors, II: Factors influencing the formation of resting cysts. Physiol. Zool. **12**: 219–30.

Tibbs, J. 1968. Fine structure of *Colpoda steini* during encystment and excystment. J. Protozool. **15**: 725–32.

Tibbs, J., and B. J. Marshall. 1969. Electron transport and phospholipase activity in encysting cells of the ciliate *Colpoda steinii*. Biochem. Biophys. Acta **172**: 382–88.

———— 1970. Cyst wall protein synthesis and some enzyme changes on starvation and encystment of *Colpoda steinii*. J. Protozool. **17**: 125–28.

van Wagtendonk, W. J. 1955. Encystment and excystment in Protozoa. *In* Biochemistry and physiology of protozoa (S. H. Hunter and A. Lwoff, eds.)., II, 85–90. New York.

Young, D. 1939. Macronuclear reorganization in *Blepharisma undulans*. J. Morph. **64**: 297–353.

CHAPTER ELEVEN

The Pigment Blepharismin
and Photosensitivity

The pigment of *Blepharisma* was first extracted by Arcichovskij (1905), who noted its absorption bands and named it zoopurpurin. The pigment's absorption of visible light was later measured by Emerson (1930), who also noted that zoopurpurin changed color when acid or alkali was added to it, much like an indicator. The pigment is present to varying degrees in most *Blepharisma*; some species are red, some are only slightly pink, and one (*B. lateritium* v. hyalinum) has been reported to lack the pigment entirely. A short-lived albino mutant of a pink strain of *B. stoltei* v. narai has been isolated in Japan (Inaba et al., 1957). Perhaps the presence of blepharismin would have given the form more vitality. However, the albino mutant of a large red species from India, *B. japonicum* v. intermedium (isolated by Henry Penner; Chunosoff et al., 1965), appears to be as viable as any of the colored strains. Another vigorous albino mutant derives from the pink Federsee strain (see Chapter 12), and still another from cysts of a pink strain of *B. americanum*, which remained pigmentless for only three months, and then became pink again (Giese, unpublished).

In view of the fact that *Blepharisma* can be completely bleached by exposure to light, the color of field specimens should not be used for determining classification. A "true" color description can be attempted only after specimens have been cultured under controlled conditions. For example, one cannot be sure that *B. lateritium* v. hyalinum, reported as colorless, is truly without pigment until the species has been grown in a laboratory culture.

Each of the pigments in the hypericin group, to which the pigment of *Blepharisma* is thought to belong (Møller, 1962; Sevenants, 1965), has a name derived from the genus of organism in which it is found (hypericin from *Hypericum,* fagopyrin from *Fagopyrum,* stentorin from

Stentor, etc.). Hence this study uses the name blepharismin rather than zoopurpurin for the red pigment of *Blepharisma,* and oxyblepharismin for the blue pigment.

Sensitization to Light by Blepharismin

Photosensitivity induced by dyes is not uncommon among ciliates and was first observed by Otto Raab (1900). Studying the toxic effect of acridine dyes on a suspension of *Paramecium,* Raab found that even a very dilute solution of dye in the medium, though not harmful in the dark, was lethal to *Paramecium* in light; the same intensity of light was harmless when the dye was not present. Only wavelengths of light actually absorbed by the dye were effective: a solution of the dye interposed between the light source and the culture medium protected the cells completely, even though considerable light of other wavelengths reached the cells. When oxygen was excluded photosensitization did not appear, and the phenomenon was therefore called photodynamic sensitization (for summary see Blum, 1964). Later experiments indicate that the light-absorbing dye activates oxygen, which then damages the cell surface of the protozoans (Wilson and Hastings, 1970).

Most studies of photodynamic action have used synthetic dyes. However, some naturally occurring pigments also sensitize cells to light, notably porphyrins, hypericins, and furocoumarins. Porphyrins (e.g., cytochromes) are present in all aerobic cells, but only mutants or otherwise deranged cells allow them to accumulate in quantities that will induce photosensitivity. Hypericins and furocoumarins, which are secreted to serve other functions in some families of plants, are photosensitizers in animal cells that accidentally acquire them by contact or ingestion. The pigment of *Blepharisma* is hypericinlike in its general characteristics (Giese, 1971).

Photodynamic action is easily demonstrated in pigmented *Blepharisma,* which are readily killed in the presence of oxygen by a brief exposure to visible and near UV light of high intensity (2,000 foot-candles). By contrast, colorless cells (*Paramecium,* invertebrate eggs, etc.) show no apparent injury even after prolonged exposure to the same light (Giese, 1946). The reaction that kills *Blepharisma* is a photooxidation, brought on by the cells' increasing oxygen consumption during illumination (Fig. 11.1; Giese and Zeuthen, 1949).

As we have seen (Chapters 1 and 3), *Blepharisma's* pigment is con-

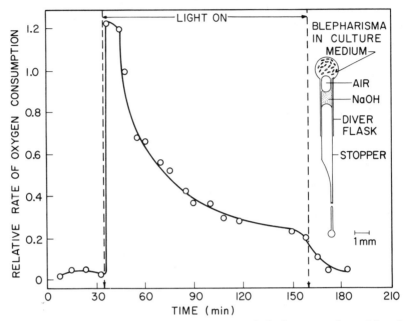

Fig. 11.1. Rise in oxygen consumption of pigmented *Blepharisma* under visible and near UV light. Insert shows the diver used. After Giese and Zeuthen, 1949; by permission of the Rockefeller Press.

centrated in subpellicular granules arranged in groups of 6–10 between each two ciliary rows (Fig. 11.2). The granules are about 0.5 μm in diameter, and electronmicrographs (see Fig. 3.2) reveal a membrane about 0.05 μm thick around each granule. The pigment granules of dark red strains (*B. japonicum* v. intermedium, *B. japonicum* v. microstomata, *B. stoltei*, *B. brevifiliformis*, and *B. stoltei* v. narai) contain fine particles or tubules. In an albino mutant of *B. japonicum* v. intermedium the granules are either large and vacuolar with few particles or irregular and honeycomblike in structure. In the pale pink *B. musculus* v. wardsi the granules contain fine particles of the same honeycomb structure (Utsumi and Yoshizawa, 1957; Inaba et al., 1958; Kurita, 1969).

The pigment can be extracted from *Blepharisma* by exposing the cells to 0° C for 30 seconds to a few minutes. A suspension of *Blepharisma* is concentrated by hand centrifuge (about 10 g), and the centrifuge tube containing the suspension is then plunged into an ice-water mixture.

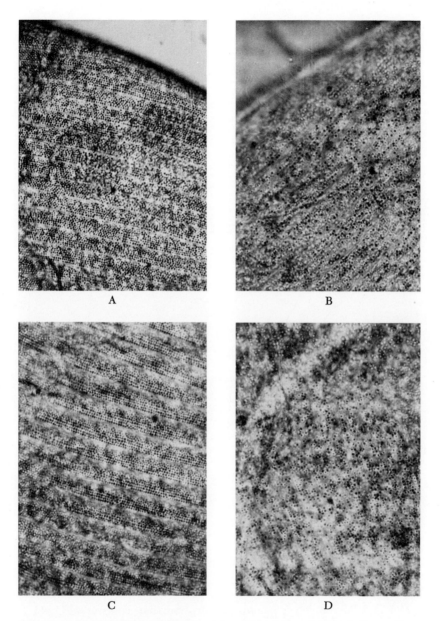

Fig. 11.2. Arrays of pigment granules in *B. japonicum* v. intermedium before and after extrusion. *A*, red form; *B*, diminished array in red form after cold extrusion; *C*, blue form; *D*, diminished array in blue form after cold extrusion. From Giese and Grainger, 1970; by permission of Pergamon Press.

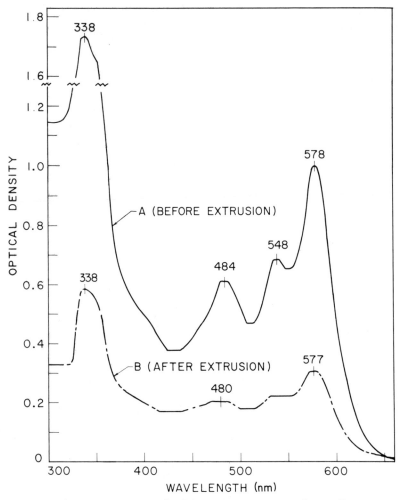

Fig. 11.3. Absorption spectrum of red *B. japonicum* v. intermedium cell suspension before and after shedding of pigment in an aqueous solution at 0° C for 30 seconds. The blepharismas were centrifuged after extrusion and washed in a fresh suspension medium free of pigment before the second absorption spectrum was taken.

Treated cells, having shed much of their pigment, are much lighter in color and have a lower-peaking absorption than controls (Fig. 11.3). If the cells are brought to room temperature quickly thereafter, they survive the treatment and multiply when fed. Prolonging their exposure to cold causes additional pigment shedding, but exposure much beyond two minutes is fatal to many of the cells (Giese and Grainger, 1970).

The extruded pigment has an absorption spectrum much like the whole cells, but with sharper peaks (Fig. 11.4). It looks slightly murky, suggesting a colloidal solution, but is evidently stable, since the pigment remains in solution. A diagnostic protein test of the solution (Lowry et al., 1951) gives positive results, but this does not necessarily prove that the pigment in the granules was complexed with protein. The protein may derive from the cytolysis of some blepharismas in the culture, since at least a few cells always cytolyze no matter how much care is taken during extraction. There may also be protein in the granular membranes, some of which are shed in response to light or other irritants (Kennedy, 1966). Boiling the extruded pigment solution, however, does not develop the coagulum of protein that might be expected, perhaps because protein is present only in minute amounts (Giese, unpublished).

When colorless cells (e.g., *Paramecium*) are suspended in dilute solutions of blepharismin, they are not affected while in the dark but are quickly killed if exposed to a light of 2,000 foot-candles or more (Giese, 1946). Blepharismin, which is an endogenous photosensitizer in *Bleph-*

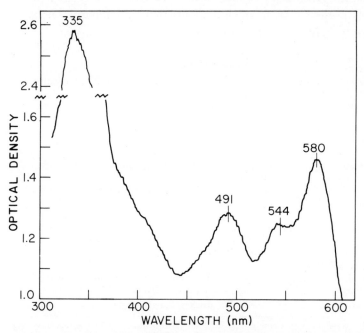

Fig. 11.4. Absorption spectrum of the red pigment of *B. japonicum* v. intermedium after extrusion in an aqueous medium. The cells were centrifuged off and the pigment suspension used for the measurement.

arisma, is thus an exogenous photosensitizer for a variety of other color-less cells (see Table 11.1; Giese, 1953, 1957).

In general, *Blepharisma's* susceptibility to light is correlated with the amount of red pigment present, the darker species being more suscep-tible (Table 11.2). By the ice-water treatment it is possible to reduce the pigmentation of one species and thus mimic a less pigmented species with phenotypic copies that are now less susceptible to visible and near UV (310–390 nm) light than the deeply pigmented controls. Even a true phenotypic albino can be produced by illuminating a red *Bleph-arisma* with dim light for 100–150 hours; this gradual treatment causes bleaching, perhaps by a very slow extrusion of the pigment (Giese, 1938). Phenotypic albinos, as one would expect, are also relatively in-sensitive to visible and near UV light. The genotypic albino mutant of *B. japonicum* v. intermedium is not really completely devoid of pig-ment, and when an albino culture is concentrated its pink coloration becomes evident; it is even possible to extract pigment from a dense culture with ethanol, and the extract has the same absorption spectrum as pigment from the deeply colored form of the species. Nevertheless, the pigment is present in such small amounts that the albino is relatively insensitive to light that will kill the red form.

TABLE 11.1

Photosensitization of Colorless Cells to Visible Light by Blepharismin

Reaction	Cell
Sensitivity to cytolysis:[a]	
Susceptible	*Frontonia leucas*
	Urocentrum turbo
Intermediate	*Paramecium multimicronucleatum*
	Stylonychia curvata
	eggs of *Strongylocentrotus purpuratus* (sea urchin)
Resistant	*Paramecium bursaria*
	Chilomonas paramecium
	Amoeba proteus
	Blepharisma americanum, bleached
	Blepharisma japonicum, albino mutant
Change in excitability:[b]	
Loss in spike height and heightened threshold	neurons of *Cancer magister* (crab) and unsheathed neurons of *Rana catesbiana* (bullfrog)
No change	sheathed neurons of *R. catesbiana*

NOTE: Light passed through Corning filter #3389; intensity about 1,000 ergs/mm²/sec. Pig-mented blepharismas are killed in 6–10 minutes. *Frontonia*, *Urocentrum*, *Paramecium*, and *Sty-lonychia* are ciliate protozoans, *Chilomonas* a flagellate, and *Amoeba* a rhizopod.

[a] Giese, 1949, 1953.

[b] Giese, 1957.

TABLE 11.2

Comparative Resistance of Various Ciliates to Visible and Near
UV Light in the Presence or Absence of Blepharismin

Species and condition	Parts pigment added to one part medium[a]	Appr. time to 1st cell immobilized by light[b]	Appr. time to 50% of cells immobilized by light
B. japonicum v. intermedium:			
Red	0	5 min	7 min
Albino	0	30	48
Albino	3	13	17
Bleached (24 hr)[c]	0	15	35
Bleached (48 hr)	0	35	50
Bleached (48 hr)	3	20	31
Gray-pink (accl. to 40 × UO)[d]	0	95	105
Gray-pink (accl. to 24 × UO)	0	45	75
B. japonicum Suzuki #5:			
Deep red	0	3	5
Pink	0	5	7
B. americanum, lt. pink	0	30	35
Paramecium multimicronucleatum:			
Colorless	0	65	90
Colorless	1	2	3

[a] Pigment solution extracted by mashing 15,000 blepharismas in 1 ml water at 50° C and centrifuging to remove detritus.

[b] Visible and near UV light from a GE CH-4 100-watt mercury spotlamp placed 46 cm from the specimen. Light passed through a 0140 Corning glass filter (cutoff at 318 nm) and 10 cm distilled water; intensity 2,700 foot-candles as measured with a Weston 703 Sight-Lite meter and Kodak density filters at position of specimen.

[c] Cells were bleached with a Lite-Mite fluorescent lamp containing two 4-watt cool white bulbs and placed 10 cm from specimen.

[d] UO is unit osmolality (4.35×10^{-3} osmolal), as present in the standard balanced salt solution described in Chapters 4 and 6.

Localization of Photosensitization

Photosensitization is presumably localized at the surface of *Blepharisma*, since the pigment granules are located there. Photooxidation, at least, seems to be confined to this area (Inaba et al., 1957). When acidified silver nitrate is applied to pigmented blepharismas and the cells are subsequently exposed to light, the salt is reduced and metallic silver is deposited in the pigment granules as the pigment oxidizes. This does not happen in darkness, and albino mutants show no reaction to silver nitrate even in light. Clearly, the photooxidizing response appears only in the blepharismin of the pigment granules.

Violent pigment extrusion following a very strong stimulus (intense light, for example) always kills the cell. We have seen that exposure to light causes the extrusion of pigment granules and the membranes sur-rounding them (Kennedy, 1966). The extrusion apparently damages the cell membrane proper, and the cell may be unable to repair the damage fast enough to avoid lethal injuries resulting from the changed permeability of its surface.

Blepharismas that have been acclimated to an abnormally high con-centration of salts have proved more resistant to light than controls, and the higher the level of acclimation the greater the resistance (Table 11.2). Entry of water through the surface is slow in these cells, as evi-denced by the infrequent systole of the contractile vacuole. We might suppose that surface entry of water hastens the destruction of the cell by light; however, salt-resistant cells also have less pigment than con-trols, which may in part account for their lesser photosensitivity (Giese, unpublished).

The contractile vacuole itself slows or stops functioning after expo-sure to light, suggesting that its membranes are also affected by the photodynamic reaction. When a *Blepharisma* is in strong light, the vac-uole enlarges, often hanging from the posterior end of the cell by a pedicel and sometimes breaking completely away. When this happens the posterior tip of the *Blepharisma* usually heals, and a new vacuole appears. Several successive vacuoles may be lost in this way, and the cell may eventually cytolyze. In other cases, the vacuole simply fails to contract, in which case the whole cell enlarges and cytolyzes without seeming to lose any vacuoles. If a cell is returned to a dimly lit medium as soon as a pedicel containing the contractile vacuole develops, it seems to recover completely and will grow and divide normally thereafter. Apparently, surface photooxidation and injury to the contractile vacuole membrane are quickly repaired (Giese, unpublished; cf. Giese and Crossman, 1946, for similar studies on *Paramecium*).

A light of relatively low intensity (150 foot-candles), which evokes a slow extrusion of the pigment in *Blepharisma*, decreases the rate of re-generation in cells from which the peristome has been removed (Giese and Lusignan, 1961). Possibly, this indicates some damage to the cell surface: the formation of an oral anlage during regeneration requires the multiplication of surface kinetosomes of the V-area, and these may be affected by the photoreaction of nearby pigment granules.

In general, photosensitization by hypericins and porphyrins appears to be localized at the surface of cells (Giese, 1971a–b). Colorless cells

(*Paramecium, Colpidium,* etc.) sensitized to light by the application of blepharismin become "blistered" or vesiculated; like blepharismas, they lose the ability to eject water from their contractile vacuoles and cytolyze soon thereafter (Giese, 1967). Light also hinders the development of nervous impulses in crab and (unsheathed) frog nerve fibers sensitized by blepharismin, since the conduction of these impulses depends on the integrity of the cell surface (Giese, 1957). However, some natural photosensitizers to visible and near UV light, such as the furocoumarins, have been shown to be specific to nucleic acids, forming adducts with the thymine moiety of the acids; thus they can affect only the interior of cells (Giese, 1971b).

The Photodynamic Effect of Various Wavelengths

By the use of a series of Corning glass filters it was shown that a wavelength of 450 nm is more effective in photosensitization than 550 nm, and that wavelengths from 310 nm to 360 nm are maximally active (Table 11.3) (Longerbeam and Giese, unpublished). Tests with the monochromatic visible and near UV light were unsuccessful because the intensity of the light was too low to photolyze the cells; nor did it delay the division or regeneration rates of the cells to any degree that could be accurately measured. Perhaps if the cells could be exposed to monochromatic light throughout the regeneration process or during an entire division interval the effects could be measured with accuracy; but the proper equipment was not available for this series of experiments. It was noted, however, that the qualitative effects of visible light and near UV are somewhat different. Near UV induced pedicel formation to a much more striking degree than visible light, which more frequently induced cells to enlarge without the formation of a pedicel.

Color Changes Induced by Light and Oxygen

When red blepharismas are exposed, in the presence of oxygen, to low-intensity visible or near UV light for two to eight hours they change color. Single cells of the small, lightly pigmented *B. americanum* appear to be bleached, but en masse they appear blue (Giese, 1938); cells of the larger and more deeply pigmented *B. japonicum* (v. intermedium and v. Suzuki #5) show a change from red to gray-blue even when viewed singly. The time required for the color change depends on the physiological state and initial pigmentation of the *Blepharisma*. But as

TABLE 11.3

Absorption Peaks of Pigment from Various Species of *Blepharisma*

Species and pigment preparation	Blepharismin		Oxyblepharismin	
	UV peaks	Visible peaks	UV peaks	Visible peaks
B. americanum				
Suspension	285	330/485/540/572	245/275	330/560/605
Water extract	240/280	330/480/540/575	245/280	330/560/602
Ethanol extract	—[a]/—	330/485/537/575	—/—	330/545/590
B. japonicum v. intermedium				
Suspension	250/280	330/487/537/575	255/280	330/562/605
Water extract	250/285	330/485/545/580	255/280	330/560/600
Ethanol extract	—/—	330/480/535/575	—/—	335/545/590
B. japonicum v. intermedium albino[b]				
Suspension	—/—	—/—/—/—	—/—	325/560/600
Ethanol extract	—/—	—/472/536/576	—/—	335/555/600
B. japonicum				
Suspension	255/280	320/480/535/575	245/280	335/560/600
Water extract	255/280	325/482/535/575	245/280	335/560/600
Ethanol extract	—/—	330/480/535/575	—/—	340/550/592
Acetone extract	—/—	335/485/540/580	—/—	334/552/598

SOURCE: Giese and Grainger, 1970. About 6,000 cells/ml were used to measure absorption by suspensions of *Blepharisma*.
[a] UV absorption for all ethanol extracts is generally strong below 300 nm, and peaks are difficult to resolve. After chromatography on kieselguhr paper a band appears that is lacking after chromatography on other papers or after purification by washing. Because it is impossible to exclude all light during preparation of suspensions or extracts, some of the red pigment is always photooxidized, and the variability in peaks from time to time (several nm) is probably a consequence of this. In the case of the blue pigment, variability in peaks may be a consequence of slight differences in the degree of photooxidation, since some pigment granules seem to be less readily photooxidized than others.
[b] The albino appears to show only blue pigment unless great care is taken to concentrate the cells and extract them in red or yellow light.

long as the light intensity is low, the pigment granules retain their characteristic arrangement. Although some granules are extruded, most of them simply change color and remain in place.

Blue *Blepharisma* (as well as bleached ones) are not killed by intense visible or near UV light. True, blue cells still absorb considerable light (Table 11.3), though at different wavelengths; they absorb less total energy than red cells owing to their loss of some pigment granules, but the absorption of the two is still on the same order of magnitude. However, the oxidized pigment of blue cells seems to have lost the destructive photochemical reaction of the red form. Presumably, the energy absorbed by the blue pigment is mostly degraded to heat and lost to the surrounding medium. Blue cells also show a far less striking increase in oxygen consumption when exposed to bright visible light, since most of their pigment is already oxidized.

Blue blepharismas retain some sensitivity to dim visible and near UV light, and will continue to lose pigment if they are kept in such light for prolonged periods. After 96–150 hours the cells are completely bleached, containing almost exclusively empty granules, and they cannot be distinguished from genotypic albinos. (Kennedy, 1965, has demonstrated this extrusion with electron micrographs.) Bleached cells kept in dim light will eventually begin to divide at the same rate as controls kept in darkness, though remaining to all appearances albino.

The pigment of a blue *Blepharisma* can be extracted by immersion in ice water just as easily as the pigment of a normal cell, and the process of extrusion seems to be much the same. The extruded pigment is pale blue in color and absorbs longer wavelengths of light than the red pigment. The blue solution is slightly murky, presumably because some protein is extruded along with the pigment; but it does not coagulate on boiling any more than red solution does, indicating that the amount of protein is slight in this case as well. Colorless cells suspended in blue pigment and exposed to intense light are unaffected; that is, the blue pigment is not a photosensitizer. Since this pigment has already been oxidized, it might appropriately be called oxyblepharismin.

It is usually not possible to change the color of blepharismas from red to blue with bright (2,000+ foot-candles) visible and near UV light without killing the cells. However, I have sometimes observed the change in surviving cells that had been briefly exposed to very intense visible light from an argon plasma arc with UV radiation filtered out. At other times the cells changed color but were killed, shedding a blue-pigmented capsule (see Chapter 7).

When oxygen is removed from an ethanol solution of blepharismin (by repeatedly freezing with liquid nitrogen, exhausting to a vacuum of 10^{-2} μm Hg, and substituting pure nitrogen) prolonged exposure to intense visible and near UV light has no effect: the blepharismin retains its characteristic color and shows the same absorption bands as before. When oxygen is admitted, however, the blepharismin quickly photooxidizes (Giese and Grainger, 1970).

Oxidizing agents (e.g., potassium ferrocyanide, potassium chlorate, or hydrogen peroxide) have no effect on blepharismin in ethanol solution, but a split-second exposure to ozone in darkness will quickly convert it to oxyblepharismin. If exposed to ozone for more than an instant, the pigment becomes a yellow oxidation product, and a still longer exposure converts it to a completely colorless form. We have also attempted to reduce oxyblepharismin, in ethanol or water solutions, to blepharismin by adding various reducing agents (hydrogen sulfide, hydrosulfite, and hydrogen with a platinum or zinc catalyst), all without success (Giese and Grainger, 1970). Yet the blue pigment eventually disappears from a living cell, and the red form reappears after a lapse of time, suggesting some enzymatic reduction inside the cell. There is always the possibility that the new pigment is synthesized from other substances.

The general effects of these various treatments are summarized in Figure 11.5; and Figure 11.6 presents the resulting color changes.

Blepharismin in solution changes color with changes in pH (Emerson, 1930; Utsumi, 1953). A living *Blepharisma* can tolerate only a relatively narrow range of pH externally (5.5 to 8.0), and no one has ever measured the internal change. However, the extracted red pigment turns blue in alkaline solution and pink in acid, whereas the blue pigment turns green in alkaline solution and pink in acid. These changes, which probably reflect the chemical nature of the pigment, are reversible with changes in pH, unlike the color changes induced by light (Giese and Grainger, 1970). It is especially interesting to observe the changes in pigment color and distribution in the aging cells of a culture that has exhausted its nutrient supply. The pigment first becomes patchy and brownish red. Then, as the cells grow thinner, the pigment turns a greenish gray and finally almost black. In some species (e.g., *B. americanum*), it then aggregates in patches in the middle of the body, which by this

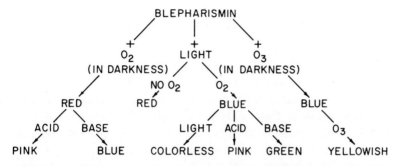

Fig. 11.5. Changes in color of blepharismin subjected to a variety of treatments. The yellowish pigment on the lower right becomes colorless on further ozonation. From Giese, 1971a: by permission of the North Holland Press.

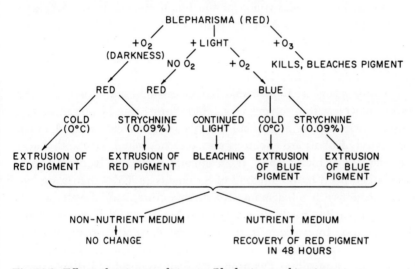

Fig. 11.6. Effects of various conditions on *Blepharisma* and its pigment.

time is flattened and leaflike. These changes in color probably result from the oxidation of the pigment already present and an inability to produce new red pigment without food. The change is accelerated by light as already described.

The red pigment in newly formed cysts turns blue, and is sometimes extruded into the ectocyst walls. Though insoluble at room temperatures, it will dissolve in boiling ethanol and show the characteristic absorption spectrum (J. Grainger, unpubl.). It is not yet certain that cyst pigment is altered in any way from pigment in the vegetative cell.

Absorption Spectra of Blepharismin and Oxyblepharismin

It is possible to measure the absorption spectrum of a suspension of living *Blepharisma*, provided the suspension is so dense that the sieve effect (light passing around the cells) does not vitiate the measurement. Our measurements (using a Cary #15 recording spectrophotometer) show definite peaks at the visible wavelengths 570–575 nm, 540 nm, and 480–485 nm, a peak in the near UV at 330 nm, and shoulders in the far UV at 280–285 nm and 240 nm (Giese and Grainger, 1970). After the pigment has been extruded, the absorption (optical density) of the suspended cells decreases to a fraction of its former value at each peak (Fig. 11.3). Extrusion does not occur to the same degree in each experiment, but the absorption of the blepharismas always decreases considerably. The absorption spectrum of the extruded blepharismin itself, by contrast, is comparable to absorption by the intact cell, although the peaks are sharper; this is true for both visible and UV ranges (Table 11.3; Fig. 11.4).

If a suspension of *Blepharisma* is concentrated and dried, and the lipids removed with a solvent (e.g., chloroform), the blepharismin can easily be extracted by an alcohol or other polar solvent (methyl, ethyl, and t-butyl alcohols are effective; also acetone, toluol, xylol, ethyl acetate, and 1-2 dichlorethane). If an ethanol extract of blepharismin is chromatographed by the method of Sevenants (1965)—that is, on kieselguhr paper with 88% acetone, 10% diethyl ether, and 2% water as solvent—it is possible to obtain a single red band, provided one forestalls photooxidation by working in red light and passing a stream of nitrogen over the chromatogram. The red band, eluted from the filter paper, has the same absorption spectrum as a suspension of red *Blepharisma* cells.

If the pigment is handled without taking precautions against oxidation, two reddish purple bands develop on the chromatograph; in most cases these are preceded by two faint yellow bands, and a faint grayish band remains at the point of application. Both the prominent bands, when eluted, show absorption peaks located somewhere between the peaks characteristic of red and blue pigments, the outer band being more displaced toward the blue peaks. Evidently, blepharismin is being photooxidized to oxyblepharismin during the time it moves on the chromatograph. The two yellow bands probably represent *Blepharisma* pigment that is even more oxidized than the blue form, since both red and blue forms turn completely yellow under ozone treatment. Chromatographs of the pigment extracted from blue *Blepharisma* generally show some of the yellow pigment, as do solutions of blepharismin that have been stored for prolonged periods.

The blepharismin from various species of *Blepharisma* tested in our laboratory shows essentially the same absorption spectra when extracted in similar manner (Table 11.3). The differences previously reported between the spectra of *B. americanum* and *B. japonicum* v. intermedium (Seshachar et al., 1957) or *B. japonicum* (Utsumi, 1953) are probably a result of differences in handling.

Blue *Blepharisma*, in dense suspension, show little absorption at 480–

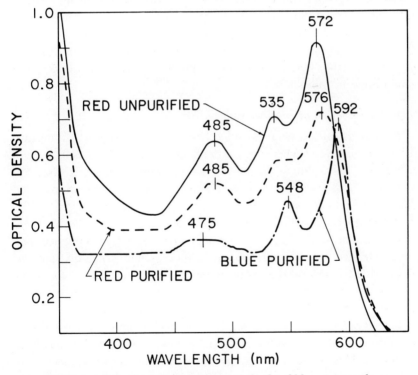

Fig. 11.7. Absorption spectra of ethanol extracts of red and blue pigments from *B. japonicum* v. intermedium. Unpurified pigment is an ethanol extract of the cells; purified pigment is the chromatographed band of an acetone extract of pigment from dried blepharismas washed with lipid solvents. From Giese and Grainger, 1970; by permission of the Pergamon Press.

485 nm, and the other peaks in the visible spectrum characteristic of the red forms are shifted toward longer wavelengths, namely 560 and 600 nm (Table 11.3). As I mentioned earlier, they also have a slightly lower optical density than red *Blepharisma*. The absorption spectrum of extruded oxyblepharismin is comparable to that of an intact blue cell, but the peaks are sharper. Again, there is little absorption at 480–485 nm but strong peaks at 550–560 and 590–605 nm. The absorption of oxyblepharismin in the near and far UV is comparable to that of blepharismin (Fig. 11.7). Similarly, purified oxyblepharismin in ethanol shows the same absorption peaks as a suspension of blue *Blepharisma* or a pigment solution extruded in ice water.

Since the peaks of an ethanol solution of blepharismin are at approximately the wavelengths characteristic of a suspension of living cells, or extruded pigment, the linkage of the pigment to cellular protein is probably not a covalent one. Otherwise, there would probably be a greater difference in absorption peaks between the alcohol extract and the cell suspension (like that between chlorophyll in a green plant cell and chlorophyll in solution).

The Regeneration of Blepharismin

After pigment has been extruded from a *Blepharisma* it will eventually be regenerated whenever nutrients are available, but cells kept in a balanced salt solution do not regenerate their pigment. It takes approximately 48 hours for the optical density of a suspension of extruded *Blepharisma* to regain its original value (Giese and Grainger, 1970). One might wonder whether cell division is necessary in order to regenerate pigment. When I irradiated *B. japonicum* from which pigment had been extruded (wavelength 265 nm, 3,200 ergs/mm^2), cell division was suspended for several days; but as long as the cells carried on active metabolism and ultimately recovered, the pigment was slowly regenerated and the cells became deep red without dividing.

Blue *Blepharisma* will regenerate their red pigment, but more slowly than do cells of either color from which most of the pigment has been extruded. This suggests either that the cell reduces the pigment more slowly than it can replace it or that the oxidation of pigment in the cell is irreversible (Giese and Grainger, 1970). When the pigment is completely extruded by prolonged treatment with dim light, forming phenotypic albinos, pigment recovery takes three or four cell generations. If no food is present in the medium, there are no cell divisions, and only enough pigment is regenerated to turn the cells a faint pink.

The slowness of pigment regeneration in all species of *Blepharisma* is puzzling, since even the complex mouthparts are usually regenerated within 5–6 hours at room temperature. Perhaps the synthesis of blepharismin depends on secondary reactions not associated with the main metabolic reactions. The pigment may even be a metabolic waste product, for we would expect something important to the survival of the cell to be replaced more quickly. It is interesting in this regard that the cysts of some *Blepharisma* species appear to synthesize red blepharismin during their activation (McLoughlin, 1955; Suzuki, unpublished). In *B. americanum*, by contrast, the cell turns blue even in the dark within 24 hours of forming a cyst, extrudes its pigment into the ectocyst, and becomes essentially colorless; when one stock of this species emerges from the cyst it is essentially albino and requires about six generations to redevelop its red pigment. If such cells are made to encyst while still colorless, they form colorless cysts. Apparently, the pigment is not required for encystment or excystment any more than it is for division or regeneration.

The Structure of Blepharismin

Information on the chemical nature of blepharismin was first presented by Møller (1962), who showed that its properties resembled those of hypericin, a plant pigment known to cause photosensitivity in range animals. Sevenants (1965) extended Møller's work and confirmed that blepharismin was indeed a hypericinlike substance (Table 11.4).

Both Møller and Sevenants were aided by the beautiful work of Brockmann (1952, 1957) on the isolation and synthesis of hypericin. The pigment occurs naturally in some 160 species of the genus *Hypericum*, or Saint-John's-wort (Mathis and Ourisson, 1963). For over a decade Brockmann tested many of these, finally selecting *H. hirsutum* for detailed study because under appropriate conditions it develops only one of the hypericins. He extracted enough hypericin from flowers of this species to determine its empirical formula by organic analyses, and from other diagnostic tests he was able to establish its structural formula. After that it was only a matter of time before he synthesized the molecule (Brockmann et al., 1957).

Brockmann proved that the synthetic hypericin, like the natural one,

TABLE 11.4

Experimental Evidence for the Hypericinlike Nature of Blepharismin

Datum	Hypericin	Blepharismin
Fluorescence emission (in nm)[a]		
In 95% acetone	593	598
In diethyl ether/HCl	580	575
In pyridine	600	597–600
Infrared absorption peaks (in μm)[b]	3–9	3–9
Visible-light absorption peaks (in nm)		
In acetone	350/551/593	350–51/551–52/593
In diethyl ether /HCl	325/455/567/580	320/455/563/575
In pyridine	335/557/600	340/557/600
In acetic anhydride	475/512/552/593	495/509/552/592
Light absorption peaks (in nm) after pyroboroacetate reaction[c] (boiled 2 min)	416/440/488/ 548/587/631	398/488/547/ 560/587/603
Ammonium molybdate reaction	Green (meta-oriented hydroxyls)	Blue (ortho-oriented hydroxyls)
Cochromatography (R_f)	R_f values similar for both pigments	

SOURCE: Møller, 1962; Sevenants, 1965.

[a] The fluorescence of hypericin is much greater than that of blepharismin.

[b] There are some significant differences at all positions of carbon to hydrogen response in infrared spectra, according to Sevenants (1965).

[c] Indicates possession of two hydroxy groups.

would photosensitize unpigmented hairless skin in cattle to visible and near UV light. He also showed that hypericin is one of a family of compounds present in various species (possibly all) of the genus *Fagopyrum* (buckwheat) and in the mold *Penicilliopsis clavariaeformis*. The members of the hypericin group differ from one another only in having different substituents in two methyl groups of the hypericin molecule (Fig. 11.8). A brief review of the effects of hypericin is available (Giese, 1971b), as well as a more extended historical account (Blum, 1964).

The evidence that blepharismin is one of the hypericins is indirect (Table 11.4), primarily because no one has yet been able to grow cultures of *Blepharisma* large enough to provide enough pigment for organic chemical analysis. Large cultures of *Blepharisma* invariably grow poorly, but when a more satisfactory axenic medium is developed, growth in large containers may be possible.

In Figure 11.8 the substituents at the methyl groups of blepharismin

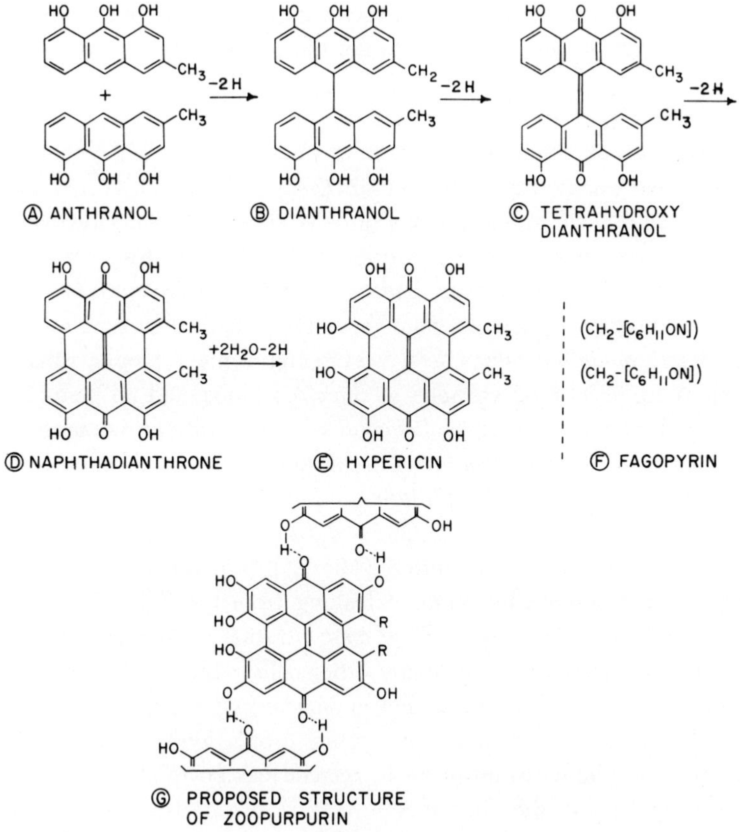

Fig. 11.8. *A, B, C,* and *D* are steps in the laboratory synthesis of hypericin (*E*). Such precursors have also been identified in *Hypericum perforatum,* a weed causing photosensitization in white range animals ingesting it. In fagopyrin, a sensitizer found in buckwheat, the radicals shown in parentheses in *F* are substituted for a hydrogen in the methyl groups of hypericin. (After Brockmann, 1952, 1957.) *G* is a proposed structural formula for blepharismin. From Sevenants, 1965; Giese, 1971b; by permission of the Academic Press.

are designated *R*, since no one has yet tried to determine the nature of this radical. Possibly, the substituent at the *R* group may be what makes blepharismin less fluorescent than hypericin, gives it a different infrared spectrum, and so on.

No one has yet tested the photosensitizing action of blepharismin on human skin. However, hypericin applied directly to human skin will sensitize it to light (Chaplinska et al., 1965). Man is not likely to be affected by hypericin because he neither eats the plants containing it nor contacts them in such a way as to get the pigment on his skin.

Possible Functions of Blepharismin

The discharge of blepharismin granules under stress might possibly be a protective reaction against predators, since the pigment in high concentrations is toxic to many kinds of cells (Giese, 1949). However, blepharismas grown in a mixed culture with other ciliates—such as *Colpidium, Paramecium, Stentor, Didinium,* and *Actinosphaerium*—do not seem to discharge pigment when they collide with their neighbors. *Actinosphaerium eichhorni* has been seen to engulf many blepharismas, which show up in its food vacuoles as dark red blobs, and no pigment is discharged. However, *Actinosphaerium* will not multiply indefinitely when fed only on *Blepharisma*, even in darkness, whereas thriving cultures can be maintained on *Colpidium campylum* alone.

When placed in bright light *Actinosphaerium* quickly "regurgitates" the *Blepharisma* previously engulfed (Giese, 1953), the reaction presumably being triggered by pigment leaking from the light-disrupted *Blepharisma*. Under light, even a low concentration of blepharismin is damaging to *Paramecium* (and many other cells); but if *Blepharisma* and *Paramecium* are cultured together in darkness or in dim light, *Paramecium* divides as rapidly as it does when grown alone (Fig. 11.9). Apparently, the blepharismin in an intact cell has no inhibiting effect on other organisms in the same medium. Wild blepharismas may possibly encounter predators that evoke a discharge of the pigment and are repelled by it, but no data are available on this point.

It has been suggested (Møller, 1962) that *Blepharisma* pigment may enable the organism to orient itself to light, much as stentorin mediates the negative phototropism of *Stentor coeruleus* (Tartar, 1961), and stentorol the positive tropism of *S. niger* (Tuffrau, 1957). However, no convincing data have been presented to substantiate this claim. In dim light blepharismas appear to swim without relation to the light, often aggregating at the surface of a culture tube until food gives out and then hovering over the particulate material at the bottom of the tube; they will do much the same in darkness. Although bright light is quite harmful to *Blepharisma*, the cells will not immediately seek refuge (e.g., in bottom debris) and may remain in the light until killed. If exposed to a gradually increasing light, however, the cells often move to the bottom of a culture and hide in the debris.

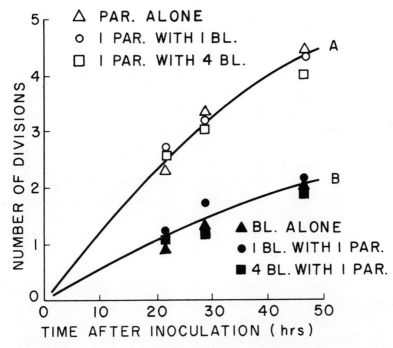

Fig. 11.9. Division rates of *Paramecium multimicronucleatum* (Curve A) and *Blepharisma americanum* (Curve B) in each other's presence (averages of three series of cultures of eight tubes each). Experiments with two of each organism per tube in one case and eight per tube in another gave similar results. From Giese, 1949; by permission of the *Biological Bulletin*.

A test-tube culture, of course, has no perceptible light gradient through which *Blepharisma* can react as it might in a sunlit natural pond, and experiments with such lighting remain to be tried. Perhaps cells that move to the bottom of a tube for other reasons stay within the debris when the sunlight becomes bright enough to drive them back if they venture out; to this extent, the pigment would prevent movement into bright light and thus protect the cells from death. Since the bacterial food in nature tends to be richest among the decomposing vegetation at the bottom of a pond or stream, such a reaction might well be adaptive.

Blepharismin might well screen a cell against far UV radiation to some extent. *Blepharisma*, like all cells, is sensitive to far UV radiation (the UV wavelengths 310–290 nm occur in sunlight at the earth's surface; shorter wavelengths are screened out by the earth's atmosphere).

After large doses of far UV the cells are immobilized and killed (Fig. 11.10); and smaller doses retard cell division.

The retardation of *Blepharisma*'s division rate by far UV has two phases: a delay of the first cell division, and a period of stasis after the first division during which the cells neither grow nor degenerate. Stasis may last for a few hours to many days, and once it ends the irradiated cells divide at approximately the rate of controls. The stasis is longer if the blepharismas are irradiated at higher temperatures, and it practically disappears at low temperatures (Fig. 11.11). Furthermore, the cells are more affected by a UV dose applied in flashes than by the same dose applied continuously (Fig. 11.12). Raising the temperature while flashing the light further amplifies the effect (Fig. 11.13). These data clearly indicate that the stasis results from thermochemical reactions following the absorption of light in the cell: the intervals between flashes allow time for the reaction to occur undisturbed, and the increased temperature speeds them up.

Does *Blepharisma*'s pigment have any part in these reactions? The absorption of far UV radiation by blepharismin (Fig. 11.5) will cause a chemical decomposition of the pigment (Giese, 1953), and it is possible that this decomposition would retard cell division. On the other hand, the similar photochemical breakdown of blepharismin under near UV and visible light does not retard division but merely alters the cell surface much as some synthetic photodynamic pigments do (Giese and Crossman, 1946; Giese, 1967). Moreover, the division of albino *Blepharisma* is also retarded by far UV radiation (Giese, unpublished). It is thus likely that the division-retarding action of far UV results from a reaction by cell constituents other than the pigment.

Since action spectra have been widely used to indicate the kind of compound mediating a particular effect of radiation (Jagger, 1969), we attempted to determine the action spectrum for retarding cell division (see Fig. 9.10). As will be noted, it suggests an absorption by nucleoproteins; in fact, most of the effects of far UV radiation, from which recovery is slow, are localized in the nucleic acids. Far UV forms pyrimidine dimers in the nuclei, which reduce or halt the replication of DNA, and the available DNA is damaged by the same radiation. Damaged DNA is probably inadequate as a template, and the transcribed messenger RNA that is needed to initiate protein synthesis becomes either abnormal or insufficient. It is probable that the delay in cell divi-

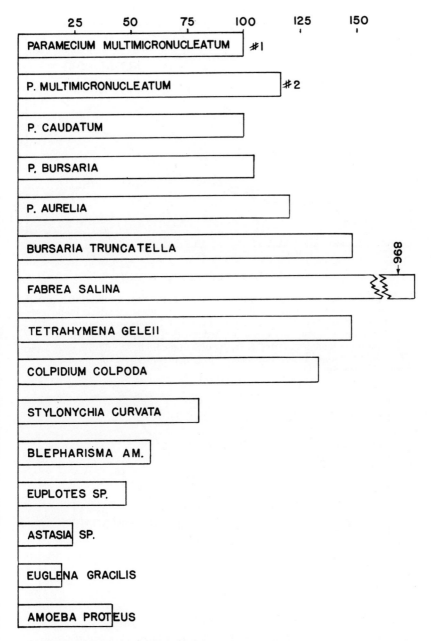

Fig. 11.10. Histogram comparing resistance of various protozoans to far UV radiation (quartz mercury resonance lamp, principal radiation 254 nm). The dose required to immobilize 50% of the *P. multimicronucleatum* was taken as 100, and the other species were compared to this value. From Giese, 1953; by permission of the University of Chicago Press.

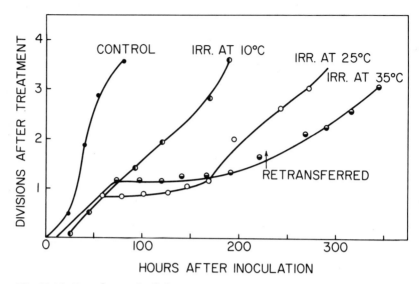

Fig. 11.11. Retardation of cell division in *B. japonicum* v. intermedium by a dose of 4,000 ergs/mm^{-2} at wavelength 265 nm. Note that division stops after a single post-irradiation division. Note also that stasis is greatest for blepharismas exposed to UV at 35° C and unnoticeable for those irradiated at 10°. The arrow shows where the blepharismas were transferred to fresh nutrient medium. All cultures were grown at 25° after irradiation. From Giese et al., 1963; by permission of the *Journal of General Physiology.*

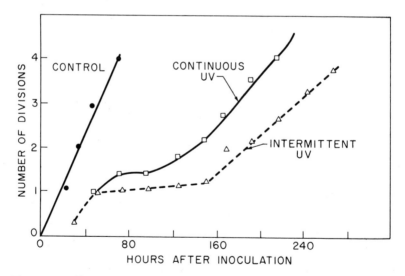

Fig. 11.12. Effectiveness of intermittent UV radiation (265 nm) after a dose of 4,025 ergs/mm^{-2} in retarding division of *B. japonicum* v. intermedium. Note that the stasis is markedly increased and division is resumed later in the sample exposed to intermittent UV. From Giese and Lusignan, 1961a; by permission of the *Journal of General Physiology.*

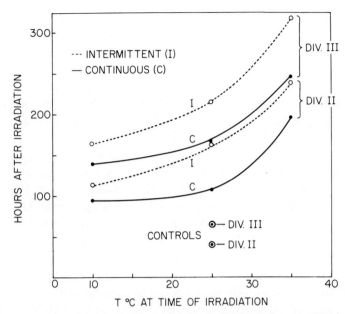

Fig. 11.13. Greater effectiveness of intermittent UV radiation (254 nm, 4,000 ergs/mm^{-2}) in retarding division of *B. japonicum* v. intermedium when the temperature is raised. Irradiation at 10°, 25°, and 35° C, and incubation of all cultures thereafter at 25°. Westinghouse Sterilamp radiation, 90% 254 nm; intensity 25 ergs/ mm^{-2}/sec^{-2}. The division rate of controls is given only at 25° because they were unaffected by exposures to 10° and 35° for periods comparable to those during which the experimental cells were irradiated. From Giese et al., 1963; by permission of the *Journal of General Physiology*.

sion under UV is the time needed for a cell to reestablish normal DNA and RNA syntheses. The effectiveness of UV varies when it is applied at different stages in the division cycle of *Blepharisma* (Schorr, 1958).

Although blepharismin decomposes under far UV radiation, the process is a slow one. Meanwhile, the pigment absorbs radiation that would otherwise reach the cellular nucleoproteins, which are vital to the economy of the cell. When irradiated by a wavelength of 265 nm, which is near the point of maximum absorption by nucleic acids, a wild-type *Blepharisma* from which the pigment had been partially removed by ice water, a laboratory albino, and a genotypic albino are all far more vulnerable than the deeply pigmented wild type (Fig. 11.14). The genetic albino is always more sensitive than the phenotypic (light-bleached) albino, though both appear alike to the eye. Perhaps some genetic alteration in the mutant other than the absence of pigment accounts for this; or perhaps the bleaching of the phenotypic form does not remove the blepharismin completely (Giese, unpublished). The regeneration of a pigmented *B. japonicum* exposed to far UV is also retarded less than that of an albino mutant (Fig. 11.15; Giese, 1965).

Since blepharismas in nature may well turn blue in dim sunlight, as they do when exposed to it in test tubes, it is of interest to know whether the blue oxyblepharismin will protect the cells from far UV radiation as red blepharismin does. *A priori*, it would be expected to do so, since the difference in color between the two pigments is due to their absorption in two different parts of the visible spectrum, whereas their absorption in the far UV is much the same (Fig. 11.16). Observations of the division rate of blue *B. japonicum* v. intermedium irradiated with far UV radiation in fact show that blue cells are about as resistant to far UV as red ones. Also, the delay of regeneration in blue *Blepharisma* induced by a given dose of far UV radiation does not differ appreciably from that in red *Blepharisma*, and is far less than the delay produced in albino cells by the same dose (Giese and Norman, unpublished).

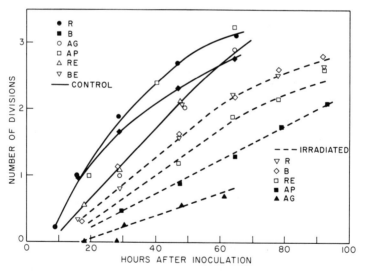

Fig. 11.14. Relative sensitivity of pigmented and unpigmented stocks of *B. japonicum* v. intermedium to a small dose (800 ergs/mm^{-2}) of far UV radiation (265 nm). Red (R) and blue (B) clones are equally sensitive. Cold extrusion of red (RE) or blue (BE) pigment retards division; therefore, the irradiated extruded sample appears to be more sensitive to UV radiation. Most sensitive are the albino clones, the genotypic (AG) more so than the phenotypic (AP). Similar results were obtained with higher doses of UV radiation, including those (9,600 ergs/mm^{-2}) that completely prevent division (i.e., cause genetic death).

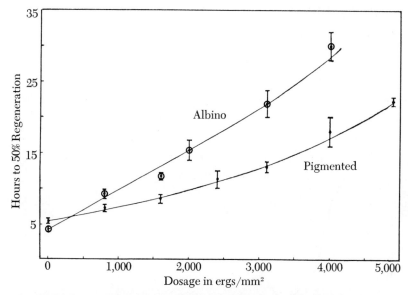

Fig. 11.15. Regeneration time for albino and pigmented stocks of *B. japonicum* v. intermedium irradiated with the indicated doses of UV radiation (265 nm). Points are for a series of 3–6 experiments; vertical lines indicate one standard deviation. At zero dose regeneration takes about 5 hours (control). From Giese, 1965; by permission of Science Press.

Apparently *Blepharisma* in nature is protected from far UV radiation equally well by both blue and red pigment, although neither pigment can protect against a very large dose of radiation. Since other freshwater species of ciliates seem to get along without a protective screen against far UV radiation, why has *Blepharisma* developed one? The pigment may only be a chance mutation; but its prevalence in the genus suggests that it gives *Blepharisma* a selective advantage, perhaps by compensating for some other defect.

Most cells possess enzymatic systems that carry out both photoreversal repair and dark repair of far UV radiation damage; cells lacking these systems (e.g., some bacterial mutants) are probably laboratory curiosities (Smith, 1971). Dark repair of far UV radiation injury has not been studied in *Blepharisma*, but photoreversal has.

Photoreversal repair of far UV damage, achieved by subsequent exposure to near UV and visible light, is thought to monomerize the thymine and other pyrimidine dimers formed by a cell's exposure to far UV radiation. Photoreversal has been demonstrated in most cells (Jagger, 1960), with some curious exceptions (Cook, 1970). In *Blepharisma*

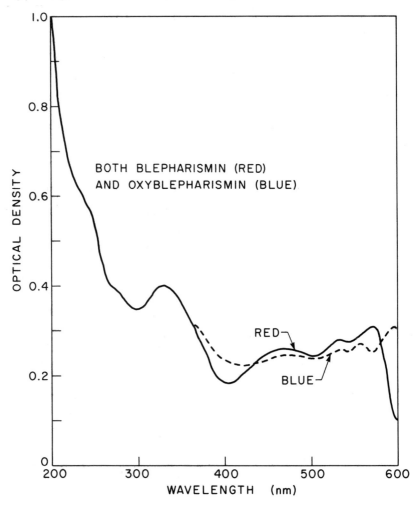

Fig. 11.16. Absorption spectrum of blepharismin (red pigment of *B. japonicum*) and oxyblepharismin (blue pigment), showing schematically the differences in the visible wavelengths and the general similarity in the UV spectrum. Based on measurements of chromatographically purified pigments using a Cary #15 recording spectrophotometer.

the division delay resulting from exposure to far UV (mainly the stasis phase) is to some extent photoreversible; that is, stasis is reduced or eliminated by visible and near UV light applied soon afterward (Giese and Lusignan, 1961a; Fig. 11.17). However, photoreversal in *Blepharisma* is at best about 30%, whereas it reaches about 95% in other protozoans tested (Giese, 1967). The albino *B. japonicum* v. intermedium shows no better photoreversal than the pigmented strain (E. M. Smith, unpublished). In bacteria, it is known that some strains show different degrees of photoreversal or lack it entirely, and that several genes determine the photoreversing enzymes (Hanawalt, 1968). Photoreversal studies in *Blepharisma* have so far used only *B. americanum* and *B. japonicum,* and it would be interesting to test other species of the genus. Under natural conditions *Blepharisma,* like all unicells, is subjected to the far UV radiation present in sunlight, and protection against this would obviously have survival value, especially when the organism lacks an effective photoreversing system. Little published information is available on the penetration of far UV radiation in pond water. Although the data of Hulbert (1928) suggest that the far UV radiation in sunlight would pass through many centimeters of water, considerable absorption occurs in 10 cm of lake water in which numerous protozoans are present (Fig. 11.18).

It is evident that *Blepharisma*'s pigment imposes some limitations that do not exist for colorless cells. *Blepharisma* cannot live if it is suddenly exposed to bright visible and near UV light, and will tolerate

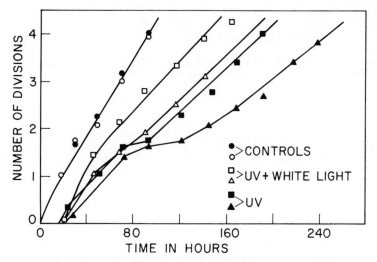

Fig. 11.17. Photoreactivation by visible light of UV damage in *B. japonicum* v. intermedium. Squares indicate an original dose (265 nm) of 2,475 ergs/mm^{-2}, triangles a dose of 3,700 ergs/mm^{-2}. Photoreactivation of irradiated cells by exposure for an hour to two 90-watt daylight fluorescent lamps one foot away (through water cell to remove heat). Redrawn from Giese and Lusignan, 1961a.

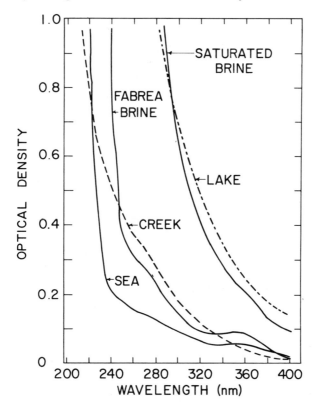

Fig. 11.18. Relative absorption of far UV radiation by filtered water containing various solutes, measured against distilled water in a Cary #14 recording spectrophotometer using a 10-cm-path quartz-faced cell. Protozoans can live in all but the saturated brine. Sea water is equivalent in solute concentration to .55 M NaCl; the brine in which *Fabrea* lives is twice this, and saturated brine is ten times this concentration. The amount of salt in creek and lake water is slight; but both contain unknown concentrations of a variety of organic materials, which for our samples were much higher in Lake Lagunita water than in San Francisquito Creek water (both taken near the Stanford campus). Data courtesy of Dr. Peter Rushbrook, NASA-Ames Research Laboratory, Moffett Naval Air Station, California.

them only after its pigment is photooxidized by prolonged exposure to very dim light. Perhaps this is why blepharismas seem less common in the field than other protozoans (Noland, 1925; Wang, 1928). Possibly, *Blepharisma* simply cannot travel to certain pools; but since cysts have not been observed in many species of the genus, it seems likely that the cells either die under unfavorable conditions or remain hidden deep in the bottom muck and are not observed.

It will be recalled that some blepharismas can live under anaerobic conditions for several days (Beadle and Nilsson, 1959). A systematic survey of pools with this in mind might uncover *Blepharisma* more frequently. It must be kept in mind that under laboratory conditions of dim light or darkness the cells accumulate blepharismin more rapidly than they would in nature, becoming deep pink or even red; and it is when the pigment is so concentrated that *Blepharisma* is especially sensitive to visible and near UV light. Furthermore, the pigment is especially abundant after periods of rapid growth not likely to be experienced in most natural environments. All in all, the hazards from visible and near UV light that *Blepharisma* encounters in nature are probably less than one would presume from laboratory experience.

Three albino strains of *Blepharisma* (two species) have been obtained in laboratories, and two of these are still in healthy culture; hence it seems likely that albino strains occur in nature. Why, then, are albinos never found in the field? Perhaps the most important factor is their lower resistance to the far UV radiation in sunlight, which gives selective advantage to the pigmented *Blepharisma* (Table 11.5). Or they

TABLE 11.5

Relative Effectiveness of Visible Light, Near UV, and Far UV on Blepharismas with Diverse Amounts of Pigment

State of pigment in *Blepharisma*	Effect of intense visible and near UV light (750–320 nm)	Effect of dim visible and near UV light (750–320 nm)	Effect of far UV radiation (310–250 nm)
A. Deeply pigmented (stationary state after log phase of culture)	quickly killed	pigment photooxidized to blue	most resistant to far UV
B. Well pigmented (log phase culture)	less quickly killed than A	more quickly photooxidized to blue form than A	less resistant than A
C. Log phase culture, extruded by exposure to 0° C	less sensitive than B	turns blue even more quickly than B	somewhat less resistant than B
D. Blue pigment (from log phase)	relatively insensitive (bleaching occurs)	very slow bleaching	about as resistant as B
E. Phenotypic albino	relatively insensitive[a]	insensitive	quite sensitive to far UV
F. Genotypic albino (mutant)	relatively insensitive[a]	insensitive	most sensitive of all to far UV

NOTE: All experiments at room temperature. At 5–7.5° C even dim visible light may kill red-pigmented cells.

[a] No albino is completely free of pigment, but all contain a very much reduced amount.

may be more susceptible to some other factor in the environment not disclosed by experiments. For example, albinos might be more palatable to predators, although there are no data on this point. Finally, albinos could easily exist in the wild without being noticed by collectors, especially if they were resting among debris at the bottom of a pond.

Blepharismin and Other Natural Photosensitizers

It is interesting to consider blepharismin in relation to the hypericin-like pigments found in other ciliates and to other photosensitizing pigments found in a variety of cells. Hypericinlike pigments are found in a number of ciliates, but the discussion here is limited to the pigments of *Blepharisma, Stentor,* and *Fabrea,* since more is known about them. When these three pigments are compared, they show differences suggesting a possible evolution.

Briefly, blepharismin is produced continuously whenever a cell is actively metabolizing, and it accumulates when the cell is no longer dividing. Under such circumstances it serves as an excellent screen against far UV radiation. It is an endogenous photosensitizer to visible and near UV light, and can also photosensitize colorless cells if extruded into the medium. In dim light it can be photooxidized to oxyblepharismin, which no longer functions as a photosensitizer to visible or near UV light, but still screens out far UV radiation fairly well (Giese and Grainger, 1970).

The stentorin of *S. coeruleus* filters out far UV, but studies on the sensitivity of this species to far UV radiation and the possible photoreversal of damage inflicted by such radiation have not been made. Only the strains of *S. coeruleus* that fluoresce can be photosensitized to visible and near UV light by stentorin. It is possible that the capacity to produce nonfluorescent stentorin is an advantageous survival adaptation acquired by the species, immunizing it against photosensitization by visible and near UV light while protecting it from far UV radiation. Nothing is known of the photosensitizing or photoprotective properties of the pink hypericinlike pigment (stentorol) of *S. igneus* (Barbier et al., 1956), the related yellow pigment of *S. niger* (Tartar, 1961), or the bluish pigment in *Folliculia* (another spirotrich; Sjogren, 1964).

The fabrein of *Fabrea,* another hypericinlike pigment (Henneguy, 1890; Møller, 1962), being black (broad absorption 570–687 nm: Donnasson and Fauré-Fremiet, 1911; Fauré-Fremiet, 1911), is also an excellent screen against far UV radiation; consequently, *Fabrea*'s resistance to far UV is of an entirely different order of magnitude than that of all other protozoans tested (Giese, 1938b; Fig. 11.10). This genus occurs in brine pools that few living things can tolerate (Ellis, 1939), and hence must live in unclouded water and suffer prolonged exposure to sunlight. *Fabrea*, it seems, has managed better than *Blepharisma*, developing an effective far UV radiation screen without risking the photosensitization by visible and near UV light that occurs in *Blepharisma*.

Blepharisma is a unique animal cell that in the wild type has incorporated into its genome a liability: blepharismin. This pigment subjects the cell to a lethal photooxidation on exposure to bright light; but by absorbing some of the far UV in sunlight it prevents this damaging radiation from reaching the nuclei. The blue form of the pigment is not a photosensitizer but absorbs far UV radiation about as well as the red form; hence it would seem that *Blepharisma* can adapt to strong light gradually if conditions permit. The capacity to produce the pigment in quantity is lost in albino mutants, but these have not been observed in nature.

The endogenous photosensitization present in *Blepharisma* and fluorescent strains of *Stentor* has not been found in any other wild-type animal cell. Something akin to it occurs in certain mutant strains of stock animals and in man, where the condition is known as hematopoietic porphyria. The red blood cells may become loaded with porphyrins and quite sensitive to the visible and near UV light absorbed by those pigments; however, hemolysis does not occur *in vivo*, but only *in vitro*. In some forms of the disease the cells of the skin absorb the porphyrin and are sensitized to visible and near UV light (summary in Giese, 1971b).

Many other animal cells contain pigments that respond to light: e.g., the retinal cells of the eye; the cells of certain invertebrates, which discharge gametes after exposure to light; and the photoreceptor cells of plants (summary in Giese, 1971b). But in all these cases the cells are not injured in the process. In green plant cells chlorophyll acts as a photosensitizer; but generally the effects of photosensitization are not evident because the cells also have carotenoids containing numerous conjugate unsaturated bonds that protect the cells against the photooxidation of chlorophyll. (Photosensitization does occur in mutants that lack the carotenoids; see Giese, 1971b.)

During the stationary phase in some species of bacteria (e.g.,

Myxococcus xanthus, supposedly the wild type) porphyrins accumulate to a level 16 times greater than that present in a logarithmically growing culture. Such cultures are quickly killed by visible and near UV light in the presence of oxygen, and the action spectrum for this lethal effect resembles the absorption spectrum of the porphyrins (protoporphyrin in this case). The protoporphyrin extracted from these bacteria will also photosensitize other types of cells to light in the presence of oxygen. The photosensitization here might seem to resemble that found in *Blepharisma.* However, all aerobic cells produce porphyrins, which are important in certain of the characteristic enzyme systems for activating oxygen (e.g., cytochrome, cytochrome oxidase), and most cells can regulate the synthesis of porphyrins as needed. The strains of *Myxococcus* reported here simply fail to regulate the synthesis, much like a reported strain of *Tetrahymena gelei.* Perhaps there are actually wild-type *Myxococcus xanthus* in which the regulation of synthesis is adequate.

Interestingly, brine-pool bacteria have sometimes developed carotenoid pigments to prevent photooxidation by the light-absorbing porphyrin constituents of their enzyme systems. Some of these bacteria are even chromogenic: that is, they develop the carotenoid pigment under the influence of light, but lack it when grown in the dark and are then highly sensitive when suddenly exposed to light (Krinsky, 1968). Ciliates do not seem to use this protective device, although one strain of *Tetrahymena* accumulates porphyrins and is killed on exposure to light (Rudzinska and Granick, 1953).

In *Blepharisma* it is possible that blepharismin is produced in quantity because, as a screen, it is useful only if a large quantity of it is present. We have seen that species of *Blepharisma* with little blepharismin, in general, are less resistant to far UV radiation than controls. And the albino mutant, as well as the phenotypic albino, is most sensitive of all.

LITERATURE CITED

Arcichovskij, V. 1905. Über das Zoopurpurin, ein neues Pigment der Protozoa (*Blepharisma lateritium* Ehrb.). Arch. Protistenk. **6**: 227–29.
Barbier, M., E. Fauré-Fremiet, and E. Lederer. 1956. Sur les pigments du cilié *Stentor niger.* C. R. Acad. Sci. Paris **242**: 2182–84.
Beadle, L. C., and J. R. Nilsson. 1959. The effect of anaerobic conditions on two heterotrich ciliate Protozoa from papyrus swamps. J. Exp. Biol. **36**: 583–89.

Blum, H. F. 1964. Photodynamic action and diseases caused by light. New York.

Brockmann, H. H. 1952. Photodynamically active natural pigments. *In* Progress in organic chemistry (J. W. Cook, ed.), I: 64–82.

———— 1957. Centenary lecture: Photodynamically active plant pigments. Proc. Chem. Soc. 1957: 304–12.

Brockmann, H. H., F. Kluge, and H. Muxfeldt. 1957. Total Synthese des Hypericins. Ber. Deuts. Chem. Gesell.: 2302–18.

Chunosoff, L., I. R. Isquith, and H. I. Hirshfield. 1965. An albino strain of *Blepharisma*. J. Protozool. **12**: 459–64.

Chaplinska, M. H., M. A. Shilinberth, and Z. H. Trybuldsk. 1965. A study of photodynamic properties of *Hypericum* extract applied externally. Farm. Zh. **20**: 47–53.

Cook, J. 1970. Photoreactivation in animal cells. *In* Photophysiology (A. C. Giese, ed.), V, 191–233. New York.

Donnasson, J., and E. Fauré-Fremiet. 1911. Sur le pigment de *Fabrea salina* Henneguy. C. R. Soc. Biol. Paris **71**: 515–17.

Ehrenberg, C. G. 1838. Die Infusionsthierschen als volkommene Organismen. Leipzig, 612 pp.

Ellis, J. M. 1939. The morphology, division and conjugation of the marine ciliate *Fabrea salina* Henneguy. University of California dissertation.

Emerson, R. 1929–30. Some properties of the pigment of *Blepharisma*. J. Gen. Physiol. **13**: 159–61.

Fauré-Fremiet, E. 1911. La structure intime de *Fabrea salina* Henneguy. Compt. Rend. Acad. Sci. **71**: 419–20.

Giese, A. C. 1938a. Reversible bleaching of *Blepharisma*. Trans. Amer. Microsc. Soc. **57**: 77–81.

———— 1938b. Differential susceptibility of a number of protozoans to ultraviolet radiations. J. Cell. Comp. Physiol. **12**: 129–38.

———— 1946. An intracellular photodynamic sensitizer in *Blepharisma*. J. Cell. Comp. Physiol. **28**: 119–27.

———— 1949. A cytotoxin from *Blepharisma*. Biol. Bull. **97**: 145–49.

———— 1952. A note on a pigment extract of *Holosticha rubra*. Anat. Rec. **113**: 108–9 (abstr.).

———— 1953. Some properties of a photodynamic pigment from *Blepharisma*. J. Gen. Physiol. **37**: 259–69.

———— 1957. Photodynamic effect of *Blepharisma* pigment on nerve. J. Cell. Comp. Physiol. **49**: 295–302.

———— 1965. *Blepharisma intermedium*: Ultraviolet resistance of pigmented and albino clones. Science **149**: 540–41.

———— 1967. Effects of radiation upon Protozoa. *In* Research in protozoology (T. T. Chen, ed.), II, 267–357. New York.

———— 1971a. Nucleic acid and protein synthesis, as measured by incorporation of tracers, in ultraviolet-treated *Blepharisma*. Exp. Cell Res. **64**: 218–26.

———— 1971b. Photosensitization by natural pigments. *In* Photophysiology (A. C. Giese, ed.), VI, 77–129. New York.

———— 1972. Natural photosensitizers and photosensitization with special reference to *Blepharisma*. *In* Research progress in organic-biological and medicinal chemistry, III, 1–28. Amsterdam.

Giese, A. C., and E. B. Crossman. 1946. Sensitization of cells to heat by visible light in presence of photodynamic dyes. J. Gen. Physiol. **29**: 193–202.

Giese, A. C., and R. M. Grainger. 1970. Studies on the red and blue forms of the pigment of *Blepharisma*. Photochem. and Photobiol. **12**: 489–503.

Giese, A. C., and M. W. Lusignan. 1960. Stimulation of post-irradiation recovery of cells by cutting. Science **132**: 806–7.

———— 1961a. Retardation of regeneration and division of *Blepharisma* by ultraviolet radiation and its photoreversal. J. Gen. Physiol. **44**: 543–54.

———— 1961b. Regeneration and division of *Blepharisma* following X-irradiation. Exp. Cell Res. **23**: 238–50.

Giese, A. C., B. K. McCaw, and R. Cornell. 1963. Retardation of division of three ciliates by intermittent and continuous ultraviolet radiation at different temperatures. J. Gen. Physiol. **46**: 1095–1108.

Giese, A. C., B. K. McCaw, J. W. Parker, and J. T. Recher. 1965. Comparative ultraviolet sensitivity of regeneration in the genus *Blepharisma*. J. Protozool. **12**: 171–77.

Giese, A. C., D. C. Shepard, J. Bennett, A. Farmanfarmaian, and C. L. Brandt. 1956. Evidence for thermal reactions following exposure of *Didinium* to intermittent ultraviolet radiation. J. Gen. Physiol. **40**: 311–25.

Giese, A. C., and E. Zeuthen. 1949. Photo-oxidations in pigmented *Blepharisma*. J. Gen. Physiol. **32**: 525–35.

Hanawalt, P. C. 1968. Cellular recovery from photochemical damage. *In* Photophysiology (A. C. Giese, ed.), IV, 203–51. New York.

Henneguy, L. F. 1890. Sur un infusoire heterotriche *Fabrea salina* (nov. sp.). Ann. Micrographie **3**: 118–35.

Hulbert, E. O. 1928. Penetration of UV light into pure water and seawater. J. Opt. Soc. Amer. **17**: 15–27.

Inaba, F., R. Nakamura, and S. Yamaguchi. 1958. An electron-microscopic study of the pigment granules of *Blepharisma*. Cytologia (Tokyo) **23**: 72–79.

Jagger, J. 1960. Photoreactivation. Rad. Res. Suppl. **2**: 75–90.

Johnson, L. P. 1948. A symbiotic *Blepharisma*. Proc. Iowa Acad. Sci. **55**: 391–93.

Kennedy, J. R., Jr. 1966. The effect of strychnine and light on pigmentation in *Blepharisma undulans* Stein. J. Cell Biol. **28**: 145–53.

Krinsky, N. I. 1968. The protective function of carotenoid pigments. *In* Photophysiology (A. C. Giese, ed.), IV, 123–95. New York.

Kurita, M. 1968. Electron microscopy of the pigment granules in *Blepharisma*. Biol. J. Nara Women's Univ. **18**: 50–52 (Jap., with Engl. summary).

Lowry, O. H., N. J. Roseborough, A. L. Farr, and R. J. F. Randall, 1951. Protein measurement with the Folin phenol reagent. J. Biol. Chem. **193**: 265–75.

McLoughlin, D. K. 1955. Cystic phenomena in the ciliate *Blepharisma undulans*. J. Protozool. **2**, Suppl. 11 (abstr.).

Mathis, C., and G. Ourisson. 1963. Etude chimio-taxonomique du genre *Hypericum*, I: Répartition de l'hypéricine. Phytochemistry **2**: 157–71.

Møller, K. M. 1962. On the nature of stentorin. Compt. Rend. Lab. Carlsberg **32**: 471–98.

Noland, L. E. 1925. Factors influencing the distribution of freshwater ciliates. Ecology **6**: 437–52.

Pace, N., and G. MacKinney. 1941. Hypericin, the photodynamic pigment from Saint-John's-wort. J. Am. Chem. Soc. **63**: 2570–74.

Parker, J. W., and A. C. Giese. 1966. Nuclear activity during regeneration in *Blepharisma intermedium* Bhandary. J. Protozool. **13**: 617–22.

Raab, O. 1900. Über die Wirkung fluorescierender Stoffe auf Infusorien. Zeitschr. Biol. **39**: 534–46.

Rudzinska, M. A., and S. Granick. 1953. Porphyrin production in *Tetrahymena geleii*. Proc. Soc. Exp. Biol. Med. **83**: 525–26.

Schorr, L. 1961. An action spectrum of ultraviolet effects on dividing *Blepharisma undulans*. Dissertation Abstr. **22**(3): 899–900.

Seshachar, B. R., A. V. S. P. Rao, and P. B. Padmavathi. 1957. Properties of the pigment of an Indian species of *Blepharisma*. J. Sci. and Indus. Res. India **16C**: 201–4.

Sevenants, M. R. 1965. Pigments of *Blepharisma undulans* compared with hypericin. J. Protozool. **12**: 240–45.

Sjogren, L. 1964. On the existence of stentorin II in folliculinids. Acta Zool. **44**: 293–97.

Tartar, V. 1961. The biology of Stentor. New York, 413 pp.

——— 1972. Caffeine bleaching of *Stentor coeruleus*. J. Exp. Zool. **181**: 245–52.

Tuffrau, M. 1957. Les facteurs essentials du phototropisme chez le cilié heterotrich *Stentor niger*. Bull. Soc. Zool. France **82**: 354–56.

Utsumi, K. 1953. Some properties of the pigment in *Blepharisma*. J. of Sci. Hiroshima Univ., Ser. B., Div. 1, **14**: 35–38.

Utsumi, K., and K. Yoshizawa. 1957. Intracellular structure of *Blepharisma* as revealed by electron microscope. Zool. Mag. (Tokyo) **66**: 234–39.

Wallengren, H. 1900. Zur Kenntnis der vergleichende Morphologie der hypotrichen Infusorien (*Holosticha rubra* Ehrbg.). Beih. Svenska Vet. Akad. Handl. **26** (Ser. 4, No. 2): 1–31.

Wang, C. C. 1928. Ecological studies on the seasonal distribution of Protozoa in a freshwater pond. J. Morph. Physiol. **46**: 431–78.

Weisz, P. B. 1950. On the mitochondrial nature of the pigmented granules in *Stentor* and *Blepharisma* (*B. undulans*). J. Morph. **86**: 177–84.

CHAPTER TWELVE

Classification, Distribution, and Evolution

When Perty first established the genus *Blepharisma* in 1849, his description was incomplete, considering only body shape, ciliation, and buccal apparatus. Stein (1867) presented a relatively complete definition: "The animals are free-swimming, persistent in form, and compressed and pointed in the anterior region. The body is roughly sickle-shaped, bending to the left. The peristomal field consists of a long, deep, fissurelike cleft situated on the left-hand border of the body. The peristome extends along the border for about one-half the body length and then continues inward as a short, funicular pharynx. The outer (or left-hand) margin of the peristome bears larger adoral cilia. There is a short undulating membrane on the basal portion of the right-hand margin." To this, Kent (1881–82) added: "The macronucleus is ovate or elongate; the contractile vacuole is single and subterminal, and the anal aperture is postero-terminal. The genus inhabits fresh water and is usually brightly colored."

Later workers added to the genus various species that possessed traits not previously included. For example, Anigstein (1912) described *B. clarissimum*, which was contractile, marine, and possessed a contractile vacuole with a dorsal collecting canal. Kahl, in his monumental work of 1932, included the species described by Anigstein, as well as *B. vestitum*, which is also contractile. The species of *Blepharisma* that have a filiform macronucleus were not included because they were still unknown. Unfortunately, Kahl's inclusion of widely divergent forms made the genus no longer a relatively homogeneous aggregate of species, and his lack of information on species with a filiform macronucleus made it incomplete. In 1965 Hirshfield, Isquith, and Bhandary redefined the

By Henry I. Hirshfield, Irwin R. Isquith, and Ann M. DiLorenzo.

genus to include filiform species and to take into account some other very diverse forms: *B. clarissimum, B. salinarum,* and *B. candidum.* Some of these forms are now excluded, making the genus somewhat more homogeneous. In addition, some synonyms have been recognized.

As the genus is now defined, all of its members share the following characteristics. The cells are lenticular, with a slightly compressed oral region and a rounded posterior end, although they may be attenuated posteriorly by starvation and rendered almost ovoidal by appropriate feeding (see Chapter 1). The body length ranges from about 50 μm in some species to more than a millimeter in others. The oral apparatus, located on the ventral surface, consists of an adoral zone of membranelles (AZM; referred to as membranellar band elsewhere in the text) on the left peristomal border, an undulating membrane (UM) on the right, and a concave oral groove between. The conspicuous membranellar band begins near the anterior end of the cell, spirals to the right at the widest region of the peristome, and terminates at the cytostome in the vicinity of the undulating membrane. The undulating membrane lies on the right border of the oral groove and progresses forward for about one-third to one-half of the peristomal length; individual cilia continue forward on the right margin from the point where the undulating membrane terminates. The peristome is divided into a narrow oral groove and fan-shaped vestibulum. The oral groove covers about half the anterior length of the peristome and then widens into the vestibulum, which curves to the right, forming the cytopharynx, and terminates in the cytostome. The contractile vacuole, almost invariably located posteriorly, is more or less spherical and has no collecting canals; diastole is brought about by the fusion of smaller vacuoles (see Chapter 6).

The color of *Blepharisma* species varies from colorless to a dark red or blue. Most species are pink, the pigment being located in discrete granules arranged in broad longitudinal stripes between the ciliary rows (see Chapters 1 and 11). On the left, the ciliary rows at their origin are more or less perpendicular to the AZM; they curve posteriorly across the dorsal region and end at the cytopyge. On the right, pigment stripes and ciliary rows start at the anterior tip of the organism and proceed dorsally back to the cytopyge.

The literature on the species of *Blepharisma* is confusing, in part because some of the early descriptions of species are too vague to identify the strains of *Blepharisma* that have since been isolated.* Moreover, instead of relegating an inadequate species to the status of *nomen nudum* (naked or useless name) many workers, even recently, have instead altered the descriptions of species in an attempt to redefine them. Further confusion was added by Stolte (1924), who, by varying the nutrition of a strain of *Blepharisma* normally possessing a filiform macronucleus, showed that in some cases the macronucleus fragmented into several ovoidal pieces. From this he concluded that macronuclear structure was not a valid taxonomic criterion. Subsequent workers, noting the apparent polymorphism displayed by Stolte's "*B. undulans*," assumed that almost any blepharismas they isolated were simply morphological variants of "*B. undulans*." Consequently, the literature is replete with various morphological types of *B. undulans* that bear little resemblance to the species originally described by Stein. Other authors, for their part, identified new species that were differentiated by minor morphological differences.

A review of the taxonomy of *Blepharisma undulans* was initiated by Suzuki (1954), who clearly differentiated three morphological types, chiefly on the basis of macronuclear differences, and accordingly split the species into three subspecies: *B. u. undulans*, with a binodal macronucleus; *B. u. americanus*, with a multinodal macronucleus; and *B. u. japonicus*, with a filiform macronucleus. Bhandary (1962) elevated Suzuki's subspecies to species level and added additional species. Hirshfield, Isquith, and Bhandary (1965), using Kahl as a guide, enumerated some of the major species of the genus and attempted to show the relationship between them, establishing four subgroups or megakaryotypes (originally called subgenera) distinguished largely by whether the macronucleus is compact, binodal, multinodal, or filiform in shape. (Bracketed species are questionable until verified in culture.)

I. Single compact macronucleus (formerly subgenus *Compactum*). Species with spherical or ovoid macronucleus: *B. lateritium*, [*B. coeruleum*], [*B. falcatum*], [*B. lentis*], [*B. seculum*], [*B. tardum*]. Species with macronucleus somewhat elongated: *B. halophilum*, *B. violaceae*.

---

* A *strain*, as used here, is a culture of protozoans collected at a known geographical location. A *stock* is a similar culture of unknown geographical origin. *Variety* is used loosely (i.e., not as a taxon) to designate a stock or strain with distinctive characteristics insufficient to warrant species or subspecies status. Some of the varieties listed were considered valid species until intergrading forms were observed. The authors of this chapter prefer to avoid the term, but it is retained to identify stocks or strains used in experiments described elsewhere in this book.

II. Binodal macronucleus (formerly subgenus *Halteroides*). Species with two spherical nodes: *B. undulans, B. tropicum, B. ichthyoides.* Species with one spherical and one elongated node: *B. semifiliformis.*

III. Multinodal macronucleus (formerly subgenus *Blepharisma*). *B. americanum, B. musculus, B. multinucleata, B. melana, B. dileptus.*

IV. Filiform macronucleus (formerly subgenus *Filiformis*). *B. japonicum, B. stoltei, B. brevifiliformis.*

Others dealing with the *Blepharisma* species problem have approached it by examining the degree of variability displayed in different strains. Dingfelder (1962) found a wide variation in general body shape and concluded that the described species were too strictly defined. He stressed the necessity for growing the organisms in the laboratory for taxonomic studies. Isquith (1966) demonstrated macronuclear variation in several filiform species, and Isquith, Repak, and Hirshfield (1968) showed that in some species the oral apparatus varied. Finally, Dragesco (1970), on the basis of data provided by Isquith for filiform species, has suggested that the species *B. japonicum* contains too many diverse strains.

Inasmuch as some of the morphological traits heretofore used to differentiate species of *Blepharisma* may vary with conditions, some slightly and others extensively, many of the currently named species are open to question. It is therefore mandatory: (1) to broaden the species definitions and take into account such variability as occurs under different external conditions; (2) to eliminate invalid species from the genus. In compiling the catalog of descriptions presented here, we have used the earliest species name created to identify a group of species found to be synonymous, differentiating the later names as "varieties." This is particularly common in polymorphous species (e.g., *B. japonicum*).

Macronuclear Morphology as the Basis for Classification

Although our proposed subdivision of the genus *Blepharisma* into megakaryotypic groups takes into account the known characteristics of the various species, it fails to come to grips with one basic taxonomic problem of this genus—namely, the relationship between the species. In asexual organisms it is impossible to test the validity of a biological species. Conjugation does occur sporadically in *Blepharisma*, but no one has been able to induce it at will, so that the interfertility of various strains cannot be tested. All that the taxonomist can do at present is to decide, subjectively and arbitrarily, how wide a range of phenotypic variation is permissible within a species, basing his conclusions on a careful study of the available members of the genus.

If there were only a few strains, each distinct from the other and with little variability, the delineation of species would be simple. However, many strains of *Blepharisma* have been described, some of them quite variable in characteristics and overlapping with other strains. Polymorphic strains of *Blepharisma* are therefore difficult to classify into valid species. The groupings given above and the listing of species thereunder attempt to meet the first function of a scheme of classification—namely, to pigeonhole valid species. The term "group" is noncommittal, and is preferable until more information allows a classification based on relationship. Our discussion of the various groups of species attempts to meet the second function of a scheme of classification—namely, to establish possible relationships between groups and species.

Geographical Distribution

Blepharisma appears to be worldwide in distribution. Freshwater strains have been found in Europe, the Americas, Africa, and Asia; and marine strains have been reported from Europe, North America, India, and Australia. Information from Oceanic areas is sparse, and the Australian species is the only one reported to date.

Blepharismas with a compact interphase macronucleus (Megakaryotype I) are abundant in Europe, including Russia, and are occasionally found in eastern North America. Marine strains have been reported from Portugal, India, and South Australia; and some of these will tolerate changes in salinity (Ruinen, 1938).

Blepharismas with a binodal interphase macronucleus (Megakaryotype II), the nodes connected by a strand, have been found in Europe (Germany), North America (United States), and Asia (Japan, India).

Blepharismas with a multinodal interphase macronucleus (Megakaryotype III) are also widely distributed, possibly because many of them form cysts. They are abundant in North America, are found in South America (Brazil), are very common in Europe (including some in Russia), and have been reported from India. The majority of the reported marine strains fall into this group. Freshwater strains are of medium size; marine strains are large. No strains in this group have been found in Japan.

Blepharismas with a filiform interphase macronucleus (Megakaryotype IV) are the largest freshwater forms known, some reaching 700 μm in length; they are also the most brilliantly colored when grown in darkness or dim light in the laboratory, though paler in the field, where they are exposed to sunlight (see Chapter 11). These strains are quite abundant in Asia (Japan and India); they have been reported from Africa and are common in Europe (Germany). Strangely, none have been found in North or South America.

Evolutionary Considerations

Nuclear morphology is likely to be more stable than cytoplasmic morphology, and so provides a somewhat better basis for classification and the determination of evolutionary relationships. Much information is available on macronuclear morphology and behavior during division, conjugation, regeneration, and encystment in *Blepharisma*. Far less is known about micronuclear morphology, mainly because the structure of a micronucleus during division cannot be resolved with a light microscope, and few studies have been made with the electron microscope. However, micronuclear fine structure, including chromosome numbers, might help to resolve some of the enigmas in *Blepharisma*'s classification (see Chapter 3). Since there is so little information for developing a scheme of evolutionary relationships in the genus *Blepharisma*, much that we shall say on the subject is pure conjecture or is based on only a few facts.

Assuming that *Blepharisma*'s morphology can suggest possible evolutionary pathways in the genus, the compact macronucleus is perhaps the most primitive type (Bhandary, 1962). Moreover, blepharismas with a compact macronucleus also have the simplest division pattern, and on this account also might be regarded as closest to the genetic type from which all the others originated. In fact, the macronucleus in the other three megakaryotypes returns to the compact form during cell division, regeneration, and conjugation—possibly a form of recapitulation, but in any case the sign of a general similarity between the macronuclei in all four megakaryotypes. The binodal macronucleus might be considered a variant of the compact type, in that the macronuclear material is simply separated into two knobs connected by a filament. The multinodal macronucleus is only a step beyond the binodal, and in the same direction (Isquith, 1966). And the filiform macronucleus is another extended form of the compact type; it may be knobbed or not, and under some conditions it develops nodes.*

These facts indicate a close relationship between all the strains of *Blepharisma*, a point reinforced by the seeming intergradation between the different types of macronuclei in various strains, which creates a real nightmare for the taxonomist. The variation of the macronucleus under diverse nutritional conditions may have unsettled the classification of various species of *Blepharisma*; and a closely controlled nutrition in axenic culture (for example, on a fully defined medium), though unnatural, might allow one to define species boundaries in this respect. This difficult objective has not been achieved (see Chapter 4). At present, it is perhaps most accurate to describe a given stock or strain simply as closely resembling one of the species so far described.

The presence of all four megakaryotypes in India suggests this area of the globe as the center of origin of the genus. But it may be that South Asia simply offers the most favorable conditions for the genus as a whole, whatever the origin of particular types. It is also interesting to speculate on whether *Blepharisma* as presently defined had a marine or freshwater origin. A marine origin could place the genus very far back in biologic time, since seawater has not changed much in salt composition or content since the beginning of life (Rubey, 1951). However, too little is known of marine blepharismas, which are far outnumbered by the strains and species found in fresh water. It is quite possible, of course, that this simply reflects a rapid evolution under the more variable environments presented by fresh water. But a marine origin would suggest that freshwater strains might adapt to saline solutions more readily than they do in the laboratory (Finley, 1930; Hilden and Giese, 1969).

Catalog of the Species of *Blepharisma*

We could increase our knowledge of the distribution and classification of *Blepharisma* if individuals who found pink protozoans anywhere in the world would ship a culture to Dr. Henry I. Hirshfield, Biology Department, New York University, Washington Square, New York, N.Y.

---

* The possible advantages of an elongate or noded macronucleus are not apparent, but these types do present a larger surface area for the diffusion or release of materials such as messenger RNA. The increase in area may therefore facilitate the housekeeping chores that are performed by the macronucleus during the cell's normal cycle of feeding and growth.

10003. These would be placed in a permanent central reference collection of cultures and slides. This central repository might also be consulted for help in identifying the strain of *Blepharisma* used in a particular study—a practice that would eliminate much of the unavoidable confusion now present in the literature.

As it is, this catalog seems to us the most accurate that can be assembled from the available data. Drawings are about × 300, except as noted.

I. *Species with a Compact Macronucleus*

It is evident from our earlier synopsis of the genus that many species in this megakaryotype are of questionable validity. Until they can be obtained in culture and studied carefully, their status cannot be resolved. They are tentatively accepted here only because there is no good reason to exclude them.

1. Blepharisma lateritium (Ehrenberg, 1831) Kahl, 1932. First species described. Length, 60–200 μm; width, 38–50 μm. The body is long, pointed anteriorly and rounded posteriorly. The species is usually pale pink, but sometimes colorless (Roux, 1901). There is a short, narrow undulating membrane (André, 1912), with a peristome extending half the total body length (Isquith et al., 1965). The macronucleus is ovoid and centered in the anterior half of the body (André, 1912). There are five or six micronuclei and a large contractile vacuole (Penard, 1922). *B. lateritium* is common in Europe and the United States, similar strains being reported from both areas.

The following nine entries, originally described as separate species, are now recognized as types synonymous with *B. lateritium*.

2. B. lateritium v. **botezati** (Lepși, 1926) Kahl, 1932. Length, about 150 μm. Anterior body beaked, posterior swollen.

3. B. lateritium v. **elongatum** (Stokes, 1884) Kahl, 1932. Length, 73–85

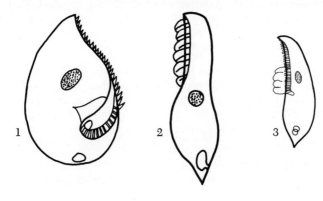

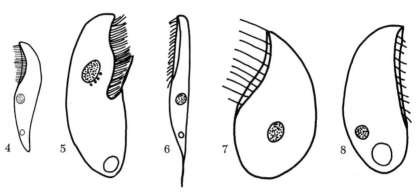

μm. Tail about one-fifth body length and may be contractile. Two contractile vacuoles, alternating in action. Wide undulating membrane and small cytopharynx. × 300.

4. B. lateritium v. hyalinum Perty, 1849. Length, 43–130 μm. Colorless. Thin, flexible body with 4–5 ciliary rows when young and up to 18 when mature. Oval macronucleus. × 300.

5. B. lateritium v. steini Kahl, 1932. Length, 100–176 μm. Bluish-red to blue, with thin, scalpel-shaped body. AZM about two-thirds body length and covered by right ventral margin. Short oval macronucleus and many micronuclei.

6. B. lateritium v. sphagni (Lepşi, 1926) Kahl, 1932. Length, 150 μm. Thin posterior half, with tail about one-fifth body length. Contractile vacuole lying one-third body length from posterior end. Small undulating membrane.

7. B. lateritium v. minima Lepşi, 1926. No distinctive characters reported.

8. B. lateritium v. navicula Lepşi, 1926. No characters reported.

9. B. lateritium v. ovata (Stokes, 1884) Kahl, 1932. Length, 127 μm; length is 1.5 to 2.1 times the width. Anterior end beaked and flattened; posterior enlarged with short tail. Two contractile vacuoles, contracting alternately. Peristome two-thirds body length. Narrow AZM and undulating membrane, with undulating membrane two-thirds peristome length.

10. B. lateritium v. bimicronucleata Villeneuve-Brachon, 1940. Length, 100–150 μm; width, 30–40 μm. Pale pink. Lateral surface widens and grows thinner at extremities; 17–18 ciliary rows. The undulating membrane is twice the width of the narrow AZM but only one-quarter as long. Peristome is two-thirds body length. Macronucleus spherical, with two flattened micronuclei nearby.

11. Blepharisma coeruleum Gajevskaja, 1927. From 90 to 130 μm in length and bilaterally symmetrical, blunt anteriorly and rounded posteriorly. It is

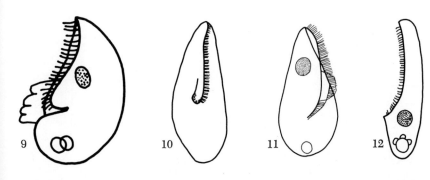

light gray, gray-blue, or greenish-blue in color. The cilia lie closely together, with 25–30 rows clustered on each side of the body. The peristome, two-thirds body length, has long, closely set membranelles that cover its exterior margin. The gullet, which merges with the peristome and reaches the middle of the ventral side, contains shorter membranelles. The undulating membrane is located on the posterior third of the inner peristomal margin and forms a transparent triangular disc. The macronucleus is spherical and lies in the anterior third of the body. The contractile vacuole is terminal. The organism is almost always found on the alga *Tetraspora* on the south shores of Lake Baikal, Siberia.

12. Blepharisma falcatum Gelei, 1954. About 120 μm long and usually 35 μm wide, with cylindrical anterior and posterior ends 15–20 μm thick. Dirty gray in color. The gullet lies on the margin of the posterior third of the body. Ciliary rows, 45 in number, run toward the "spinning organ" (peristomal structures beneath the surface) on the left side of the cell, and in a longitudinal direction on the right. The spinning organ comprises two-thirds of the body volume and includes 60 double-layered membranelles. The AZM is short, covering the oral opening. The macronucleus is spherical.

13. Blepharisma lentis Gelei, 1954. About 150 μm long; normal vegetative interphase length/width ratio of 3:2 changes to 2:1 in dividing organisms and 4:3 in well-fed specimens (they feed on small flagellates and ciliates). The body is rounded dorsally and narrows ventrally and posteriorly. Faintly gray-blue in color ("dove-colored"). The 60–70 ciliary rows lie in the body indentations and are unevenly distributed (about 38 on the right side and 22 on the left). The spinning organ, a powerful system of two-layered membranelles (about 100 lamellae), runs spirally from the left side over to the right to a depression at the margin of the last third of the body, and ends in a broad oral opening or funnel. Just in front of the mouth is a short but broad membrane arranged anteriodorsally and six ciliary rows in width; this covers the oral opening and the spinning organ and participates in swallowing. The spherical macronucleus and the terminal contractile vacuole are large.

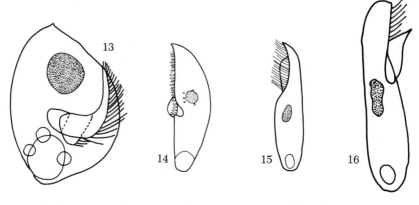

14. Blepharisma seculum (Isquith, 1965) Isquith et al., 1965. From 60–110 μm in length, 20–30 μm in width. Slightly pink in color. When well fed the organism is stubby, but when starved it is thin and forms a tail. The dorsal border is curved, giving the cell a sickle-shaped appearance. The somatic ciliary rows, 10–14 in number, are arranged in the typical *Blepharisma* pattern. The AZM does not reach the anterior tip, but begins behind a slight beak. The undulating membrane extends for one-third of the peristomal length, which is, in turn, half the body length. The macronucleus is spherical and about 10 μm in diameter. Two to eight micronuclei about 2 μm in diameter are located near the macronucleus. Encystment has been observed only once, and giantism and conjugation not at all (Isquith et al., 1965). This species may be a synonym of *B. lateritium*. × 300.

15. Blepharisma tardum Kahl, 1928. This small species ranges in length from 100 to 120 μm. The body is very thin, the length/width ratio being 14:1. The peristome is one-quarter to one-third the total body length, and the undulating membrane is three-quarters of the peristomal length. The terminal contractile vacuole is small. The body is loosely striated with short cilia. The macronucleus is a small ellipsoid lying in the middle of the body (see Kahl, 1928, 1932, 1933).

16. Blepharisma halophilium Ruinen, 1938. From 100 to 250 μm in length, 15–20 μm in width, and faintly yellowish to reddish; variable in shape, often half as wide anteriorly as posteriorly. The peristome, one-third to one-half the body length, has on the right margin an undulating membrane one-half to two-thirds the length of the peristome and preceded by thick, powerful cilia 10–15 μm long. The macronucleus varies in shape from an elongated ellipsoid to a short rod. The contractile vacuole is terminal.

The species has been reported to grow in 3% NaCl solution, 15% NaCl solution, and even saturated NaCl solution. Strains have been found in South Australia, India, and Portugal.

17. Blepharisma violaceae Tucolesco, 1962. About 200 μm long and violet or red-violet in color. The body is flattened laterally and pointed at the extremities, with about ten ciliary rows. Digestive vacuoles are found only in the posterior third of the body and often contain red bacteria of the genus *Cromatium*. The peristome extends two-thirds the body length and a short, fibrillar undulating membrane is present at the edge of the oral opening. The oral cavity leads into a thin pharyngeal passage. A nearly rectangular but elongated terminal contractile vacuole is present. The macronucleus is oval and one or two micronuclei are present. Found on the Romanian coast.

II. *Species with a Binodal Macronucleus*

The species in this megakaryotype appear acceptable, in part because they are not as variable as some of the others.

18. Blepharisma undulans Stein, 1867 (syn. *B. undulans undulans* Suzuki, 1954). The length of this pink, spindle-shaped *Blepharisma* varies from 70 to 250 μm. The anterior half of the organism is flat, tapering to a round, expanded posterior end. The peristome is a narrow groove generally situated in the anterior third of the body, but at times reaching midbody. The undulating membrane, on the right side, occupies the entire posterior half of the peristomal border and 12–15 somatic ciliary rows are present on one side of the body. The macronucleus is binodal, with one node anterior and the other posterior. The two nodes, which have an intense Feulgen-positive reaction, are connected by a thin strand. The micronuclei, which number 1–12, are located near the macronuclear membrane.

Cysts are almost ovoid in shape and are dark brown in color. The outer ectocyst is 48–71 μm in diameter, the endocyst 36–40 μm. The macronucleus of the cyst retains its two connected nodes, which may contract to a dumbbell shape. There are 4–11 micronuclei scattered within the cytoplasm of the cyst. In division, the connecting strand of the macronucleus contracts without breaking, and a condensed macronucleus is formed. This elongates into a filiform body before dividing, and the vegetative macronuclear condition reappears in the daughter cells (Suzuki, 1954).

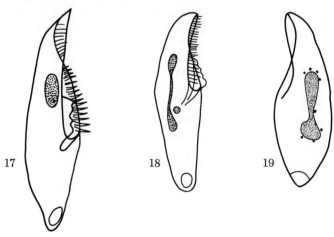

17   18   19

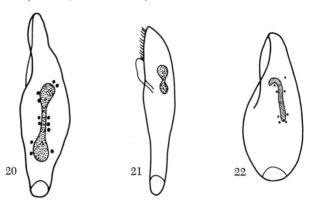

19. Blepharisma semifiliformis Isquith, 1966. This strain, from Andhra, India, is probably a synonym for *B. undulans*. It ranges from 100 to 180 μm in length, averaging 150 μm, and is pale pink with no apparent order in the pattern of pigment granule arrangement. Ciliary rows number 10–14. The AZM membranellar band extends to the anterior tip, and the undulating membrane is more than half the peristomal length. The peristome itself is less than half the total body length. The bipartite macronucleus generally has one round node, which is joined to an elongated node by a strand of varying thickness.

20. Blepharisma tropicum Bhandary, 1962. The organism is 135–200 μm in length and pink in coloration. The peristome extends for one-third the total body length, and the undulating membrane is not prominent. The macronucleus is binodal, the nodes being connected by a thick strand. There are 6–18 micronuclei, each about 1.6 μm in diameter. During conjugation the macronuclear anlagen divide before fission of the cell.

21. Blepharisma ichthyoides Gelei, 1933. This coppery red to colorless species is 150 μm in length and 30–45 μm in width. The posterior portion of the body is cylindrical, with the terminal end swollen near the contractile vacuole. The oral groove points posteriorly. The peristomal region is extremely narrow. The spinning organ is short and stops at the rear marginal swelling of the oral funnel; the undulating membrane is short and low. The binodal macronucleus is described as being elliptical or biscuit-shaped; four micronuclei are present. The author, von Gelei, considered that *B. lateritium*, *B. steini*, and *B. ichthyoides* might be variations of one species but provisionally established *B. ichthyoides* as a distinct species.

22. Blepharisma biancae Lepși, 1948. This species is considered a *nomen nudum* because the original description is insufficient to characterize it.

III. *Species with a Multinodal Macronucleus*

Because the number of macronuclear nodes at first seemed characteristic of *Blepharisma* species in this group, several new species were de-

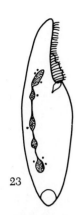
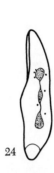
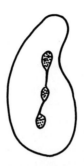
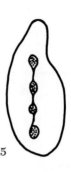

23   24   25

scribed on this basis. However, this number was found to vary within a strain under different conditions of culture (Table 12.1); and as a result, several species were found to be invalid and were reclassified as synonyms of *B. americanum* or *B. musculus*.

23. Blepharisma americanum Suzuki, 1954 (syn. *B. undulans americanus* Suzuki, 1954). Pink. Length, 115–220 μm. Peristome nearly half this length, with a conspicuous undulating membrane. The macronucleus is multinodal with 3–7 nodes; these are of different sizes and are connected by slender strands, the nodes at either end being the largest. There are 6–20 micronuclei, each about 0.9 μm in diameter. Nutritional giantism is found in this species. The species is widespread in North America, and many strains are known.

In conjugation, the macronuclear and micronuclear anlagen differentiate prior to conjugant separation. The exconjugant macronuclear anlagen develop connections with one another to produce the multinodal structure characteristic of the vegetative state. The old macronucleus persists until the exconjugant assumes the vegetative form. Many exconjugants are nonviable (Bhandary, 1962).

The two entries following are now considered synonyms for *B. americanum*, since the macronuclear characters by which they were differentiated are not as constant or diagnostic as first supposed. Until more distinctive differences are shown there seems to be no reason to give them species status.

24. B. americanum v. **trinodatum** Hirshfield et al., 1965. Length, 100–120 μm. Three-noded macronucleus, except in cannibal giants, which have six or more nodes and reach a length of 300 μm. Conjugation pattern typical of *B. americanum*. There are 4–16 micronuclei, each about 1 μm in diameter.

25. B. americanum v. **dawsoni** Christie and Hirshfield, 1967. Length, 115–130 μm; width, 40–50 μm. Macronucleus with 3–5 nodes, terminal nodes largest. Conjugation differs in detail from typical *B. americanum*, and during division the macronucleus forms a two-noded rather than a compact structure. There are 8–13 micronuclei 1–2 μm in diameter. This strain has been in culture longer than any other known to us.

TABLE 12.1
Variability of Macronuclear Nodes in Two Species of *Blepharisma*

Organism	Species	Cells counted	Mean nodal number	Standard deviation	Range	Mode
Americanum N.Y.U.	B. americanum	104	4.2	0.91	3–6	4
Trinodatum 665	B. americanum	100	3.3	0.54	3–6	3
Trinodatum 611	B. americanum	104	3.5	0.71	2–6	3
Sinuosum	B. musculus	66	4.6	0.095	3–7	5
Seshachari	B. musculus	105	5.2	1.06	3–7	5
Giesei 653	B. musculus	105	5.5	0.78	—	5–6
Giesei 622	B. musculus	102	5.4	0.73	—	5

26. **Blepharisma musculus** Penard, 1922. Length, 120–140 µm. Body very pale pink, spindle-shaped, and elongated posteriorly into a long caudal point. The macronucleus has 5–8 (generally 6) spherical nodes, arranged as a bent string of equal-sized beads; it is accompanied by several very small micronuclei. The contractile vacuole is large and forms directly behind the peristome.

The following six varieties are now considered too little different from *B. musculus* to warrant a separate species status and are placed in synonymy with *B. musculus*.

27. **B. musculus** v. **wardsi** Hirshfield et al., 1965. Length, 100–200 µm. Macronucleus with 4–6 nodes connected by a thin strand, terminal nodes largest. A few very small micronuclei.

28. **B. musculus** v. **seshachari** Bhandary, 1962. Length, 120–160 µm. Macronucleus with 4–7 equal nodes; 8–12 micronuclei 1.7 µm in diameter. Conjugation pattern quite distinctive.

29. **B. musculus** v. **sinuosum** Sawaya, 1940. Length, 140–300 µm, averaging 200–220 µm; width, one-quarter to one-third the length. Peristome about one-half body length and very delicate on left margin. Undulating membrane about one-third body length. There are 5–6 micronuclei.

30. **B. musculus** v. **giesei** Hirshfield et al., 1965. Length, 150–200 µm. Macronucleus with 4–8 nodes, usually 6–7 equal size. Also 3–16 relatively large micronuclei. Conjugation resembles that in *B. musculus* v. seshachari. Cyst formation and conjugation are common.

31. **B. musculus** v. **multinodatum** Hirshfield et al., 1965. No observations on size or oral structures. Macronucleus with 10–12 nodes. This type may be a *nomen nudum*.

32. **B. musculus** v. **persicinum** Perty, 1849. Length, 118–176 µm. "Peach-

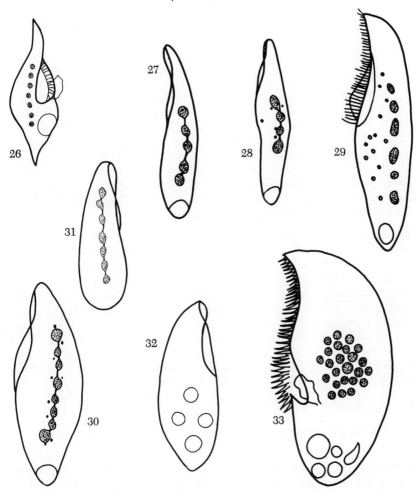

blossom" color, and about 15 ciliary rows. No data on oral structures or nuclei. Best considered a *nomen nudum*.

33. **Blepharisma multinucleata** Dragesco, 1960. Average length, 200 μm. Flat, leaflike body with a sharp anterior beak. About 52 somatic ciliary rows, with rows of brownish-red pigment granules interspersed. The posterior region contains numerous contractile vacuoles, and the cytoplasm appears fibrous. There is a well-developed AZM, which penetrates into the pharynx, and a well-developed undulating membrane that has a tendency to separate into its constituent cilia. The macronucleus consists of about 20–28 discrete ovoids, with nucleoli, scattered in the cytoplasm; no micronuclei described or illustrated.

34. Blepharisma melana Borror, 1963. This marine organism ranges in length from 450 to 640 µm, and in width from 64 to 100 µm. The body is widest in the midsection, tapering to a rounded posterior and prolonged in a narrow anterior snout for about half the body length. The cilia are 10–12 µm long and set about 3 µm apart. The ciliary rows number 30 to 35, are 7 µm apart at midbody, and spiral slightly counterclockwise. There is a large contractile vacuole in the posterior region. The membranellar band, 161–200 µm long, is overhung in its anterior portion by a bill-like lip; posteriorly, it follows the left edge of the oral cavity, ending abruptly near the cytostome. The membranelles number about 115, and are 8 µm wide by 1 to 2 µm thick. The undulating membrane is 16 µm long. The macronucleus is central, many-noded, and 100 µm long. The two micronuclei are adjacent to the macronucleus. (The mismatch between the figure and the description given here is in accordance with the original description; × 125.)

35. Blepharisma dileptus Kahl, 1928. This species ranges from 200 to 260 µm in length (Kahl, 1932) and is narrowly striated, with ciliary rows running diagonally to the left. Two-fifths of its total length is a thin, flexible neck or proboscis that bears the oral groove and membranelles. The undulating membrane, not easily seen, extends along three-quarters of the peristome on the right margin. The posterior body may be linear or swollen, depending on its food content. Brownish, lenticular storage granules occur in the cytoplasm and color the cells, and this species often contains large food vacuoles filled with Rhodobacteria. The macronucleus has 10–12 nodes (Kahl, 1932). *B. dileptus* swims in a snakelike manner, or lies still and waves its neck back and forth like its namesake, the ciliate *Dileptus*.

IV. Species with a Filiform Macronucleus

In this megakaryotype the macronucleus is always filiform, but it may take various shapes in cells undergoing unusual conditions. In some strains the ends of the macronucleus may become enlarged; and it can also appear knobbed, thin, coiled, split, doubled, compacted, or noded. But in a bacterized medium and under an approximation of natural conditions, it regains its filiform appearance.

36. Blepharisma japonicum Suzuki, 1954 (syn. *B. undulans japonicus* Suzuki, 1954). In this species, one of the largest known, the body ranges from 150 to 500 µm in length. The cell is spindle-shaped and blunt at each end. There are 25–35 ciliary rows on one side. Under dim light (the natural condition) the cells acquire a deep red color from the 6–10 longitudinal rows of pigment granules located between each two ciliary rows. Cannibal giants may attain a length of over 700 µm and a width of 300 µm (Suzuki, 1954).

Some strains resembling *B. japonicum* in many characters seemed sufficiently different at one time to make valid species, e.g., *B. intermedium*

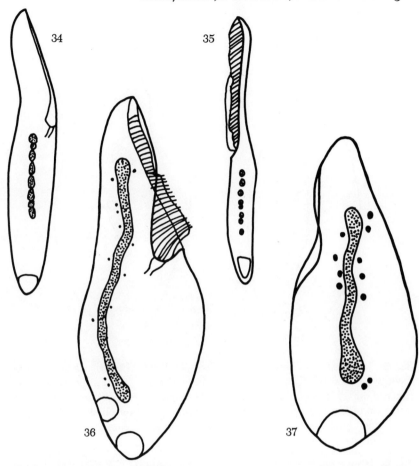

Bhandary, 1962. But the accumulation of strains with many of the characters of *B. japonicum* made evident a graded series between *B. japonicum* and *B. intermedium*, e.g., the Niigata strain (formerly *B. microstomata*) and the Nagpur strain from India. These are reclassified below as types of *B. japonicum*, which has been redefined to include more variability in characters than originally proposed.

37. B. japonicum v. intermedium Bhandary, 1962. Length, 200–350 μm. Cannibal giants may reach 600 μm. Well-organized dark pink pigment granules. Peristome is one-third body length, with an inconspicuous undulating membrane. Macronucleus cylindrical with inconspicuous terminal swellings. Micronuclei 6–30 in number and about 2 μm in diameter. Conjugation similar to other types in genus (see Chapter 2), although Padmavathi (1962) claims to have identified a peculiar pattern.

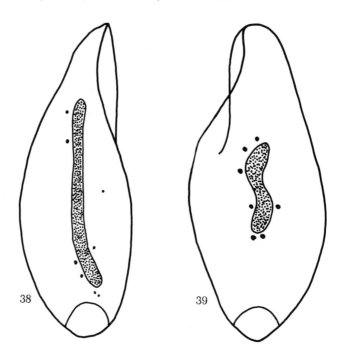

38. B. japonicum v. **microstomata** Isquith, 1966. Length, 200–350 μm. Deeply pigmented. The peristome is quite narrow (microstomatous). The somatic ciliary rows spiral around the body, and the AZM reaches the anterior tip of the cell. Macronucleus without taper or terminal swellings. The 6–14 micronuclei are relatively large. Conjugation, encystment, and giant formation have not been observed.

39. B. japonicum v. **nilssoni** Repak, 1967. Length, 250–400 μm. Deeply pigmented with 5–8 rows of granules. Pear-shaped body with anterior end flattened and terminal contractile vacuole at posterior; there are 60–100 ciliary rows. The AZM occupies the entire left side of the oral groove, and the undulating membrane extends along two-thirds of the length on the other side. The knobbed macronucleus is about two-thirds the length of the body. Cannibalism is frequent, usually producing giants. Conjugation has been seen.

40. Blepharisma stoltei Isquith, 1966 (syn. *B. undulans* Stolte, 1924). This species has the typical *Blepharisma* shape, with color ranging from pale pink to pale red. In darker strains (six in culture, four from Japan and two from Germany) the pigment granules are arranged in short longitudinal rows 3–6 granules long, with up to five rows of pigment granules between each two ciliary rows. The body is 100–280 μm in length, and giants grow to 300 μm. The peristome extends about half the body length, and the AZM extends to the anterior end of the cell. The macronucleus has marked terminal swellings. The 4–18 micronuclei are 1.5 to 2.0 μm in diameter.

Division in this species is typical for *Blepharisma*, except that two macronuclear spheres form before they merge into one compact mass (Isquith, 1966, 1967). The nuclear events during conjugation are also the same as in other species of *Blepharisma* with a filiform macronucleus (Isquith, 1966). Encystment and excystment are readily induced and have been studied (Repak, 1968).

41. B. stoltei v. **narai** Isquith, 1966. Length, 90–210 μm, averaging 170 μm. This type is pale pink, with 14–18 ciliary rows. Morphologically, the cell resembles the typical *B. stoltei*. However, the AZM does not extend all the way to the anterior tip of the cell, and the macronucleus develops terminal swellings only during division (Isquith, 1966, 1967). Encystment, conjugation, and giant formation have not been observed.

42. Blepharisma brevifiliformis Isquith, 1966. From 120 to 195 μm long, averaging 160 μm. Each side of the body has about 20 ciliary rows. The AZM extends half the body length. The filiform macronucleus is quite short, extending when straight to about one-third the body length; it does not taper toward the middle, and only on rare occasions do terminal swellings occur. Usually, the macronucleus is bent or twisted, presenting an even shorter appearance. Four to ten micronuclei are present. Encystment and conjugation have not been observed, and giantism is rare.

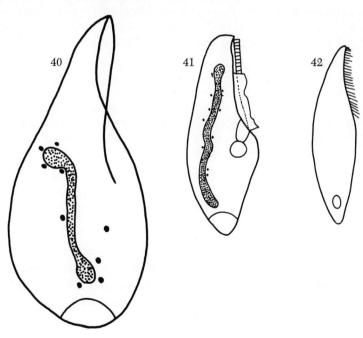

Species Removed from the Genus Blepharisma

Since the keys in some textbooks are likely to list these species as members of the genus *Blepharisma*, they are listed here. The characters given are quite different from those listed for the genus at the beginning of this chapter.

43. B. salinarum (Florentin, 1899) Kahl, 1932. Length, 160–360 μm. Not contractile. Body light yellow in color and elongated. The anterior tip is beaklike, and the entire body is flattened laterally, swelling in the middle and widening to a truncated posterior end. There are 8–9 ciliary rows. The long AZM contains 60–170 membranelles, and the undulating membrane is about one-fifth the length of the peristome. The contractile vacuole lies at the posterior terminal and is associated with a dorsal canal. The nucleus is divided into 50–75 separate particles scattered through the cytoplasm. This species differs from the *B. salinarum* of Dragesco (1960), which is also excluded from the genus *Blepharisma*.

44. B. vestitum Kahl, 1932. Length, 159–189 μm. Reddish color. Contractile, with a necklike structure two-thirds the body length. Ovoid macronucleus.

45. B. clarissimum Anigstein, 1912. Length, 160–380 μm; width about one-tenth length. Body slightly contractile and compressed laterally. Peristome half body length; AZM present, but no undulating membrane. Moniliform macronucleus with 44 nodes. Contractile vacuole present. The varieties *arenicola* and *longissimum* (Kahl, 1932) are also described by Dragesco (1960). This species is now placed in the genus *Anigsteinia* (Isquith, 1968).

46. B. candidum Yagiu and Shigenaka, 1956. Length, 330–520 μm; width about one-tenth length. Body tapers to the right, and has a beak at the anterior end. There are 22–27 ciliary rows. Those on the dorsal surface start at the margin of the peristome and run obliquely; those on the ventral surface run longitudinally. Both an AZM and an undulating membrane are present. The macronucleus resembles a string of 182–287 loose beads. Species now placed in *Anigsteinia* (Isquith, 1968).

47. B. tenuis Kahl, 1932. Since transferred by Kahl (1935) to genus *Pseudoblepharisma*.

A Tentative Key to Blepharisma

At present, it is not possible to establish a comprehensive key for the genus, given the questionable status of so many species and types. However, we have prepared a key to those strains actually in culture at New York University, since it was possible to observe these in detail. Table 12.2 and the key that follows may illustrate for the reader some of the

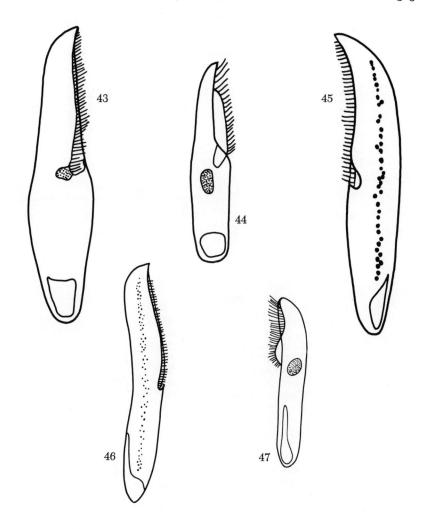

difficulties involved in classifying *Blepharisma* from the descriptions available. The various strains are listed in the table under the species that they most closely resemble, although in some cases a strain differs markedly from the description for that species. Pigmentation has not been used in the key, since it can vary greatly under different environmental conditions; and although we have used giantism to distinguish types in some cases, this character, too, has not been established as a consistently reliable one.

TABLE 12.2
Strains of *Blepharisma* in Culture at New York and
Fairleigh Dickinson Universities

Mega-karyo-type	Species	Strain	Date collected	Habitat
I	B. seculum[a]	Parkville, Md.	1964	Sewage runoff
II	B. undulans	Augusta, Ga.	1961	Pond
	B. tropicum	New Delhi, India	1960	Yamuna R.
	B. semifiliformis	Andhra Pradesh, India	1964	
III	B. americanum	Hingham, Mass.	1961	Stream
		New Brunswick, Can.	1961	Riv. du Vin
		Halifax, N.S.	1922	
		Urbana, Ill.	1956	
		Stanford, Calif.	1933	Pond
		Monterey, Calif.	1965	Ward's Biol. Supply
		Bloomington, Ind.	1963	
		N.Y.U.	—	Possible Calif. origin
		C.C.N.Y.	—	" " "
		N. Carolina (old)	1962	N.C. Biol. Supply
		N. Carolina (new)	1970	" " "
		McManus (Calif.)	1969	
		Williamsburg, S.C.	1968	
		Savannah, Ga.	1968	
		Hardee County, Ga.	1968	
		Cypress Swamp, Fla.	1968	
		South Florida	1968	
	B. musculus	Bangor, Me.	1961	
		Leningrad, Russia	1965	
		São Paulo, Brazil	1939	
		Bangalore, India	1957	
		Stella, Wash.	1960	
		Perlmutter (Curaçao?)	1968	
IV	B. japonicum	Bangalore, India	1956	
		Bangalore (albino)	1964	
		Nagpur, India	1963	
		Suzuki #3, Yamagata	1962	
		Suzuki #5, Yamagata	1962	
		Uganda, Africa	1967	Papyrus swamp
		Niigata, Japan	1954	Rice paddy
		Cameroun, Africa	1969	
	B. stoltei	Nara, Japan	1962	
		Federsee, Germany	1963	Lake
		Federsee (albino)	1968	
		Fukuchiyama, Japan	1957	
		Komatsushima, Japan	1957	
	B. brevifiliformis	Kyoto, Japan	1969	

NOTE: All descriptions are based on organisms grown on 0.3% (N.Y.U.) or 0.15% (Isquith) Cerophyl at 18° C (N.Y.U.) or 20° C (Isquith); giants and dwarves are excluded from the description of megakaryotypes.

[a] Slides only are available. Culture lost in 1969.

With these cultures actually under observation, it has been possible to establish reasonably reliable standards for differentiating them. They can be assigned to the various species and "varieties" given in our catalog according to the following key. (The reader should remember that variety, as we use it, is not a formal unit of classification, but simply a convenient means of identifying a species for those who may be familiar with its older name.)

Partial Key to the Genus

1. Macronucleus noded 2
   Macronucleus not noded 10
2. Macronucleus usually consists of two nodes 3
   Macronucleus usually consists of at least three nodes 5
3. Two macronuclear nodes are usually connected by a thick strand; micronuclei are large; no giantism observed . . . .*B. tropicum*
   Two macronuclear nodes usually connected by a thin strand 4
4. Thin connecting strand is occasionally broken; micronuclei small; inconspicuous undulating membrane . . . .*B. undulans*
   One macronuclear node is frequently elongated; large micronuclei; conspicuous undulating membrane . . . .*B. semifiliformis*
5. Usually three macronuclear nodes; the terminal nodes are larger than the middle node; small micronuclei; giantism frequent . . . .
   . . . .*B. americanum* v. trinodatum
   Usually more than three macronuclear nodes 6
6. Usually four macronuclear nodes 7
   Usually more than four macronuclear nodes 8
7. Four nodes connected by a thin filament; small internodes present in some strains . . . .*B. americanum* v. dawsoni
   Nodes almost always randomly distributed in the cytoplasm . . . .
   . . . .*B. americanum* v. wardsi
8. Nodes are of unequal size; usually about five nodes; the two terminal nodes are the largest; micronuclei are small; giantism is common . . . .*B. americanum*
   Nodes are all of approximately equal size; micronuclei are large; giantism rare 9
9. Usually five nodes, range four to six . . . .
   . . . .*B. musculus* v. sinuosum (includes seshachari, etc.)
   Usually seven nodes, range five to eight . . . .*B. musculus* v. giesei
10. Macronucleus consists of one sphere; large micronuclei; body acutely curved . . . .*B. seculum*
    Macronucleus consists of a filament 11
11. Large average vegetative length of 250 μm; giants 450 μm 12
    Animals small to moderate length, average less than 200 μm; giants not more than 350 μm 14

12. Small micronuclei; AZM does not extend all the way to the anterior
    tip; giantism present ....*B. japonicum*
    Large micronuclei; AZM extends all the way to the anterior tip......13
13. Capable of giant formation.............*B. japonicum* v. intermedium
    No giantism; somatic ciliary rows tend to spiral around the body....
    ....*B. japonicum* v. microstomata
14. Macronucleus has prominent terminal swellings and tapers toward its
    middle; macronucleus extends about half the body length; large
    micronuclei; giantism common; membranellar band reaches the
    anterior tip ....*B. stoltei*
    Macronucleus does not taper; terminal swellings not obvious.........15
15. Macronucleus extends only about one-third the body length; giant-
    ism common; AZM extends to the anterior tip......*B. brevifiliformis*
    AZM does not extend to the anterior tip.............*B. stoltei* v. narai

Conclusions

1. The genus *Blepharisma* is worldwide in distribution, and representative species are present in both fresh and salt water.

2. Investigators have not fully agreed on which characters, nuclear or
cytoplasmic, to emphasize for classification of the species; both have
been used, but the emphasis has been on macronuclear characters.

3. The present classification of the genus *Blepharisma* must be considered tentative, since satisfactory criteria have not been adduced to
distinguish what appear to be an almost intergrading series of strains
collected from various parts of the world. Furthermore, many of the
characters, both cytoplasmic (e.g., color) and nuclear (e.g., number of
nodes or filaments) change with altered cultural conditions. It is suggested that investigators receiving cultures from the field or from other
laboratories describe these characters at once, and then again after subculture. It is necessary to culture each species with some degree of environmental control, and to study its variability before confirming its
species status. This is not possible with species described long ago, or
with those from distant regions. Often, descriptions of either kind are
incomplete and based on a limited observation of blepharismas collected
rather than grown in culture. To define a species, it would be desirable
to study division, conjugation, and encystment, as well as cannibalism
and giant formation; obviously, this cannot be done by collecting wild
specimens.

4. Four nuclear megakaryotypes have been distinguished among the
many strains of *Blepharisma* now in culture: compact, binodal, multi-

nodal, and filiform. In all these forms, however, the macronucleus condenses to a compact unit during division, conjugation, and regeneration, suggesting a common ancestry.

5. A study of the fine structure of the micronucleus and chromosomes might provide information of use in classifying *Blepharisma*, inasmuch as the ultimate master plan for the cell is contained in the micronuclei (see Chapter 3). Differences in behavior of the micronuclei during conjugation have already been observed in a few species (see Chapter 2).

6. Differences in the tendency for conjugation, encystment, and cannibal giant formation have been observed in different species, and even in different strains of the same species. If all species can in fact conjugate, encyst, and form cannibal giants, then the conditions for inducing these phenomena must differ between species and strains.

7. In this catalog many species of *Blepharisma* are declared synonymous with other species that they resemble in major characters and are thus considered invalid, although their names and characteristics are listed. A few species described in insufficient detail are considered *nomen nudum*, and should be disregarded from a listing of species in the genus. Still other species differ so markedly from the definition established for *Blepharisma* that they are placed in other genera.

8. The presence of all four megakaryotypes of *Blepharisma* in India suggests that the genus may have originated in this area, perhaps from a common ancestor that presumably possessed a compact macronucleus.

LITERATURE CITED

André, E. 1912. Catalogue des invertébrés de la Suisse. Infusoires. Fascicule 6: 1–228. Mus. Hist. Nat. Genève. Geneva.

Anigstein, L. von. 1912. Über zwei neue marine Ciliaten. Arch. Protistenk. 24: 127–40.

Bhandary, A. V. 1962. Taxonomy of the genus *Blepharisma*, with special reference to *Blepharisma undulans*. J. Protozool. 9: 435–42.

Bhandary, A. V., and H. I. Hirshfield. 1964. Comparative studies of RNA synthesis in two strains of cannibal giant *Blepharisma*. J. Cell. Comp. Physiol. 63: 217–24.

Borror, A. C. 1963. The morphology and ecology of benthic ciliated Protozoa of Alligator Harbor, Florida. Arch. Protistenk. 106: 465–534.

Calkins, G. N. 1912. The paedogamous conjugation of *Blepharisma undulans*. J. Morphol. 23: 667–91.

Christie, S. L., and H. I. Hirshfield. 1967. Macronuclear variations during

the life cycle of *Blepharisma dawsoni* n. sp. and *B. wardsi*. J. Protozool.
14: 759–62.

Chunosoff, L., I. R. Isquith, and H. I. Hirshfield. 1965. An albino strain of
Blepharisma. J. Protozool. 12: 459–64.

Dingfelder, J. H. 1962. Die Ciliaten vorubergehender Gewässer. Arch. Protistenk. 105: 509–658.

Dragesco, J. 1960. Cilies mésopsammiques littoraux: Systématique, morphologie, écologie. Trav. Stat. Biol. Roscoff (N.S.) 12: 1–356.

———— 1970. Cilies libres du Cameroun: Annales de la Faculté des Sciences
de Yaoundé, Numero Hors Série, Université Fédérale du Cameroun, pp.
88–92.

Ehrenberg, C. G. 1831. Über die Entwicklung und Legensdauer der Infusionstiere. Abh. Berlin Akad., p. 1.

———— 1838. Die Infusionstierchen als vollkommene Organismen. Leipzig,
612 pp.

Finley, H. E. 1930. Toleration of freshwater Protozoa to increased salinity.
Ecology 11: 337–47.

Florentin, P. R. 1899. Etudes sur la faune des mares salées de Lorraine. Ann.
Sci. Nat., 8me Série, Zool. 10: 209–349.

Gajevskaja, N. 1927. Zur Kenntnis der Infusorien de Baikalsees. Compt.
Rend. Acad. des Sci. USSR 19: 313–18.

Gelei, J. von. 1933. Adatok szeged környékének ázalékállatka világához, III:
Nehany *Blepharisma* szeged környékérol. Acta Lit. Sci. Univ. Hung. Francisco-Josephinae, Sect. A, Biol. Sci. Nat. 2: 169–94.

———— 1954. Über die Lebensgemeinschaft einiger temporärer Tümpel auf
einer Bergwiese im Börzsonygebirge (Oberungarn), III: Ciliaten. Acta
Biol. Magyar Tudományos Akadémia Biologiai Közlemenyei 5: 259–343.

Hilden, S., and A. C. Giese. 1969. Effect of salt concentration on regeneration rate in *Blepharisma* acclimated to high salt levels. J. Protozool. 16:
419–22.

Hirshfield, H. I., I. R. Isquith, and A. V. Bhandary. 1965. A proposed organization of the genus *Blepharisma* Perty and description of four new species.
J. Protozool. 12: 136–44.

Isquith, I. R. 1966. Inheritance and speciation in *Blepharisma*. Doctoral dissertation, New York University. 125 pp.

———— 1967. Three new *Blepharisma* species and criteria for establishing a
species. J. Protozool. 14 (supplement): 27.

———— 1968. *Anigsteinia* g. n., a member of family Spirostomatidae.
J. Protozool. 15 (supplement): 26.

Isquith, I. R., A. J. Repak, and H. I. Hirshfield. 1965. *Blepharisma seculum*
sp. nov., a new member of subgenus (Compactum). J. Protozool. 12: 615–
18.

———— 1968. Studies of doublet *Blepharisma* intermedium (Protozoa: Ciliata) Notulae Naturae, No. 413, May 20, 1968.

Kahl, A. 1926. Neue und wenig bekannte Formen der holotrichen und heterotrichen Ciliaten. Arch. Protistenk. **55**: 197–438.

—— 1928. Die Infusorien (Ciliata) der oldesloer Salzwasserstellen. Archiv. für Hydrobiol. **19**: 189–246.

—— 1932. Urtiere oder Protozoa, I: Wimpertiere oder Ciliata (Infusoria), 3, Spirotricha. *In* Die Tierwelt Deutschlands, 25 Teil. Jena.

—— 1933. Ciliata libera et ectocommensalia. *In* Die Tierwelt der Nord- und Ostseen (G. Gripe and E. Waglar, eds.), pp. 29–146. Leipzig.

Kent, S. W. 1881–82. A manual of the Infusoria, II, 585–86. London.

Lepşi, J. 1926. Die Infusorien des Süsswassers und Meeres. Berlin, 100 pp.

—— 1948. Protozoen aus Boden und Laubstreu eines Eichenwaldes. Not. Biol. **6**: 149–59.

McLoughlin, D. 1957. Macronuclear morphogenesis during division of *Blepharisma undulans*. J. Protozool. **4**: 150–53.

Moore, E. L. 1924. Regeneration of various phases in the life history of *Spathidium spathula* and *Blepharisma undulans*. J. Exp. Zool. **39**: 249–315.

Nilsson, J. 1967. An African strain of *Blepharisma japonicum* (Suzuki). A study of morphology, giantism and cannibalism, and macronuclear aberration. Compt. Rend. Trav. Lab. Carlsberg **30**: 1–24.

Padmavathi, P. B. 1959. Studies on the cytology of an Indian species of *Blepharisma* (Protozoa: Ciliata). Vestnik Ceskoslov. Zool. Spokcnosti Acta Soc. Zool. Bohem. o Slovenicae **23**: 193–200.

Penard, E. 1922. Etudes sur les infusoires d'eau douce. Geneva, 331 pp.

Perty, M. 1849. Mikroskopische Organismen der Alpen und der italienischen Schweiz. Mitt. Naturforsch. Gesell. Bern, **164/165**: 151–76.

—— 1852. Zur Kenntnis kleinster Lebensformen nach Bau: Funktionen, Systematik mit Spezialverzeichnis der in der Schweiz. Bern, 228 pp.

Repak, A. J. 1967. Cortical studies on *Blepharisma* and associated phenomena. Doctoral dissertation, New York University. 248 pp.

—— 1968. Encystment and excystment of the heterotrichous Ciliate *Blepharisma stoltei* Isquith. J. Protozool. **15**: 407–12.

Roux, T. 1901. Faune infusorienne des eaux stagnants des environs de Genève. Geneva, 148 pp.

Rubey, W. W. 1951. Geological history of seawater. Bull. Geol. Soc. Am. **62**: 1111–48.

Ruinen, J. 1938. Notizen über Ciliaten aus konzentrierten Salzegewassern. Zool. Mededielingen. **20**: 243–56.

Sawaya, M. P. 1940. Sobre um Ciliado novo de S. Paulo: *Blepharisma sinuosum* sp. n. (Ciliata, Heterotricha) e sobre a sub-ordem Odontostomata, nom. nov. Bul. Fac. Fil., Cien. Letr. Univ. S. Paulo **19**: 303–8.

Sevenants, M. R. 1965. Pigments of *Blepharisma undulans* compared with hypericin. J. Protozool. **12**: 240–45.

Stein, F. 1859. Der Organismus der Infusionstiere, I. Leipzig, 206 pp.

———— 1867. Der Organismus der Infusionstiere, II. Leipzig, 355 pp.

Stokes, A. C. 1884. Notes on some apparently undescribed forms of fresh water Infusoria. Am. J. Science **28**: 38–49.

Stolte, H. A. 1924. Morphologische und physiologische Untersuchungen an *Blepharisma undulans* Stein. Arch. Protistenk. **48**: 245–301.

Suzuki, S. 1954. Taxonomic studies on *Blepharisma undulans* Suzuki, with special reference to the macronuclear variation. J. Sci. Hiroshima Univ., Ser. B, Div. 1. **15**: 205–20.

Tucolesco, J. 1962. Espèces nouvelles d'infusoires de la mer Noire et des Bassins sales Paramarins. Arch. Protistenk. **106**: 1–36.

Villeneuve-Brachon, S. 1940. Recherches sur les cilies heterotriches. Arch. Zool. (exper. gen.) **82**: 1–180.

Wilfert, M. 1972. Zytologische Untersuchungen an dem Ciliaten *Blepharisma americanum* Suzuki 1954, Stamm Berlin (Heterotrichida, Spirostomatidae) sowie Bemerkungen zur Taxonomie und Systematik der Gattung *Blepharisma* Perty 1849. Arch. Protistenk. **114**: 152–230. [Received too late for text discussion, but bears closely on some of the problems treated in this chapter.]

Woodruff, L. L., and H. Spencer. 1922. Racial variation in *Blepharisma undulans*. Proc. Soc. Exp. Biol. Med. **19**: 339–40.

Yagiu, R., and Y. Shigenaka. 1956. A new marine ciliate, *Blepharisma candidum*, n. sp. J. Sci. Hiroshima Univ., Ser. B., Div. 1. **16**: 81–86.

CHAPTER THIRTEEN

Conclusion

Although *Blepharisma* has been studied for some time, many aspects of its biology present problems for future research. The previous chapters have dealt with a wide variety of topics, some of which have not been thoroughly studied in any protozoan; but obviously, there are equally glaring omissions. Nothing has been said about *Blepharisma*'s behavior, motility, genetics, or metabolism, for example—not always because data are lacking, but because all information on these topics has so far been incomplete or questionable. It should be clear from the discussion throughout this study that *Blepharisma* is an ideal experimental subject for investigating many aspects of cellular biology. Its large size and vivid color make it easy to see, and its slow movement makes it easy to handle for studies of single cells. For example, it is easy to cut with a needle, and is therefore suitable for studies of parts of cells and their regeneration. But it would be useful at this point to sum up what we presently know about the organism.

The exact classification of species within the genus *Blepharisma* is still uncertain, although the limits of the genus itself are fairly well defined. Under different conditions of culture the same stock will show differences in macronuclear structure and shape, even though the macronucleus is often used as one of the key characters for classification. An axenic (and therefore uniform) culture has been achieved in one strain. But the medium used in this case was complex; and even so the blepharismas did not divide as rapidly as they do in wild cultures or cultures reared on a single strain of bacteria. Until we can establish standard conditions for the laboratory growth of *Blepharisma*, the taxonomic identity of a good many strains will still be questionable. Lacking this, a study of the fine structure of the chromosomes during mitosis might do much to resolve the species affinities of various strains.

There is a general agreement on the characters that distinguish *Blepharisma* from other ciliates. Most species are large, slow-moving, and noticeably pigmented. Like most ciliates, *Blepharisma* has complex and distinctive feeding organelles—in this case an oral groove lined on one side by a membranellar band and on the other by an undulating membrane. The genus has both micronuclei (always multiple) and a macronucleus that is quite large and sometimes multiple. The macronuclei appear to govern trophic events, whereas the micronuclei presumably act as carriers of the genome and participate in an exchange of genomes during conjugation. The macronucleus varies in shape from species to species, taking one of four principal forms: compact (and often spheroid), binodal, multinodal (beaded), or filiform. In all species, however, the macronuclei become compact at some stage during the life cycle.

Little has been done with the genetics of *Blepharisma*, largely because no one has found a way of inducing conjugation at will. This would be a particularly interesting area of research, since albino mutants have appeared in the laboratory and could be used to study color inheritance.

At the fine-structural level it has been demonstrated that in *Blepharisma*, as in other ciliates, the various systems of organelles typical of eukaryotic (nucleated) cells are present, and that the nuclei in interphase show little internal structure. When the micronuclei undergo mitosis, small but distinct chromosomes appear and can be counted on the spindles. The study of these chromosomes, though difficult, would be desirable, since it might resolve some of the controversies regarding classification. Also, no one has yet studied the internal fine structure of any *Blepharisma* during regeneration or encystment.

Although *Blepharisma* has been found on all continents except Antarctica, little is known of its ecology. In temperate regions blepharismas are usually collected from ponds, though not very frequently; but in warmer habitats, such as the rice paddies of Asia, they are present most of the time. Although we sometimes think of protozoans as ubiquitous, no one has yet found a *Blepharisma* species with a filiform macronucleus in the United States or Canada; yet some of these species, and possibly all of them, form cysts that are apparently capable of surviving and spreading from continent to continent. An intensive ecological study is needed, since investigators reporting blepharismas in nature have usually obtained them by chance and have little or no information about the microhabitat from which the samples came. What we know of *Blepharisma's* food preferences and resistance to environmental factors such as temperature changes or salts comes almost entirely from experimental work conducted in the laboratory. No one appears to have studied circadian or other rhythms in *Blepharisma.*

Cannibalism has been found in many species of the genus cultured in the laboratory; and the cultures in which cannibalism occurs have been observed to outlast those in which all the cells become smaller and die for lack of food. The "lifeboat" hypothesis explains this survival in the laboratory, but whether blepharismas ever become cannibalistic in nature has not been shown. Cannibalism leads to giantism, the cannibal growing until it is several times as large as the prey. Blepharismas are usually bacterial feeders; but cannibals will also eat other protozoans, or even small rotifers, and thrive on them. A nonselective diet like this should be particularly useful for survival under natural conditions. However, there is no reported correlation between the size of blepharismas found in nature and the type and amount of available food.

Because their feeding organelles are so well differentiated, blepharismas have been favorite objects for morphogenetic studies. It has been demonstrated that the macronucleus, the pattern and polarity of the ectoplasm, and the multiplication of kinetosomes to form oral anlage all play a role in morphogenesis during cell division, conjugation, regeneration, etc. The kineties subtending the peristome are dominant in all these events; if they are removed, regeneration and reorganization will still occur, but much more slowly. The "growing zone" is important in morphogenesis or cell division; and the polarities of the oral area, the V-area, and the anal area all influence morphogenesis. There are many morphogenetic parallels between *Blepharisma* and the metazoans.

Blepharisma has been useful in studying the factors that govern cellular polarity, especially the role of the cell cortex in morphogenesis during division, conjugation, and regeneration. Along with Tartar's parallel studies on *Stentor*, the findings for *Blepharisma* show how much alike are the factors that control morphogenesis in protozoans and in a developing multicellular animal. In ciliates the macronucleus is needed to initiate and maintain cell structures in their differentiated form, but the cortical layer determines polarity and other details of development. A comparison of the experimental findings on *Blepharisma* and *Stentor* and their significance to the principles of morphogenesis is a theme so extensively developed by Tartar (1961) in his book on *Stentor* that additional comment is hardly necessary here.

Studies of the molecular events during regeneration indicate that the macronucleus of *Blepharisma* probably produces both messenger RNA and other kinds of RNA. Chemical agents that are known to stop RNA production will stop a cell's regeneration (and probably other morphogenetic events as well, though these have not been studied). Many of the same agents also stop the cyclic macronuclear changes that accompany morphogenetic events in *Blepharisma*, but it is not known whether these cyclic changes are primary or secondary. An outline of probable macromolecular events during regeneration can be constructed, but a detailed account of the molecular sequence is still in the future.

Encystment has been observed in a number of species of *Blepharisma*, although some laboratory strains do not encyst. How the species that do not encyst manage to disperse themselves in nature is an interesting and unsolved problem. Little work has been done with *Blepharisma* cysts, and no one has yet developed a satisfactory procedure for inducing excystment. Therefore, little is known about the resistance of cysts to unfavorable environmental factors in natural ponds, which must undergo seasonal changes such as drying out.

One of the most interesting characteristics of *Blepharisma* is its pigmentation, which is of a type unique to a small number of spirotrichs. The pigment is localized in granules lying just under the cell surface, and these are easily shed when the cells are shocked by physical or chemical agents—e.g., low temperature, bright light, salts, or alkaloids. For this reason, *Blepharisma* might be a sensitive detector of traces of noxious materials in the environment—for example, oxides of nitrogen— though no work has been done in this regard. Some chemicals, such as the alkaloids, induce a shedding of pigment associated with sufficient other material to make a capsule that reproduces the shape of a *Blepharisma* even to the point of having openings corresponding to mouth and cytopyge. After shedding pigment, cells become lighter in color; but they recover their normal pigment content in one or two days. The pigment granules are membrane-bound, suggesting origin in the endoplasmic reticulum, but this has not yet been studied with the electron microscope.

The red pigment of *Blepharisma* sensitizes the cell to light, and if a deeply pigmented *Blepharisma* is exposed to the visible and near UV portion of sunlight, or to bright artificial light, it is quickly killed; an albino is not affected. This photosensitization requires the presence of oxygen. Pigment extruded from *Blepharisma* into water will also sensitize colorless ciliates, flagellates, marine eggs, and other cells to the same wavelengths. For reasons unknown, albino blepharismas are sensitized by this treatment to a lesser degree than are other ciliates (e.g., *Paramecium* or *Colpidium*).

If red blepharismas in suspension are exposed to dim light in the laboratory, they turn blue-grey. The blue cells are no longer photosensitive and can resist doses of light several times as large as those that kill red cells. It is probable that in nature the red pigment changes to the blue form in the early hours of the day; since the regeneration of the red pigment takes more than a day, the cells would remain resistant to light for at least that time. However, no species of *Blepharisma* that are red when grown in dim light or darkness have been reported to be blue when picked up by day in the field.

Albino mutants of deep red stocks of *Blepharisma* have appeared a number of times in the laboratory but have not been reported in nature. This suggests that the pigmented strain has some natural selective advantage. Since blepharismas are readily eaten by some other protozoans and by small crustaceans, the pigment does not seem to protect against predators; nor has anyone demonstrated a positive or negative phototropism mediated by the pigment, although blepharismas that move out of the light remain out. A critical experimental analysis of this reaction remains to be made. However, both the red and the blue pigment absorb far UV radiation about equally, and pigmented blepharismas are more resistant to this radiation than are albino stocks or blepharismas from which the pigment has been extruded. Perhaps the pigment forms a screen against far UV radiation and benefits the genus in this way; but if so, one wonders why it normally occurs in its more lethal red form.

The pigment of *Blepharisma*, extracted and purified, has been proved by diagnostic tests to be a hypericinlike substance. However, the complete biochemical analysis and synthesis of the pigment have not yet been accomplished, as is true of hypericin. *Blepharisma* is almost unique in producing a pigment that kills the cell containing it under bright light. If nothing else, the very survival of *Blepharisma* in nature is a testimony to its adaptability. If the acquisition of a photosensitizing pigment by *Blepharisma* appears to be a paradox in its evolution, it must be remembered that some ciliates related to *Blepharisma* have a similar hypericinlike pigment that screens out far UV but is no longer a photosensitizer. This may represent another stage in the evolution of cellular pigmentation: a pigment that has retained the desirable property of protection against far UV without the hazard of sensitization to near UV and visible light that still characterizes blepharismin.

Glossary

Glossary

Aboral. Dorsal; that is, on or near the surface (of a protozoan) that does not contain the oral organelles.

Adduct. A compound formed by the union of two compounds, like that between certain dyes and deoxyribonucleic acid (DNA).

Adoral. Ventral; that is, in or adjacent to the oral region.

Adoral zone of membranelles. *See* AZM.

Alkaloid. One of a group of organic basic substances found in plants, usually bitter in taste and physiologically active; e.g., strychnine sulfate.

Anaerobic. Without oxygen.

Anaphase. The phase of mitosis during which the split chromosomes separate from one another.

Anarchic field. An unorganized aggregation of kinetosomes that eventually migrate and develop into the organelles of a new peristome in a dividing or regenerating *Blepharisma*.

Anion. Negative ion. *See* Cation.

Anlage. Primordium or precursor; the undifferentiated state of an organelle: for example, the structures that will eventually form the new macronucleus in an exconjugant cell (pl. anlagen).

Anterior. The end of a protozoan toward which the oral opening is pointed.

Autogamy. *See* Cytogamy.

Axenic. Growing in the absence of any other living organism; said, for example, of a culture containing only *Blepharisma* and nonliving nutrients.

Axoneme. The ciliary shaft.

Axosome (or **axosomal granule**). A spherical or discoidal body about 80 nm in diameter at which the two central fibers of a cilium end.

AZM. Adoral zone of membranelles. The membranelle-bedecked ribbon that runs along one margin of the peristome in *Blepharisma* and other spirotrichs. "Membranellar band," an alternative name for this structure, is also used in the text.

Balanced salt solution. A solution generally consisting of a mixture of salts of the cations of sodium, potassium, calcium, and magnesium in about the proportions of seawater and in a concentration approximating blood, body fluid, or environmental water.

Binary fission. Division into two approximately equivalent halves.

Binodal. Said of the macronuclear type that consists of two nodes or swellings joined by a filament. *See* Filiform, Halteriform, Moniliform.

Blepharismin. The hypericinlike pigment of *Blepharisma,* formerly called zoopurpurin.

Buccal cavity. In a ciliate, the depression that surrounds the mouth (same as vestibulum).

Capsule. The film of protein and pigment shed by a *Blepharisma* when stimulated in one of several ways.

Cartwheel. A term applied to the appearance of kinetosomes in a tangential section of *Blepharisma.* The kinetosomes are arranged in regular rows, and each one in the middle row is surrounded by six others in a circular pattern. The pattern of tubules in the cross section of a cilium and in a kinetosome is also termed a cartwheel.

Cation. Positive ion. *See* Anion.

Centriole. A duplex microbody that helps to form the poles of a spindle in a eukaryotic cell. Kinetosomes are thought to be homologues of the centriole.

Cerophyl. A powder made by grinding wheat greens that is used to make infusions for growing protozoans.

Chelate. To bind divalent or multivalent ions, for example, calcium.

Chromatin. The diffuse hereditary substance (DNA) of a cell as it exists during interphase.

Chromosome. The carrier of heredity in true cells, located in the nucleus.

Chromosome aggregates. The particles in a protozoan that stain with reagents specific to deoxyribonucleic acid (DNA).

Ciliate. A protozoan characterized by possession of numerous cilia and micro- and macronuclei.

Cilium. The hairlike motile organelle of a ciliate or of ciliated epithelium.

Circumanal fiber. A contractile fiber surrounding the anal opening.

Cirrus (pl. **cirri**). In protozoans, a limblike structure formed by the fusion of several cilia; generally more rodlike than a membranelle.

Cisternae. The large, saclike cavities of the endoplasmic reticulum.

Clone. The offspring produced by the vegetative reproduction of a single cell.

Conjugation. A union of two individuals during which genetic material is exchanged; common in ciliates.

Contractile vacuole. The organelle that evacuates excess fluid from a protozoan.

Cortex. The outer portion of the cytoplasm in a cell.

Cristae. The partitions in mitochondria.

Cryptobiotic. Having the normal life processes suppressed or not in evidence, as in an encysted protozoan.

Cyst. The cryptobiotic resting stage of a protozoan, often enclosed in a heavy outer wall (ectocyst) and a more fragile inner wall (endocyst). In some ciliates, though not in *Blepharisma*, the cyst also forms an intermediate wall (mesocyst) between the other two.

Cytogamy. A cellular reorganization in ciliates that involves a fusion of the gametic haploid nuclei produced within each of the two members of a conjugating pair; in cytogamy there is no actual exchange of genetic material between the conjugants. Also called autogamy.

Cytolysis. The dissolution of cells.

Cytopharynx. The portion of *Blepharisma*'s food canal that lies just back of the cytostome. It is not ciliated and may be quite short.

Cytoplasm. The contents of a cell within the outer membrane and surrounding the nucleus.

Cytoplasmic bridge. The tube of cytoplasm between two conjugating protozoans.

Cytopyge (also cytoproct or anus). The opening through which a protozoan voids indigestible food residues.

Cytostome. The opening through which the food canal of a protozoan enters the endoplasm of the cell.

Deoxyribonucleic acid (DNA). The hereditary substance of which the genes are made.

Desmodexy, rule of. The observation that in ciliates the kinetodesma are always to the right of the kinetosomes they are associated with.

Diploid. Having twice the basic (haploid) number of chromosomes characteristic of a species. In *Blepharisma*, the micronuclei are diploid, whereas the gametic nuclei produced from them during pregamic divisions are haploid.

Distal. Away from; for example, at one or both of the extreme ends of a cell.

Divalent. Ion of double charge ($2+$ or $2-$).

DNA. *See* Deoxyribonucleic acid.

DNA-ase. A hydrolytic enzyme that digests DNA.

Dorsal. In a protozoan, on or near the surface opposite the mouthparts. *See* Ventral.

Ectocyst. The outer cyst wall of a protozoan.

Ectoplasm. The outer layer, or cortex, of the cytoplasm in a cell.

EDTA. Ethylene diamine tetra-acetic acid—an agent used to chelate divalent cations, especially calcium.

Electron microscope. A microscope in which electron beams are focused by condensers as the lenses in a light microscope focus light. The resolution is over one hundred times greater than that possible with a light microscope.

Eluted. Washed out of; for example, a chromatographed substance is eluted from the filter paper on which it appears as a band.

Emacronucleate. Said of a ciliate deprived of its macronucleus.

Emergence pore. The thin, small region of a cyst wall through which an excysting protozoan leaves its cyst.

Endocyst. The inner wall of a cyst, usually quite thin.

Endoplasm. The inner cytoplasm of a cell, usually more fluid than the ectoplasm.

Endoplasmic reticulum. A series of interconnected sacs and canals in the cytoplasm of a cell; it performs various synthetic tasks. In *Blepharisma* the reticulum is poorly developed, and the endoplasm has many vacuoles.

Erythrocyte. A red blood cell.

Eukaryotic. Possessing a fully differentiated nucleus (or nuclei).

Exconjugant. A protozoan cell from the time it separates from its partner in conjugation until its first vegetative division thereafter.

Exocyst. The outer wall of a cyst.

Fabrein. The hypericinlike pigment of the brine ciliate *Fabrea salina*.

Fagopyrin. The hypericinlike pigment of buckwheat.

Far UV. The electromagnetic spectrum between the wavelengths of 190 and 300 nm. *See* UV.

Feulgen stain. A staining medium specific to DNA.

Fibrillar system. The complex of fibers that connect the kinetosomes and ramify from them to form a floor for some of the oral structures.

Fibrous lattice. A band 80 nm thick at the boundary of the endoplasm and the ectoplasm, made up of tubules 4 nm in diameter.

Filiform. Said of the macronuclear type that is threadlike. *See* Binodal, Halteriform, Moniliform.

Filopodia. The thin pseudopodia radiating from the surface of the "sun animalcules," members of the class to which *Amoeba* belongs.

Fission. In protozoology, the splitting of an entire cell into two or more parts; usually taken to mean vegetative binary fission.

Fission line. A clear, unpigmented central band evident at Stage IV in the division of a ciliate.

Gamete. A reproductive cell or nucleus with a haploid number of chromosomes; two gametes fuse to form a diploid zygote.

Gametic nuclei. Haploid micronuclei produced just before an exchange of nuclei during conjugation.

Gene. A unit of a DNA molecule that codes for the synthesis of one specific nucleotide; the basic unit of heredity.

Genotype. The hereditary type of an organism, breeding as expected from its genes.

Glycogen. A storage carbohydrate composed of glucose units.

Glycolysis. Anaerobic metabolism in which glycogen is utilized to supply energy to a cell and in which lactic acid is usually formed.

Golgi body. An organelle most commonly composed of flattened sacs (cisternae) and canals. Probably an assembly point for material synthesized in other organelles.

Growing zone. A narrow area encircling the midbody of a dividing ciliate between the two presumptive oral areas.

Halteriform. Said of the macronuclear type that is shaped like a dumbbell. *See* Binodal, Filiform, Moniliform.

Haploid. Having one chromosome of each kind characteristic of the species— as seen during certain stages of conjugation in a ciliate. *See* Diploid.

Heteropolar. Of opposite polarity, as in some transplanted anterior parts of a *Blepharisma* attached to one another in opposite directions. *See* Homopolar.

Heterotrich. One of a group of ciliates characterized by a well-developed adoral zone of membranelles; otherwise the cilia are of equal size over the whole body. One subdivision of the spirotrichs.

Histochemistry. Study of the chemical nature of cells and tissues by staining and other colorimetric or spectrophotometric methods.

Holdfast. The termination of an organism like *Stentor* or *Vorticella*, by which it attaches to the substrate while eating.

Homologous. Corresponding in structure or origin.

Homopolar. Of the same polarity. *See* Heteropolar.

Hydrolase. An enzyme that causes hydrolysis—i.e., a breakdown of a complex molecule caused by the incorporation of water.

Hypericin. A pigment present in some species of Saint-John's-wort (*Hypericum*). Hypericin is chemically a naphthadianthrone, and it will photosensitize the skin of unpigmented animals who eat the plant.

Hypertonic. Said of a medium in which solutes are more concentrated than in the cell, causing a withdrawal of water from the cell. *See* Hypotonic.

Hypostome. The oral area of a protozoan. *See* Peristome.

Hypotonic. Said of a medium in which solutes are less concentrated than in the cell, causing the cell to swell by intake of water. *See* Hypertonic.

Hypotrich. A heterotrich ciliate whose cilia are fused into ventral pencil-like organelles (cirri) that are used for walking.

Infraciliature. The organized kinetosomes that during morphogenesis give rise to cilia and to the cell structures composed of modified cilia.

Infusorian. An organism in a culture medium such as hay infusion. Sometimes this archaic term is used for a ciliate.

Internodal. Between the nodes of a macronucleus.

Interphase. A stage in the life cycle of the cell between mitoses and divisions, during which the chromosomes are in a diffuse state.

Invagination. A depression or bending inward to form a groove, pocket, or tube.

Kinetochore. The area at the junction of the two arms of a chromosome (also termed the centromere); during nuclear division the spindle fiber appears to attach itself to a chromosome at this point.

Kinetodesma. The grouped fibers lying to the right of a row of kinetosomes in a ciliate.

Kinetosome. A self-duplicating body in the ectoplasm that gives rise to a cilium, and sometimes to trichites or trichocysts.

Kinety. A ciliary row with all its parts, including kinetosomes, cilia, kinetodesma, and so on.

Lag phase. Starting phase of a culture, in which the cells divide very slowly.

Lamella. Any thin, platelike structure.

Lipase. An enzyme catalyzing digestion of fats (lipids).

Log phase. The most rapid growth phase of a culture, during which the logarithm of the number of cells plotted against time yields a straight-line graph.

Lyophilize. To dry at low temperature by subjecting frozen material to a vacuum.

Lysin. A substance that dissolves or disintegrates a specific organic structure or compound; for example, hemolysin will break down red blood cells.

Lysosome. A cellular structure that stores the hydrolases of a cell.

Macronucleus (MN). The trophic nucleus of a ciliate. It is highly polyploid —that is, it contains several multiples of the chromosome number basic to the species involved. *Blepharisma*'s macronucleus may take one of several forms, depending on the species or variety, but in all species it condenses to a spherical mass during cell division.

Megakaryotype. Macronuclear type; one of the four major subdivisions of the genus *Blepharisma.*

Meiosis. The process preceding formation of gametes or, in conjugating ciliates, gametic nuclei. During meiosis the members of a pair of homologous chromosomes are separated from one another so that each gamete or gametic nucleus gets only one. The net effect of meiosis is haploidy; that is, halving of the chromosome number. Diploidy is reestablished in sexual union.

Membranellar band. Another term for the AZM of a ciliate.

Membranelle. A flattened, membranous structure composed of (usually) three transverse rows of interdigitated cilia.

Metaphase. The stage in mitosis in which the chromosomes are lined up on the equatorial plate.

Micrometer (μm). A unit of length measuring 10^{-6} meter. This unit was formerly termed a micron and abbreviated μ.

Micronucleus (mN). A diploid nucleus that is mainly active during cell division and conjugation. *Blepharisma* usually has several micronuclei.

Microphagous. Eating minute particles, e.g., bacteria.

Microtubules. Minute structures about 6–7 nm in diameter and sometimes several micrometers in length. They give support to the cell and perhaps help it to expand or contract; they are the "9 + 2 fibrils" of a cilium.

Mitochondria. Aerobic energy-liberating organelles in a eukaryotic cell; 0.5 μm in diameter and several micrometers in length.

Mitosis. Cell division in which the chromosomes split and one of each of the products goes to each of the two cells.

Moniliform. Said of the macronuclear type that appears beaded. *See* Binodal, Filiform, Halteriform.

Monovalent. An ion of unit charge, positive or negative.

Monoxenic. Growing on or containing a single species of organism; said, for example, of a culture in which *Blepharisma* feed on one species of bacteria.

Morphogenesis. The structural development of an organism or part of it.

mRNA. Messenger ribonucleic acid; it furnishes the information that translates the genic code into protein.

Multinodal. Said of the many-noded, moniliform type of macronucleus found in some strains of *Blepharisma*.

Nanometer (nm). A length of 10^{-9} meter, equal to the old measure of 10 angstroms. This unit is now in favor for indicating the wavelength of light and for describing microstructures viewed under the electron microscope.

Near UV. The electromagnetic spectrum between 300 and 390 nm in wavelength.

Nemadesmal fibers. Fine structures that connect the bases of the cilia in the AZM and then pass down into the endoplasm.

Nucleolus. The small body in a nucleus in which ribosomes are synthesized.

Nucleoplasm. The fluid material in a nucleus around the chromosomes and other structures.

Nucleus. In eukaryotic cells, a membrane-bounded concentration of nucleic acids and proteins that controls the life processes and reproduction of the cell; in ciliates, the nuclear functions are divided between a single macronucleus and a number of much smaller micronuclei.

Opisthe. The posterior daughter cell of a dividing ciliate. *See* Proter.

Oral. Associated with the structures by which an organism ingests food.

Oral groove. The oval depression surrounding the mouth in some ciliates.

Oral replacement. Formerly called physiological reorganization. The reorganization of the mouthparts of a ciliate following physical or chemical injury; the mouthparts also reorganize in a daughter cell shortly after division.

Organelle. A specialized structure in a unicellular organism that performs functions analogous to those of an organ in a multicellular organism.

Osmolality. The potential osmotic pressure in a solution or in the protoplasm of a living cell—that is, the force that tends to push osmotically active particles (such as salt-derived ions) from an area of greater concentration to one of lesser concentration. In the context of this book, osmotic pressure is always acting across a cellular or infracellular membrane.

Osmole. The unit of osmotic pressure: one gram molecular weight of osmotically active particles.

Osmotic shock. Injury to a cell caused by exposing it to a higher or lower osmolality than obtains inside the cell.

Oxyblepharismin. The blue, oxidized form of the pigment blepharismin.

Parabiotic fusion. A physical and physiological union of two cells.

Parabiotic union. Union of two organisms (cells) by surgical means.

Paraglycogen. A substance occurring in granules about the size of mitochondria (but without membranes), which are scattered through the cytoplasm of *Blepharisma* and respond cytochemically to the same tests as glycogen.

Parthenogametes. Nuclei formed during parthenogenetic conjugation that serve as the genetic nuclei of the exconjugant.

Parthenogenetic conjugation. A type of reorganization in paired blepharismas. Only two pregamic divisions occur; and the diploid micronuclei, without fusing, multiply to form the new micronuclei and macronuclear anlagen in each of the conjugants.

Pedicel. A small stalk.

Pellicle. The stiff but elastic outer covering by which a ciliate retains its shape.

Penicilliopsin. The hypericinlike pigment of the fungus *Penicilliopsis*.

Peristome. The complex of undulating membrane, membranelles, and ciliated groove that forms *Blepharisma*'s feeding canal.

Peroral cone. A cone that forms between the oral regions of conjugating cells.

Phagocyte. A cell that eats other cells.

Phase microscope. A microscope in which peripheral and central beams of light are projected out of phase with each other by one-quarter wavelength; this phasing allows the discrimination of boundaries and objects differing only slightly in refractive index.

Phenotype. The apparent physical type of an organism, regardless of its genetic makeup. For example, an albino phenotype of *Blepharisma* can be produced by bleaching a normal cell that is genotypically red.

Photodynamic action. Injurious action resulting from the absorption of light by a cellular pigment in the presence of oxygen; photooxidation.

Photooxidation. Oxidation in light by oxygen.

Photoreactivation. *See* Photoreversal.

Photoreversal. The reversal of the injurious action of far UV light by post-illumination with visible or near UV light.

Physiological regeneration. Oral replacement owing to changes in conditions affecting the cell; occurs in *Blepharisma* and some other ciliates.

Pinocytosis. "Cell drinking," intake of environmental fluid and its contents in small vacuoles. Pinocytosis occurs chiefly in amoeboid cells.

Plasma membrane. The outer membrane of a cell, usually 7–10 nm thick.

Polyxenic. Containing several organisms; said, for example, of a culture medium for protozoans containing a variety of cells, including bacteria.

Posterior. In *Blepharisma*, the end of the cell in which the cytopyge lies; the peristomal structures face away from the posterior end.

Postgamic. Referring to the divisions of a protozoan synkaryon while conjugation is still in progress.

Postperistomal. The area of a ciliate body behind the peristome; usually referring to a cell fragment produced by experimental cutting.

Pregamic. The divisions of the micronuclei preceding the disjunctional division that forms the gametic nuclei.

Primordium. Precursor, forerunner; same as anlage.

Pronucleus. One of the haploid micronuclei that are present during conjugation in protozoans; a pronucleus is essentially gametic, like the pronucleus of a sperm in an egg.

Prophase. The first stage in mitosis of a cell, during which the chromosomes condense.

Proter. The anterior daughter cell of a dividing ciliate. *See* Opisthe.

Pseudopodia. The temporary "feet" that extend from the main cytoplasmic body of a rhizopod protozoan (e.g., *Amoeba*); used both for locomotion and for engulfing food.

Psi. Pounds (of pressure) per square inch.

Pyriform. Pear-shaped; the usual shape of *Blepharisma* after forming many food vacuoles.

Ribonucleic acid (RNA). The type of nucleic acid found in ribosomes, messenger nucleic acid, and transfer nucleic acid.

Ribosomes. The small cellular bodies, composed of ribonucleic acid and protein, on the surface of which protein is synthesized.

RNA. *See* Ribonucleic acid.

RNA-ase. A hydrolytic enzyme that digests RNA.

Scanning electron microscope. A microscope in which the image is formed by a flying spot of electrons that produces a televisionlike image, permitting observations of the topography of dried, fixed cells; of lower resolution than a normal (transmission) electron microscope.

Somatic cilia. Body cilia other than those in the mouth region.

Spindle. The fibrillar structure on which chromosomes arrange themselves during cell division.

Spinning organ. A name applied to the peristomal structures in *Blepharisma*, chiefly to the undulating membrane and the membranelles where they go below the cell surface.

Spirotrich. One of a subclass of ciliates with an extensively developed membranellar band arising on the left side of the oral area, and with simple body ciliature (if any).

Stentorin. The hypericinlike pigment of *Stentor coeruleus* (the blue *Stentor*).

Stock. A cultured organism for which the locality of origin is not known with certainty.

Stomatin. A substance formed by one ciliate that induces enlargement of the mouthparts in another.

Stomatogenesis. Structural development of the oral apparatus.

Strain. A cultured organism from a known locality.

Synapsis. The pairing-off of homologous pairs of chromosomes in a nucleus.

Synaptinemal complex. Linear structures, with fibrous projections, which appear in the micronucleus in Prophase I of meiosis. Possibly, they represent synapsed chromosomes; but in any case they are associated with synapsis.

Syngamy. The fusion of the gametes or gametic nuclei during conjugation.

Synkaryon. The diploid nucleus formed by the fusion of migratory and stationary pronuclei during conjugation.

Telobiotic union. An end-to-end union of cells (or embryos) achieved by microsurgery.

Telophase. The last stage in the mitosis of cells, during which the nuclei reform within the nuclear envelopes.

Terminal spiral. The termination of the oral groove above the cytopharynx.

Thermolabile. Altered by heat, as in the case of proteins that are denatured and coagulated by heat.

Trichocyst. An organelle underlying the surface of a ciliate (and some flagellates) and capable of suddenly discharging a slender filament; possibly of some use in attachment during feeding.

Trinodal. Said of the three-noded macronucleus found in some strains of *Blepharisma*.

Trophic. Said of the feeding or vegetative stage of a cell; fulfilling a nutritive function.

Trophont. In loose usage, a vegetative or feeding cell; in strict usage, a feeding and growing stage in parasitic protozoans.

Undulating membrane. A structure made up of three rows of interdigitated cilia forming a longitudinal, tonguelike structure used to engulf particulate food.

UO. Unit osmolal; equivalent to the balanced salt solution as used here, or 4.35×10^{-3} osmolal.

UV. Ultraviolet (100 to 390 nm: 100–190 nm, vacuum UV; 190–300 nm, far UV; 300–390 nm, near UV).

Vacuole. A fluid-filled spherical body in a cell.

Vacuum UV. *See* UV.

Variety. The term is used here loosely, and not as a formal taxon. It refers to a stock or strain with distinctive characteristics but insufficiently distinct to warrant species or subspecies status.

Vegetative stage. A stage in the life of a protozoan during which no sexual activity is evident.

Ventral. In a protozoan, on or near the oral surface. *See* Dorsal.

Vesicles. Small, fluid-filled cavities.

Vesicular. Containing small cavities; usually used to describe a nucleus with a large amount of nucleoplasm.

Vestibulum (vestibule). A ciliated depression or invaginated area on the ventral surface leading to the cytopharynx (same as buccal cavity).

Visible light. The electromagnetic spectrum between the wavelengths of 390 and 650 nm; that is, the range of wavelengths perceived by the human eye.

V-zone. The ciliary region posterior to the oral groove invagination in which the kineties from the posterior end ramify (divide) anteriorly and subtend the invagination.

Zoopurpurin. The name conferred by Arcichovskij (1904) on the pigment of *Blepharisma*. Now replaced by the term blepharismin, following the custom of naming hypericinlike compounds by the genus in which they are found.

Zygote. The stage in a protozoan, comparable to the fertilized egg of a metazoan, in which nuclei contributed by two cells have fused.

Index

Index

on nuclear behavior, 18f, 22, 34, 309; on cannibalism, 124, 128ff; on classification, 304, 306, 316ff, 321

Binary fission, 18–22, 39; morphogenesis in, 173–76, 185, 187–91. *See also* Cell division

Blepharisma: classification of, 1, 304–8, 310–29, 332; distribution of, 1, 4, 308–9, 328; molecular biology of, 5, 215–45; regeneration in, 5, 22, 102f, 110–14, 138, 145–50 *passim*, 169–70, 215–45, 274, 329, 335f; pigmentation and photosensitivity in, 5, 266–300, 336–37; morphology of, 5–15, 39–52, 128–31, 307–10; cannibalism in, 6, 9, 96, 115, 123–33, 247f, 328f, 335; nuclear behavior in, 10, 13f, 18–36, 333–36; fine structure of, 39–52; Turtox strain, 54, 72, 78, 80, 92; ecology and culture of, 54–55, 94–120, 262; electron micrographs of, 56–92; and capsule shedding, 138ff, 157–70, 278; surface properties and salt relations of, 135–55; morphogenesis of, 172–212, 335–36; Woods Hole strain, 186; encystment and excystment of, 247–62, 328f, 334, 336; evolution, 309–10; catalog of, 310–24; species removed from, 324; key to, 324–28

Blepharisma, subgenera: *Compactum*, 306; *Filiformis*, 307; *Halteroides*, 307

Blepharisma, species and varieties:

B. americanum: morphology of, 1, 9, 14; nuclear behavior in, 19, 21f, 30–31, 34; fine structure of, 45, 51, 54, 56, 60, 64, 74, 82–88 *passim*, 92; ecology and culture of, 96, 98, 100ff, 115f; Stanford stock of, 102, 167f, 326; and cannibalism, 123–31 *passim*; salt relations in, 145, 151; capsule shedding in, 164f, 167f; morphogenesis of, 187; cysts of, 247–56 *passim*, 260; pigmentation and photosensitivity in, 266, 272–95 *passim*; classification of, 307, 317f, 326f

   B. a. v. americanum, 318
   B. a. v. dawsoni, 317, 327
   B. a. v. trinodatum, 31, 317f, 327
   B. a. v. wardsi, 327
B. biancae, 316
B. brevifiliformis, 268, 307, 323, 326, 328
B. candidum, 305, 324
B. clarissimum, 304f, 324
   B. c. v. arenicola, 324

   B. c. v. longissimum, 324
B. coeruleum, 6, 306, 312–13
B. dileptus, 307, 320
B. falcatum, 306, 313
B. halophilium, 94, 306, 314
B. ichthyoides, 307, 316f
B. intermedium, 320–21
B. japonicum: morphology of, 1, 6–14 *passim*; nuclear behavior in, 18, 20ff; conjugation in, 22–35; fine structure of, 44f, 51, 58–76 *passim*, 88, 90; Suzuki # 3 strain, 54, 102, 108, 167f, 326; ecology and culture of, 101f, 115; Suzuki #5 strain, 102, 163ff, 167f, 273, 275, 326; African stock of, 115, 124, 126f, 130, 145; cannibalism in, 123f, 126–29; Niigata strain, 167f, 321, 326; morphogenesis of, 173–212; regeneration in, 216, 235f; cysts in, 247ff, 252; pigmentation and photosensitivity in, 272, 276, 281f, 292, 294f; classification of, 307, 320, 326, 328

   B. j. v. intermedium: morphology of, 2, 14; nuclei of, 14, 22; fine structure of, 54, 60, 62, 70, 82, 84; albino, 54, 60, 62, 70, 124, 178, 266, 268, 272, 276; ecology and culture of, 95–113 *passim*, surface and salt relations in, 136, 142–50 *passim*; regeneration in, 146–50, 216–25 *passim*, 232, 239f, 244; capsule shedding in, 159–68 *passim*; pigmentation and photosensitivity in, 266–76 *passim*, 281, 290f, 295; classification of, 321, 328
   B. j. v. microstomata, 268, 321f, 328
   B. j. v. nilssoni, 322
B. lateritia, 311
B. lateritium, 94, 99, 152, 247; classification of, 306, 311, 314, 316
   B. l. v. bimicronucleata, 312
   B. l. v. botezati, 311
   B. l. v. elongatum, 311–12
   B. l. v. hyalinum, 6, 266, 312
   B. l. v. minima, 312
   B. l. v. navicula, 312
   B. l. v. ovata, 312
   B. l. v. sphagni, 312
   B. l. v. steini, 312
B. lentis, 306, 313
B. melana, 307, 320
B. microstomata, 221
B. multinucleata, 307, 319

Chatton-Lwoff staining process, 166
Chen, T. T., 35n, 185, 190
Cheung Ho, M. A., 244
Child, F. M., 107, 202
Chlamydophrys, 132
Chloral hydrate, 159
Chloramphenicol, 221, 229, 256
Chlorella, 99; *C. conductrix*, 99
Chlorophyll, 299
Choline chloride, 158, 163
Choline esterase, 159
Christie, S. L., 98, 317f
Chromatin, 10, 14, 187, 261; and nuclear
  behavior, 21f, 24f; and fine structure,
  49ff, 78, 82, 84, 88, 90
Chromosomes, 176, 236f; and nuclear
  behavior, 21, 24–25; and fine struc-
  ture, 49–50, 56, 78–84 *passim*, 309,
  329, 333f
Chymotrypsin, 138
Chunosoff, L., 130, 256, 266
Cienkowsky, L., 247
Cilia, 1–10 *passim*, 304f; and fine
  structure, 41–45, 56, 58, 60, 70; and
  morphogenesis, 173, 175f, 210; and
  cysts, 251, 253, 261
Ciliary rows, *see* Kineties
Ciliates, 1, 4–5, 8–10, 159; and fine
  structure, 39, 334; and cultures, 97,
  107; and cannibalism, 123, 132f; as
  food, 125f; surface properties of, 135,
  139ff; morphogenesis in, 172–73, 187,
  202, 335; and regeneration, 215, 217,
  222, 230, 232, 236; and cysts, 257,
  261. *See also genera by name*
Circumanal fibril, 9
Cirri, 4
Cisternae, 50, 84
Classification of *Blepharisma*, 1, 304–8,
  328–29, 332; catalog of species, 310–
  24; key to species, 324–28
Cleveland, L. R., 132
Cocaine, 157f
Codeine, 157f
Colchicine, 52
Color, 5f, 305; and cysts, 254, 257–58,
  279, 283; and light and oxygen, 275–
  79. *See also by name*
Colpidium, 96, 275, 286; *C. campylum*,
  286; *C. colpoda*, 125f, 130
Colpoda, 249f, 256f, 260, 262; *C.
  duodenaria*, 248; *C. maupasi*, 258; *C.
  steini*, 248, 250, 253, 257f, 261
Condylostoma, 39, 173, 187, 194

Conjugation, 10, 22–36 *passim*, 50, 86,
  307, 328f, 334; parthenogenetic, 35–
  36, 191f; and morphogenesis, 187,
  191–92, 208, 210ff, 335; and regeneration, 234ff
Contractile vacuole, 2, 4, 14f, 48; and
  salt relations, 150–55; and morphogenesis, 174–76, 180, 183, 197, 201,
  207; and cysts, 253, 255, 261; and
  light, 274; classification and, 304f
Cook, J., 293
Cortex, 39, 210, 235, 335; structures of,
  39–43, 256
Cortical ridge, 40–41, 58, 68
Crab neurons, 272, 275
Crossman, E. B., 274, 288
Crowding, and cysts, 248–50
Crustaceans, 116–17, 272, 275
Cultures: monoxenic, 54, 96; polyxenic,
  54, 95; axenic, 95, 97ff, 108, 111f, 231,
  249; food and, 94–100; and temperature, 101–5; osmolality and, 106–14;
  and division rate, 117–20
Cyanide, 218, 255
Cysts, 4, 39, 255–60, 328f; and temperature, 101, 248, 250–51, 254, 256ff;
  wall of, 135, 248, 252; and morphogenesis, 180, 208, 211, 261–62; dedifferentiation and redifferentiation in,
  180, 235, 261; kinds of, 247–48;
  conditions for, 248–51, 296, 334, 336;
  stages in, 251–54; and color, 254, 257–
  58, 279, 283
Cytochrome oxidase, 218, 229
Cytochromes, *see* Porphyrins
Cytogamy, 31, 35f
Cytolysis, 136–38, 159, 167, 233, 274
Cytopharynx, 8, 10, 95, 305; fine
  structure of, 46, 56, 72, 74; and
  morphogenesis, 175ff, 180, 193, 195,
  201, 204, 211
Cytoplasm, 14–15, 19, 215, 219; and
  conjugation, 10, 23, 25, 50; and fine
  structure, 39, 46–47; and morphogenesis, 176, 181, 183, 188, 190; and
  cysts, 253, 256, 260f
Cytopyge, 4f, 9, 15, 153, 304f; morphogenesis of, 197, 201–9, 211
Cytostome, 8, 10, 95, 187, 305; of
  cannibals, 126–27

Dass, M. S., 187
Dawson, J. A., 94, 185, 257; on
  cannibalism, 126n, 128, 132

360 *Index*